Respiratory Medicine

Series Editors

Sharon I.S. Rounds
Alpert Medical School of Brown University
Providence, RI, USA

Anne Dixon
University of Vermont, Larner College of Medicine
Burlington, VT, USA

Lynn M. Schnapp
University of Wisconsin - Madison
Madison, WI, USA

More information about this series at http://www.springer.com/series/7665

Surya P. Bhatt
Editor

Cardiac Considerations in Chronic Lung Disease

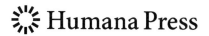 Humana Press

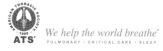

Editor
Surya P. Bhatt
Division of Pulmonary, Allergy and Critical Care Medicine
University of Alabama at Birmingham
Birmingham, AL
USA

ISSN 2197-7372   ISSN 2197-7380   (electronic)
Respiratory Medicine
ISBN 978-3-030-43437-3   ISBN 978-3-030-43435-9   (eBook)
https://doi.org/10.1007/978-3-030-43435-9

This Humana imprint is published by the registered company Springer Nature Switzerland AG
The registered company address is: Gewerbestrasse 11, 6330 Cham, Switzerland

Preface

With the reduction in mortality attributable to cardiovascular disease in the developed world, the burden of chronic lung disease is becoming increasingly apparent. Globally, respiratory diseases are amongst the leading causes of mortality. Significant challenges exist in the prevention, diagnosis, and treatment of chronic lung disease. There is now growing awareness that chronic lung disease is a distinct risk factor for cardiovascular disease, akin to immunologic diseases such as rheumatoid arthritis and systemic lupus erythematosus. Given the overlapping symptoms and signs, considerable challenges exist in the recognition of cardiovascular disease in the presence of chronic lung disease. This book aims to increase awareness of this important comorbidity in individuals with chronic lung disease. The individual chapters address important issues including the epidemiology of cardiovascular disease in the presence of chronic lung disease, as well as factors to consider when diagnosing one in the presence of the other (Chap. 1). Peak lung function is usually attained in the third decade of life, and there is now growing awareness that a substantial number of individuals never reach optimal lung function. Chapter 2 discusses the early life origins of both cardiac and pulmonary diseases and their interactions. There appear to be substantial gender differences in both lung and heart diseases, and these are discussed in Chap. 3. The pathophysiologic mechanisms of increased risk for coronary artery disease and left ventricular dysfunction are not fully understood and are discussed in Chap. 4. Chapter 5 addresses the pathophysiology of right heart dysfunction in the presence of chronic lung disease. A substantial number of individuals with chronic lung disease develop pulmonary hypertension for which there are no disease-modifying therapies at present. Chapter 6 addresses treatment considerations for these individuals with secondary pulmonary hypertension. Chapter 7 describes imaging modalities for the lung and the heart. When both cardiac and lung diseases are present in the same individual, it can be difficult to identify the predominant contributor to symptoms as well as their relative contributions. Chapter 8 discusses the nuances of cardiopulmonary exercise testing to help discern these aspects. Chapter 9 addresses heart-lung interactions and how physiologic changes in one organ system affect the other. Most guidelines recommend treating chronic lung disease and cardiac disease as they would usually be treated regardless of the presence of heart-lung comorbidity. A number of cardiac and pulmonary medications interact with each other and can result in adverse consequences. Chapter 10 addresses medication safety. Chapter 11 addresses non-pharmacologic therapy with exercise training and considerations involved in exercise prescription. The course of chronic lung disease is frequently punctuated by acute exacerbations, and a number of these are closely associated with cardiovascular derangements. Chapter 12 addresses cardiac considerations in acute exacerbations of chronic lung disease. Finally, when chronic lung disease is far advanced, lung transplantation becomes the only remaining option. Chapter 13 addresses cardiac considerations in individuals who are candidates for lung transplantation. We hope that this broad range of topics addressing cardiac manifestations and considerations in chronic lung disease will be helpful for both cardiologists and pulmonologists, as well as primary care practitioners, who treat patients with these common diseases that frequently coexist.

Birmingham, AL, USA   Surya P. Bhatt, MD

Contents

Contributors

Deepak Acharya, MD, MSPH Division of Cardiovascular Diseases, Sarver Heart Center, University of Arizona, Tucson, AZ, USA

Maria Clara N. Alencar, PhD Pulmonary Function and Clinical Exercise Physiology Unit (SEFICE), Division of Respirology, Federal University of Sao Paulo, Sao Paulo, Brazil

Flavio F. Arbex, MD Pulmonary Function and Clinical Exercise Physiology Unit (SEFICE), Division of Respirology, Federal University of Sao Paulo, Sao Paulo, Brazil

Surya P. Bhatt, MD, MSPH Division of Pulmonary, Allergy and Critical Care Medicine, University of Alabama at Birmingham, Birmingham, AL, USA

Michael J. Cuttica, MD, MS Northwestern University, Feinberg School of Medicine, Division of Pulmonary and Critical Care Medicine, Chicago, IL, USA

Mark T. Dransfield, MD Lung Health Center, Division of Pulmonary, Allergy, and Critical Care, University of Alabama at Birmingham, Birmingham, AL, USA

Birmingham VA Medical Center, Birmingham, AL, USA

Rachael A. Evans, PhD National Institute of Health Research Biomedical Research Centre, Respiratory Sciences, University of Leicester, Leicester, UK

Department of Respiratory Medicine, Thoracic Surgery and Allergy, Glenfield Hospital, University Hospitals of Leicester NHS Trust, Leicester, UK

Alicia K. Gerke, MD University of Iowa, Department of Internal Medicine, Division of Pulmonary Diseases, Critical Care, and Occupational Medicine, Iowa City, IA, USA

Christine Jenkins, MD, FRACP Concord Hospital Sydney, Concord, NSW, Australia

The George Institute for Global Health, Sydney, NSW, Australia

Faculty of Medicine, UNSW Sydney, Sydney, NSW, Australia

University of Sydney, Sydney, NSW, Australia

Ravi Kalhan, MD, MS Northwestern University, Feinberg School of Medicine, Division of Pulmonary and Critical Care Medicine, Chicago, IL, USA

Kate Milne, MD University of British Columbia (UBC) Division of Respiratory Medicine (Department of Medicine) and Centre for Heart Lung Innovation, St. Paul's Hospital, Vancouver, BC, Canada

Firdaus A. A. Mohamed Hoesein, MD, PhD Department of Radiology, University Medical Center Utrecht, University Utrecht, Utrecht, The Netherlands

David Montani, MD, PhD Université Paris-Sud, Faculté de Médecine, Université Paris-Saclay, Le Kremlin-Bicêtre, France

Service de Pneumologie, Hôpital Bicêtre, AP-HP, Le Kremlin-Bicêtre, France

INSERM UMR_S 999, Hôpital Marie Lannelongue, Le Plessis Robinson, France

J. Alberto Neder, MD Laboratory of Clinical Exercise Physiology (LACEP), Queen's University & Kingston General Hospital, Kingston, ON, Canada

Respiratory Investigation UniT (RIU), Queen's University & Kingston General Hospital, Kingston, ON, Canada

Denis E. O'Donnell, MD Laboratory of Clinical Exercise Physiology (LACEP), Queen's University & Kingston General Hospital, Kingston, ON, Canada

Respiratory Investigation UniT (RIU), Queen's University & Kingston General Hospital, Kingston, ON, Canada

Mayron Oliveira, PT Pulmonary Function and Clinical Exercise Physiology Unit (SEFICE), Division of Respirology, Federal University of Sao Paulo, Sao Paulo, Brazil

Trisha M. Parekh, DO Lung Health Center, Division of Pulmonary, Allergy, and Critical Care, University of Alabama at Birmingham, Birmingham, AL, USA

Roy Pleasants, PharmD Division of Pulmonary Diseases and Critical Care Medicine, University of North Carolina at Chapel Hill, Chapel Hill, NC, USA

Pulmonary Department, Durham VA Medical Center, Durham, NC, USA

Indranee Rajapreyar, MD Section of Advanced Heart Failure, Pulmonary Vascular Disease, Heart Transplantation, and Mechanical Circulatory Support, Division of Cardiovascular Diseases, University of Alabama at Birmingham, Birmingham, AL, USA

Tyler R. Reynolds Louisiana State University, Baton Rouge, LA, USA

Alcides Rocha, MD Pulmonary Function and Clinical Exercise Physiology Unit (SEFICE), Division of Respirology, Federal University of Sao Paulo, Sao Paulo, Brazil

Victoria Rusanov, MD Department of Medicine, University of Alabama at Birmingham, Birmingham, AL, USA

Gregory A. Schmidt, MD University of Iowa, Department of Internal Medicine, Division of Pulmonary Diseases, Critical Care, and Occupational Medicine, Iowa City, IA, USA

Don D. Sin, MD MPH University of British Columbia (UBC) Division of Respiratory Medicine (Department of Medicine) and Centre for Heart Lung Innovation, St. Paul's Hospital, Vancouver, BC, Canada

Olivier Sitbon, MD, PhD Université Paris-Sud, Faculté de Médecine, Université Paris-Saclay, Le Kremlin-Bicêtre, France

Service de Pneumologie, Hôpital Bicêtre, AP-HP, Le Kremlin-Bicêtre, France

INSERM UMR_S 999, Hôpital Marie Lannelongue, Le Plessis Robinson, France

Jason Weatherald, MD University of Calgary, Department of Medicine, Division of Respiratory Medicine, Calgary, AB, Canada

Libin Cardiovascular Institute of Alberta, Calgary, AB, Canada

Keith M. Wille, MD Department of Medicine, University of Alabama at Birmingham, Birmingham, AL, USA

Chapter 1
Cardiovascular Comorbidity in Chronic Lung Disease: Epidemiology, Clinical Manifestations, and Diagnosis

Surya P. Bhatt

Clinical Pearls
- Strong epidemiologic data exist for the association between chronic lung disease, especially chronic obstructive pulmonary disease, and the occurrence of cardiovascular disease, including atherosclerosis, coronary artery disease, cerebrovascular disease, peripheral vascular disease, heart failure, and cardiac arrhythmias.
- Chronic lung diseases and cardiovascular disease are both very prevalent, but their coexistence is not explained by chance but by the risk of atherosclerosis and deranged cardiopulmonary interactions conferred by the presence of chronic lung disease.
- A low index of suspicion should be maintained to evaluate for chronic lung or cardiovascular disease when one of these is present, especially when symptoms and functional impairment are deemed to be out of proportion for the existing diagnosis.

Epidemiology

Chronic lung diseases account for a substantial amount of morbidity and disability. They are, however, frequently under-recognized and remain undiagnosed in a significant proportion of the population. The most common chronic

S. P. Bhatt (✉)
Division of Pulmonary, Allergy and Critical Care Medicine,
University of Alabama at Birmingham, Birmingham, AL, USA
e-mail: sbhatt@uabmc.edu

© Springer Nature Switzerland AG 2020
S. P. Bhatt (ed.), *Cardiac Considerations in Chronic Lung Disease*,
Respiratory Medicine, https://doi.org/10.1007/978-3-030-43435-9_1

lung diseases include chronic obstructive pulmonary disease (COPD), bronchial asthma, and interstitial lung diseases. With significant advances made in the reduction of mortality from cancer and cardiovascular disease, mortality attributable to chronic lung disease continues to rise [1]. Between 1969 and 2013, the largest decreases in mortality were for stroke (77%) and heart disease (68%) [1]. The mortality for all cancers combined decreased by 18%. There was however a 100% increase in mortality from COPD in the same time interval [1]. Similarly, the age-standardized years of potential life lost decreased by 75% for stroke, 68% for heart disease, and 41% for cancer but without any change over this time interval for COPD [1]. The reduction in mortality due to heart disease is likely due to improvement in the detection and control of risk factors such as hypertension and hyperlipidemia, smoking cessation efforts, and improvements in medical care. The decrease in cancer deaths is also likely due to smoking cessation efforts and due to advances in screening and early detection as well as advances in therapy. The increase in COPD-related mortality is likely due to a multitude of factors: the lag between improved smoking cessation rates and disease incidence that would correspond with a decrease in the occurrence of chronic lung disease, limited efforts in tackling causes other than cigarette smoking such as environmental pollution and biomass fuel exposure, limited advances in therapies that affect the course of the disease, a direct effect of reduction in mortality due to the other chronic diseases, and a higher rate of diagnosis of these chronic lung diseases.

Both chronic lung disease and cardiovascular disease are highly prevalent. The prevalence of COPD in the United States is approximately 6.5%; 14 million adults have COPD, and approximately 10 million adults who meet criteria for airflow obstruction have not been diagnosed with COPD [2, 3]. COPD also accounted for 133,575 deaths in 2010 [3]. In 2016, approximately 19 million (8.4%) of adults in the United States had an active diagnosis of asthma. 8.4 million reported an asthma attack including 7.3 million office visits, 1.2 million emergency room visits, and 108,505 hospitalizations [4]. In the United States, 92.1 million individuals have some form of cardiovascular disease; 16.5 million adults older than 20 years have coronary artery disease (CAD), and 6.5 million have heart failure [5]. It is therefore not surprising that these conditions frequently coexist. Although math suggests that these interactions could happen by chance in 1% of the general population, multiple cohort studies suggest that the frequency of coexistence of these chronic diseases is considerably higher, underscoring the overlapping pathophysiologic links. Most of the epidemiologic data available for chronic lung disease is regarding COPD (Fig. 1.1). Recent data suggest similar associations between other chronic lung diseases and cardiovascular disease, including for atherosclerosis, coronary artery disease, cerebrovascular disease, peripheral vascular disease, heart failure, and cardiac arrhythmias. This chapter is not meant to be a systematic review or meta-analysis but will include large studies and results of meta-analyses to highlight these associations.

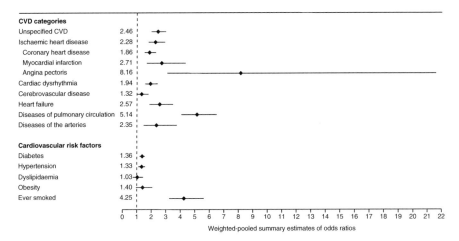

Fig. 1.1 Forest plot showing the weighted-pooled summary estimates of odds ratio (meta-OR) with 95% CI for cardiovascular disease in COPD compared with individuals without COPD. The meta-odds ratio is indicated with a black diamond, and the 95% CI are indicated by the error bars. The dash vertical line indicates threshold for significance. *CVD* cardiovascular disease, *COPD* chronic obstructive pulmonary disease. (Reproduced, with permission of the publisher, from Chen et al. [8])

Coronary Artery Disease (CAD)

There are a number of overlapping risk factors for chronic lung disease and CAD; these include cigarette smoking, environmental pollutants, advancing age, gender, and diet [6, 7]. These risk factors, however, do not fully explain the frequent coexistence of these chronic diseases. A substantial number of observational studies in the past two decades have demonstrated that CAD occurs much more frequently in individuals with COPD than is explained by the risk factors [6, 7].

Low forced expiratory volume in the first second (FEV_1) and low forced vital capacity (FVC) are both associated with poor cardiovascular outcomes. Multiple cohort studies have shown a relationship between low FEV_1 and cardiovascular mortality, even after adjustment for age, gender, and smoking burden [8]. Data from the Renfrew and Paisley population-based study ($n = 15,411$) showed that the hazard ratio (HR) for mortality in the lowest quintile of FEV_1 was 1.92 in males and 1.89 in females, compared with healthy controls after adjustment for age, cigarette smoking, serum cholesterol, diastolic blood pressure, body mass index, and social class [9]. There appears to be a dose-response relationship between the degree of lung function impairment and the occurrence of CAD. Data from the Lung Health Study showed that cardiovascular mortality rose by 28% for every 10% decrease in FEV_1 [10]. The Renfrew and Paisley study suggested that one-fourth of the attributable risk from ischemic heart disease was due to low FEV_1 [9]. In a more recent community-based international cohort study of 126,359 adults followed for a median duration of 7.8 years, the population attributable risk from mild to moderate reduction in FEV_1 was 17.3% for cardiovascular disease and 24.7% for all-cause mortality [11]. These studies suggest that a low FEV_1 is second only to hypertension when attributable risk factors for cardiac disease are ranked. Despite these findings, lung function is not included in risk scores for cardiovascular outcomes.

Although low FEV_1 is often used as a reflector of airflow obstruction, this can be due to either obstructive or restrictive lung disease. Multiple studies have also evaluated the association between airflow obstruction (low FEV_1/FVC ratio, either <0.70 or less than the lower limit of normal derived from normative population data) and cardiovascular morbidity and mortality. In a large population-based study of 341,329 individuals registered in the Health Search Database in Italy, the prevalence of CAD was 6.9% in general population and 13.6% in those with COPD [12]. In a retrospective study of 11,493 subjects, the presence of airflow obstruction was associated with a 1.61-fold higher odds of angina and myocardial infarction, and a relative risk of 2.07 for cardiovascular mortality, even after adjusting for other known risk factors [13]. In a very large retrospective cross-sectional study involving 1,204,100 subjects, Feary et al. found that the prevalence of cardiovascular disease (including CAD, congestive heart failure, peripheral arterial disease, and aortic aneurysm) was 28% in those with COPD and 7.2% in those without COPD (odds ratio 4.98, 95% CI 4.85–5.81) [14]. Mannino et al. analyzed data from 20,296 subjects enrolled in the Atherosclerosis Risk in Communities (ARIC) Study and the Cardiovascular Health Study (CHS) and found that the prevalence of cardiovascular disease was 19.7–22.1% across the range of disease severity in COPD compared with 9% in those with normal spirometry (overall odds ratio 2.4, 95% CI 1.9–3.0) [15]. In the Danish Nationwide Study of 7.4 million individuals, Sode et al. found that individuals with COPD had a higher lifetime age-standardized incidence of myocardial infarction compared to those without COPD (27.2 vs. 17.7 events per 10,000 person-years) [16].

Low FVC is also associated with cardiac disease. Results from the Framingham study of 5209 individuals aged 45–74 years, followed for approximately 20 years, suggested that there was a graded inverse relationship between FVC and cardiovascular mortality as well as for incident CAD, heart failure, intermittent claudication and stroke [17]. FVC ranked high on the list of risk factors for cardiac mortality, and these associations were seen even in those without established pulmonary disease [17]. More recent data from the ARIC study showed that individuals in the lowest FVC quartile had HR of 5.64 for incident CAD compared with the highest FVC quartile, after adjustment for age, race, study center, height, height [2], and smoking status [18].

Data from subjects referred for lung transplantation suggest that fibrotic lung diseases are associated with a greater risk of CAD than non-fibrotic lung diseases; these studies are however biased due to the variation in disease severity required for referral for transplantation [19, 20]. In the Health Improvement Network, a longitudinal primary care dataset from the United Kingdom, Hubbard et al. found a higher prevalence of history of acute coronary syndrome (8% vs. 5%) and angina (16% vs. 9%) in those with idiopathic pulmonary fibrosis (IPF) than in age- and sex-matched controls without pulmonary fibrosis [21]. On follow-up over approximately 3–4 years, the incidence of acute coronary syndrome was higher in IPF than in controls (19.3 vs. 8.5 per 1000 person-years) [21]. There are few epidemiologic studies of CAD in asthma. A large meta-analyses of 495,025 individuals enrolled in asthma cohorts revealed a higher risk of CAD in those with asthma than in those without the disease (HR 1.42, 95% CI 1.30–1.57) [22].

In summation, these studies indicate that CAD is very common in individuals with spirometric impairment, and the data is especially robust for the association of CAD with COPD. There are also similar reports of a high prevalence of COPD in studies of CAD. Although COPD frequently remains undiagnosed, its prevalence in CAD ranges from 7% to 34% [23, 24].

Cerebrovascular Disease

Given the similarities in pathophysiologic processes between CAD and ischemic cerebrovascular disease, it is to be expected that chronic lung disease would be associated with a higher prevalence of and risk for incident cerebrovascular disease. Most of the available data is for COPD; high-quality prevalence data from population studies are, however, limited. Curkendall et al. analyzed data from a longitudinal healthcare database in the Saskatchewan region of Canada and found that the prevalence of stroke in individuals with COPD was 1.47-fold higher than in those without COPD (4.8% vs. 3.3%) [13]. In 18,342 adults from the 2002 National Health Interview Survey (NHIS), Finkelstein and colleagues found that the prevalence of stroke in those with COPD was 8.6%, compared with 3.6% in those without COPD and 4.1% in smokers that did not have COPD [25]. In the National Health and Nutrition Examination Survey (NHANES), Schnell et al. analyzed 14,828 participants for prevalent comorbidities in physician-diagnosed COPD and reported that individuals with COPD had twice the risk of stroke than individuals without COPD (8.9% vs. 4.6%) [26]. In a UK primary care data study of 1,204,100 members of the general population aged ≥35 years, the presence of COPD was associated with a 3.3-fold higher odds of stroke after adjustment for age, sex, and smoking burden; the prevalence of stroke in those with COPD was 9.9% compared with 3.2% in those without COPD [14].

A number of longitudinal studies have demonstrated a relationship between the presence of airflow obstruction and incident stroke. In a study of 18,403 males followed for 18 years, individuals with FEV_1 less than 3 L had a 1.9-fold increase in HR for fatal cerebrovascular disease, compared with those with higher FEV_1 [27]. Wannamethee et al. prospectively studied 7,735 men and found that the relative risk of stroke in the lowest FEV_1 tertile was 1.4 times that in the highest tertile [28]. In the Renfrew and Paisley study ($n = 15,411$), those in the lowest FEV_1 quintile had a 1.6-fold higher mortality due to stroke compared with the highest quintile, after adjustment for age, cigarette smoking, serum cholesterol, diastolic blood pressure, body mass index, and social class [9]. In the Copenhagen City Heart Study of

12,878 individuals, the relative risk of stroke increased by 5% for every 10% decrease in FEV_1 percent predicted [29]. The risk of fatal stroke followed a similar pattern; there was an 11% increase in relative risk for each 10% decrease in FEV_1 percent predicted [29]. In the Bergen Clinical Blood Pressure Survey of 5,617 participants followed for approximately four decades, there was an inverse relationship between FEV_1 and fatal stroke (HR 1.38 in men and 1.62 in women), adjusted for age and height [30]. In the Rotterdam study, 13,115 participants were followed for approximately 9.6 years, and the risk of stroke was 1.2-fold higher in those with COPD compared to those without COPD [31].

Studies of stroke in individuals with asthma are sparse. A meta-analysis of 524,637 participants found that asthma was associated with an increased risk of stroke (HR 1.32) [32]. A more recent analysis of the Korean Health Insurance Review and Assessment Service-National Sample Cohort that included 111,364 individuals with asthma and 111,364 controls found that there was no elevated risk for hemorrhagic or ischemic stroke in asthma [33]. A large study of 446,346 Taiwanese adults however showed that asthma is associated with a 1.23-fold higher risk of fatal stroke [34]. No robust data are available for the prevalence of ischemic stroke in pulmonary fibrosis and other chronic lung diseases, but it is expected to be high.

Peripheral Arterial Disease

Given the high prevalence of atherosclerotic disease and COPD, it is not surprising that peripheral arterial disease is also frequently observed in individuals with COPD. The true prevalence of peripheral arterial disease in COPD is not known and varies widely between studies. In 2,741 individuals enrolled in the German COSYCONET (COPD and Systemic Consequences–Comorbidities Network) cohort study, and evaluated for peripheral arterial disease using the ankle-brachial index, 8.8% had peripheral arterial disease [35]. The prevalence of peripheral arterial disease increased with increasing lung disease severity, and individuals with peripheral arterial disease had a worse disease-specific health status with higher SGRQ (St. George's Respiratory Questionnaire) scores and CAT (COPD Assessment Test) scores [35]. Of those with evidence of peripheral arterial disease, 55% did not report this in their medical history [35]. This prevalence rate is consistent with a cross-sectional study from Taiwan in which 8% of 427 individuals with COPD were found to have peripheral arterial disease [36]. In a large case-control study of claims data from Taiwan, 6% of individuals with COPD had peripheral arterial disease, and COPD was associated with a 1.23-fold higher prevalence of peripheral arterial disease compared with those without COPD [37]. Analysis of 3,123 participants from the population-based Rotterdam study showed that the presence of COPD was associated with a 1.9-fold increase in incident peripheral arterial disease [38].

The reported prevalence of peripheral arterial disease has generally been higher in smaller cohorts of special populations such as hospitalized patients or outpatients with COPD. In a Swiss study of hospitalized COPD patients who were assessed for peripheral arterial disease using the ankle-brachial index and the toe-brachial index, 43% of those with spirometry-confirmed COPD had evidence of peripheral arterial disease [39]; in comparison, 24% of individuals without COPD had peripheral arterial disease. A smaller outpatient study of 412 individuals with COPD found a prevalence rate of 28% [36]. In a small cross-sectional study of 246 subjects, 36.8% of COPD patients had peripheral arterial disease [40].

There are no population-based studies of peripheral arterial disease in other chronic lung diseases such as bronchial asthma and idiopathic pulmonary fibrosis. In a large insurance claims study in Taiwan, 28,158 adults with newly diagnosed asthma were compared with 56,316 individuals without asthma [41]. The prevalence of peripheral arterial disease was 1.46 times higher in those with asthma than in controls [41]. The prevalence of peripheral arterial disease in pulmonary fibrosis remains unknown but is expected to be high based on features of inflammation and high risk of atherosclerosis similar to that seen in COPD.

Heart Failure

Heart failure, both with reduced and preserved ejection fraction, is common in chronic lung disease, especially with COPD. The mechanisms for this increased risk are described in Chap. 5. The epidemiologic data supporting this association is sparse. In a retrospective analysis of longitudinal healthcare databases maintained by the government of Saskatchewan in Canada, Curkendall and colleagues found that congestive heart failure was reported in 19% of individuals with COPD compared with 3.7% of those without COPD [13]. In a cross-sectional study of 405 elderly patients (age >65 years) with COPD, Rutten et al. found that 20.5% had presence of previously undiagnosed heart failure [42].

Lower lung function is also associated with a greater risk of incident heart failure. In the Health ABC study, in 2,125 participants without known lung disease or heart failure, FEV_1 was inversely associated with incident heart failure over the median follow-up of 9.4 years (HR 1.18) [43]. In the population-based Malmö Preventive Project that included 20,998 males with no prior myocardial infarction or stroke and with a median of 23 years of follow-up, lower FEV_1 was associated with an increased incidence of hospitalization due to heart failure (HR 1.25 in non-smokers and 1.32 in smokers) [44]. In the retrospective Saskatchewan cohort, the risk ratio for developing congestive heart failure was 4.5 in COPD compared with age-matched controls without COPD, after adjustment for other cardiovascular risk factors [13].

There is growing awareness that COPD is also associated with diastolic dysfunction and heart failure with preserved ejection fraction. Population data for this association is again sparse; prevalence rates are mostly informed by small studies that used different diagnostic approaches, and hence the prevalence varies widely. In 615 individuals with COPD in the COSYCONET cohort, 4.1% had evidence of diastolic dysfunction [45]. In a nested case-control study of 115 individuals with COPD and 115 age- and sex-matched controls, the prevalence of diastolic dysfunction was 10.5% in those with COPD compared to 9.1% in those without COPD [46]. Reflecting the high variability in small studies, a frequency of diastolic dysfunction up to 71% has been reported [47–51]. Independent of airflow obstruction, the presence of emphysema also appears to be associated with impaired left ventricular filling. Barr and colleagues used magnetic resonance imaging (MRI) in 2,816 subjects and showed that the percentage emphysema on CT was associated with impaired left ventricular filling; the study however did not provide prevalence estimates for diastolic dysfunction [52]. There are no population-based estimates of prevalence of diastolic dysfunction and heart failure with preserved ejection fraction in other chronic lung diseases.

Cardiac Arrhythmias

COPD is associated with cardiac arrhythmias, both atrial and ventricular, and these arrhythmias are found in higher frequencies in COPD than in individuals without COPD. In the retrospective Saskatchewan cohort data, Curkendall et al. found that the prevalence of cardiac arrhythmia was 11.3% in COPD compared with 5.2% in age- and sex-matched controls without COPD [13]. Multifocal atrial tachycardia (MAT) is often seen in COPD, especially at the time of an exacerbation [53]. In one review, COPD was present in 55% of individuals with MAT [53]. MAT is also associated with the use of theophylline, a phosphodiesterase inhibitor used in the treatment of COPD [54]. Other arrhythmias are less specific to COPD but more frequently seen and include premature ventricular complexes, atrial flutter, atrial fibrillation, and ventricular tachycardia [6]. In stable but hypoxemic COPD subjects, 24-hour ambulatory electrocardiography showed a high incidence of arrhythmias: ventricular premature complexes were noted in 83%, supraventricular tachycardia in 69%, ventricular bigeminy in 68%, and non-sustained ventricular tachycardia in 22% [55]. In the Copenhagen City Heart Study, 13,430 individuals without known cardiac disease were followed for approximately 13 years. A low FEV_1 was independently associated with the incidence of atrial fibrillation, independent of age, gender, smoking burden, blood pressure, and body mass index [56]. In the ARIC study, after adjustment for traditional cardiovascular risk factors, the lowest quartile of FEV_1 was associated with an increased likelihood of atrial fibrillation compared with the highest FEV_1 quartile (HR ranging from 1.37 in white women to 2.36 in black men) [57]. In a retrospective analysis of 7,441 individuals with COPD who underwent 24-hour Holter monitoring, COPD was associated with a higher rate of atrial flutter/fibrillation (23.3% vs. 11%), and non-sustained ventricular tachycardia (13% vs. 5.9%), but a lower rate of sustained ventricular tachycardia (0.9% vs. 1.6%), compared to those without COPD [58].

Many arrhythmias are paroxysmal and may not be detected on routine monitoring but confer similar cardiac risk for adverse outcomes. Using surface electrocardiographic surrogates for arrhythmias, Tutek et al. found that the dispersion of P waves, a surrogate for atrial arrhythmias, is greater in those with COPD compared to age- and sex-matched controls without COPD [59]. P-wave dispersion was also significantly greater in COPD patients who had paroxysmal atrial fibrillation compared with COPD without paroxysmal atrial fibrillation [59]. P-wave dispersion is also greater in COPD patients with frequent exacerbations [60]. Susceptibility to ventricular arrhythmias is also higher in COPD as evidenced by greater QTc dispersion than in age-matched controls without COPD [61].

Although prevalence of sudden cardiac death in COPD is hard to determine, the presence of COPD is associated with 1.4-fold greater odds of sudden cardiac death [62, 63]. Both prolonged and abnormally short QTc interval are known risk factors for sudden cardiac death. The association between a prolonged QTc interval and COPD has been inconsistent in previous studies [64]. In a large cross-sectional study of 6.4 million electrocardiographs in 1.7 million individuals, the presence of COPD was associated with 2.4-fold greater odds of a short QTc interval [65]. Heart rate variability is also a risk factor for sudden cardiac death and has been found to be reduced in COPD, a reflection of the high sympathetic tone observed in COPD [66].

Clinical Manifestations and Diagnosis

The symptoms and signs of most chronic lung and cardiac diseases have substantial overlap and hence lack specificity for either diagnosis [67]. The most common symptoms of chronic lung disease include dyspnea and cough that is either dry or productive of phlegm. Wheezing is often a symptom of airway diseases including asthma and COPD, but it can also be seen in heart failure and pulmonary edema with bronchovascular congestion where it is referred to as "cardiac asthma." Chest pain related to lung disease is pleuritic in nature as the lungs themselves do not have pain fibers. Orthopnea and paroxysmal nocturnal dyspnea, although more frequently observed with heart failure and pulmonary edema, are not specific to cardiac disease and are often noted in individuals with asthma and COPD.

Physical examination is also frequently not sufficient to distinguish heart from lung disease although there are certain pointers for each organ involvement. Inspection of the chest can reveal a barrel-shaped chest in cases of severe asthma or COPD. These individuals may also have hyper-resonant notes on percussion. Polyphonic rhonchi on auscultation indicate airway disease but are again not specific as bronchovascular congestion can result in airway narrowing. Rales on examination are also nonspecific, but "Velcro-like" crackles, especially in the bases, can point toward interstitial lung disease. Jugular venous distention and pedal edema are frequently signs of volume overload from cardiac disease but can also be seen with cor pulmonale in the presence of severe lung disease.

In individuals already diagnosed with either a cardiac or lung disease, the symptoms are frequently ascribed to the existing diagnosis [42, 68]. Although the correlation between reported symptoms and objective findings (either on clinical examination or on diagnostic testing) is not linear, efforts should be made to note whether these are reasonably proportionate. Symptoms that are disproportionate to objective findings should alert the clinician to the presence of an additional disease. In the context of chronic lung disease, out-of-proportion dyspnea is frequently due to cardiovascular disease and deconditioning. In the majority, differentiation of chronic lung disease and cardiovascular disease can be made if history and physical examination findings are complemented by appropriate laboratory tests and imaging. These include serum markers (troponin, brain natriuretic peptide, or BNP), spirometry, chest radiography, 2D echocardiography, and computed tomography (CT) imaging. Sometimes, more advanced testing is needed including right heart catheterization and cardiopulmonary exercise testing. These aspects are discussed in greater detail in Chap. 8.

Laboratory tests are frequently useful, but caution should be exercised in their interpretation. For instance, an elevated BNP can be seen in both heart failure with reduced ejection fraction as well as with cor pulmonale and right ventricular failure. Spirometry is useful for the diagnosis of lung disease and also for narrowing the differential diagnoses to predominantly obstructive or restrictive patterns. However fluid accumulation in the lungs in stable heart failure with reduced ejection fraction can result in low forced vital capacity (FVC) and normal or elevated FEV_1/FVC ratio, thus resulting in a restrictive ventilatory defect [69]. Alternatively, peribronchial edema can result in airflow obstruction [70]. The resulting airflow obstruction can also confound severity grading of airflow obstruction [71]. For these reasons, spirometry should be performed after every attempt has been made to achieve euvolemia. Lung volumes are either normal or elevated in obstructive lung disease and decreased in restrictive lung disease. The variable influence of pulmonary edema on lung parenchyma and the airways can result in a mixed obstructive and restrictive pattern, wherein spirometry shows an obstructive pattern and total lung capacity is low on lung volume testing. The diffusing capacity of carbon monoxide (DLCO) is frequently low in the case of emphysema and interstitial lung disease, whereas it can be normal or mildly low in cases of heart failure.

Additional tests with lung imaging may be required to differentiate cardiac and lung disease. Chest X-ray may show signs of hyperinflation with flattening of hemidiaphragms and obstructive lung disease and small lung volumes and restrictive lung disease. Idiopathic pulmonary fibrosis is associated with interstitial opacities that are frequently bilaterally symmetric, basal, and peripheral. Widened mediastinum, bilateral pleural effusions, and fluid in the horizontal fissures point toward a diagnosis of pulmonary edema. With diffuse interstitial markings, it can be difficult to differentiate fluid overload from interstitial lung disease. A widened vascular pedicle points toward volume overload [72, 73]. In acute care settings, lung ultrasound can be used to differentiate obstructive airway disease from congestive heart failure as pulmonary edema is frequently associated with B-lines [74]. CT of the chest with prone positioning may be required to differentiate basal fluid accumulation and Kerley B-lines from reticular opacities due to interstitial lung disease [75, 76].

Pulmonary hypertension can result from both chronic lung disease and cardiovascular disease. Differentiation frequently requires right heart catheterization, and a disproportionate increase (>12 mmHg) in pulmonary artery diastolic pressure over the wedge pressure indicates the presence of a secondary cause of pulmonary hypertension that is not purely due to left ventricular dysfunction [77]. The diagnosis and characterization of pulmonary hypertension are discussed in greater detail in Chap. 6.

All of the above-described tests are performed at rest and may not indicate the predominant pathophysiology contributing to an individual's dyspnea. The role of cardiopulmonary exercise testing (CPET) in determining the predominant cause of dyspnea is discussed in Chap. 8.

Conclusions

In summary, chronic lung diseases and cardiovascular disease are both very prevalent, and their coexistence is not explained by chance but by the risk of atherosclerosis and deranged cardiopulmonary interactions conferred by the presence of chronic lung disease. A low index of suspicion should be maintained to evaluate for chronic lung or cardiovascular disease when one of these is present.

References

1. Ma J, Ward EM, Siegel RL, Jemal A. Temporal trends in mortality in the United States, 1969-2013. JAMA. 2015;314:1731–9.
2. Mannino DM, McBurnie MA, Tan W, Kocabas A, Anto J, Vollmer WM, Buist AS, BOLD Collaborative Research Group. Restricted spirometry in the Burden of Lung Disease Study. Int J Tuberc Lung Dis. 2012;16(10):1405–11.
3. Ford ES, Croft JB, Mannino DM, Wheaton AG, Zhang X, Giles WH. COPD surveillance – United States, 1999-2011. Chest. 2013;144:284–305.
4. Mazurek JM, Syamlal G. Prevalence of asthma, asthma attacks, and emergency department visits for asthma among working adults – National Health Interview Survey, 2011-2016. MMWR Morb Mortal Wkly Rep. 2018;67:377–86.
5. Benjamin EJ, Blaha MJ, Chiuve SE, Cushman M, Das SR, Deo R, de Ferranti SD, Floyd J, Fornage M, Gillespie C, Isasi CR, Jimenez MC, Jordan LC, Judd SE, Lackland D, Lichtman JH, Lisabeth L, Liu S, Longenecker CT, Mackey RH, Matsushita K, Mozaffarian D, Mussolino ME, Nasir K, Neumar RW, Palaniappan L, Pandey DK, Thiagarajan RR, Reeves MJ, Ritchey M, Rodriguez CJ, Roth GA, Rosamond WD, Sasson C, Towfighi A, Tsao CW, Turner MB, Virani SS, Voeks JH, Willey JZ, Wilkins JT, Wu JH, Alger HM, Wong SS, Muntner P, American Heart Association Statistics Committee and Stroke Statistics Subcommittee. Heart disease and stroke statistics-2017 update: a report from the American Heart Association. Circulation. 2017;135:e146–603.
6. Bhatt SP, Dransfield MT. Chronic obstructive pulmonary disease and cardiovascular disease. Transl Res. 2013;162:237–51.

7. Sin DD, Man SF. Chronic obstructive pulmonary disease as a risk factor for cardiovascular morbidity and mortality. Proc Am Thorac Soc. 2005;2:8–11.
8. Chen W, Thomas J, Sadatsafavi M, FitzGerald JM. Risk of cardiovascular comorbidity in patients with chronic obstructive pulmonary disease: a systematic review and meta-analysis. Lancet Respir Med. 2015;3:631–9.
9. Hole DJ, Watt GC, Davey-Smith G, Hart CL, Gillis CR, Hawthorne VM. Impaired lung function and mortality risk in men and women: findings from the Renfrew and Paisley prospective population study. BMJ. 1996;313:711–5; discussion 715–6.
10. Anthonisen NR, Connett JE, Enright PL, Manfreda J, Lung Health Study Research Group. Hospitalizations and mortality in the Lung Health Study. Am J Respir Crit Care Med. 2002;166:333–9.
11. Duong M, Islam S, Rangarajan S, Leong D, Kurmi O, Teo K, Killian K, Dagenais G, Lear S, Wielgosz A, Nair S, Mohan V, Mony P, Gupta R, Kumar R, Rahman O, Yusoff K, du Plessis JL, Igumbor EU, Chifamba J, Li W, Lu Y, Zhi F, Yan R, Iqbal R, Ismail N, Zatonska K, Karsidag K, Rosengren A, Bahonar A, Yusufali A, Lamelas PM, Avezum A, Lopez-Jaramillo P, Lanas F, O'Byrne PM, Yusuf S, PURE Investigators. Mortality and cardiovascular and respiratory morbidity in individuals with impaired FEV1 (PURE): an international, community-based cohort study. Lancet Glob Health. 2019;7:e613–23.
12. Cazzola M, Bettoncelli G, Sessa E, Cricelli C, Biscione G. Prevalence of comorbidities in patients with chronic obstructive pulmonary disease. Respiration. 2010;80:112–9.
13. Curkendall SM, DeLuise C, Jones JK, Lanes S, Stang MR, Goehring E Jr, She D. Cardiovascular disease in patients with chronic obstructive pulmonary disease, Saskatchewan Canada cardiovascular disease in COPD patients. Ann Epidemiol. 2006;16:63–70.
14. Feary JR, Rodrigues LC, Smith CJ, Hubbard RB, Gibson JE. Prevalence of major comorbidities in subjects with COPD and incidence of myocardial infarction and stroke: a comprehensive analysis using data from primary care. Thorax. 2010;65:956–62.
15. Mannino DM, Thorn D, Swensen A, Holguin F. Prevalence and outcomes of diabetes, hypertension and cardiovascular disease in COPD. Eur Respir J. 2008;32:962–9.
16. Sode BF, Dahl M, Nordestgaard BG. Myocardial infarction and other co-morbidities in patients with chronic obstructive pulmonary disease: a Danish nationwide study of 7.4 million individuals. Eur Heart J. 2011;32:2365–75.
17. Kannel WB, Hubert H, Lew EA. Vital capacity as a predictor of cardiovascular disease: the Framingham study. Am Heart J. 1983;105:311–5.
18. Schroeder EB, Welch VL, Couper D, Nieto FJ, Liao D, Rosamond WD, Heiss G. Lung function and incident coronary heart disease: the Atherosclerosis Risk in Communities Study. Am J Epidemiol. 2003;158:1171–81.
19. Kizer JR, Zisman DA, Blumenthal NP, Kotloff RM, Kimmel SE, Strieter RM, Arcasoy SM, Ferrari VA, Hansen-Flaschen J. Association between pulmonary fibrosis and coronary artery disease. Arch Intern Med. 2004;164:551–6.
20. Izbicki G, Ben-Dor I, Shitrit D, Bendayan D, Aldrich TK, Kornowski R, Kramer MR. The prevalence of coronary artery disease in end-stage pulmonary disease: is pulmonary fibrosis a risk factor? Respir Med. 2009;103:1346–9.
21. Hubbard RB, Smith C, Le Jeune I, Gribbin J, Fogarty AW. The association between idiopathic pulmonary fibrosis and vascular disease: a population-based study. Am J Respir Crit Care Med. 2008;178:1257–61.
22. Liu H, Fu Y, Wang K. Asthma and risk of coronary heart disease: a meta-analysis of cohort studies. Ann Allergy Asthma Immunol. 2017;118:689–95.
23. Behar S, Panosh A, Reicher-Reiss H, Zion M, Schlesinger Z, Goldbourt U. Prevalence and prognosis of chronic obstructive pulmonary disease among 5,839 consecutive patients with acute myocardial infarction. SPRINT Study Group. Am J Med. 1992;93:637–41.
24. Soriano JB, Rigo F, Guerrero D, Yanez A, Forteza JF, Frontera G, Togores B, Agusti A. High prevalence of undiagnosed airflow limitation in patients with cardiovascular disease. Chest. 2010;137:333–40.

25. Finkelstein J, Cha E, Scharf SM. Chronic obstructive pulmonary disease as an independent risk factor for cardiovascular morbidity. Int J Chron Obstruct Pulmon Dis. 2009;4:337–49.
26. Schnell K, Weiss CO, Lee T, Krishnan JA, Leff B, Wolff JL, Boyd C. The prevalence of clinically-relevant comorbid conditions in patients with physician-diagnosed COPD: a cross-sectional study using data from NHANES 1999-2008. BMC Pulm Med. 2012;12:26.
27. Strachan DP. Ventilatory function as a predictor of fatal stroke. BMJ. 1991;302:84–7.
28. Wannamethee SG, Shaper AG, Ebrahim S. Respiratory function and risk of stroke. Stroke. 1995;26:2004–10.
29. Truelsen T, Prescott E, Lange P, Schnohr P, Boysen G. Lung function and risk of fatal and non-fatal stroke. The Copenhagen City Heart Study. Int J Epidemiol. 2001;30:145–51.
30. Gulsvik AK, Gulsvik A, Skovlund E, Thelle DS, Mowe M, Humerfelt S, Wyller TB. The association between lung function and fatal stroke in a community followed for 4 decades. J Epidemiol Community Health. 2012;66:1030–6.
31. Portegies ML, Lahousse L, Joos GF, Hofman A, Koudstaal PJ, Stricker BH, Brusselle GG, Ikram MA. Chronic obstructive pulmonary disease and the risk of stroke. The Rotterdam Study. Am J Respir Crit Care Med. 2016;193:251–8.
32. Wen LY, Ni H, Li KS, Yang HH, Cheng J, Wang X, Zhao DS, Xie MY, Su H. Asthma and risk of stroke: a systematic review and meta-analysis. J Stroke Cerebrovasc Dis. 2016;25:497–503.
33. Kim SY, Lim H, Lim JS, Choi HG. Analysis of the relationship between adult asthma and stroke: a longitudinal follow-up study using the Korean National sample cohort. Biomed Res Int. 2019;2019:8919230.
34. Strand LB, Tsai MK, Wen CP, Chang SS, Brumpton BM. Is having asthma associated with an increased risk of dying from cardiovascular disease? A prospective cohort study of 446 346 Taiwanese adults. BMJ Open. 2018;8:e019992.
35. Houben-Wilke S, Jorres RA, Bals R, Franssen FM, Glaser S, Holle R, Karch A, Koch A, Magnussen H, Obst A, Schulz H, Spruit MA, Wacker ME, Welte T, Wouters EF, Vogelmeier C, Watz H. Peripheral artery disease and its clinical relevance in patients with chronic obstructive pulmonary disease in the COPD and Systemic Consequences-Comorbidities Network Study. Am J Respir Crit Care Med. 2017;195:189–97.
36. Camiciottoli G, Bigazzi F, Magni C, Bonti V, Diciotti S, Bartolucci M, Mascalchi M, Pistolesi M. Prevalence of comorbidities according to predominant phenotype and severity of chronic obstructive pulmonary disease. Int J Chron Obstruct Pulmon Dis. 2016;11:2229–36.
37. Liao KM, Kuo LT, Lu HY. Increased risk of peripheral arterial occlusive diseases in patients with chronic obstructive pulmonary disease: a nationwide study in Taiwan. Int J Chron Obstruct Pulmon Dis. 2019;14:1455–64.
38. Terzikhan N, Lahousse L, Verhamme KMC, Franco OH, Ikram AM, Stricker BH, Brusselle GG. COPD is associated with an increased risk of peripheral artery disease and mortality. ERJ Open Res. 2018;4:00086.
39. Tschopp J, Dumont P, Hayoz D. True prevalence of COPD and its association with peripheral arterial disease in the internal medicine ward of a tertiary care hospital. Swiss Med Wkly. 2017;147:w14460.
40. Pecci R, De La Fuente Aguado J, Sanjurjo Rivo AB, Sanchez Conde P, Corbacho Abelaira M. Peripheral arterial disease in patients with chronic obstructive pulmonary disease. Int Angiol. 2012;31:444–53.
41. Yao CW, Shen TC, Lu CR, Wang YC, Lin CL, Tu CY, Hsia TC, Shih CM, Hsu WH, Sung FC. Asthma is associated with a subsequent risk of peripheral artery disease: a longitudinal population-based study. Medicine (Baltimore). 2016;95:e2546.
42. Rutten FH, Cramer MJ, Grobbee DE, Sachs AP, Kirkels JH, Lammers JW, Hoes AW. Unrecognized heart failure in elderly patients with stable chronic obstructive pulmonary disease. Eur Heart J. 2005;26:1887–94.
43. Georgiopoulou VV, Kalogeropoulos AP, Psaty BM, Rodondi N, Bauer DC, Butler AB, Koster A, Smith AL, Harris TB, Newman AB, Kritchevsky SB, Butler J. Lung function and risk for heart failure among older adults: the Health ABC Study. Am J Med. 2011;124:334–41.

44. Engstrom G, Melander O, Hedblad B. Population-based study of lung function and incidence of heart failure hospitalisations. Thorax. 2010;65:633–8.
45. Alter P, Watz H, Kahnert K, Pfeifer M, Randerath WJ, Andreas S, Waschki B, Kleibrink BE, Welte T, Bals R, Schulz H, Biertz F, Young D, Vogelmeier CF, Jorres RA. Airway obstruction and lung hyperinflation in COPD are linked to an impaired left ventricular diastolic filling. Respir Med. 2018;137:14–22.
46. Kubota Y, Asai K, Murai K, Tsukada YT, Hayashi H, Saito Y, Azuma A, Gemma A, Shimizu W. COPD advances in left ventricular diastolic dysfunction. Int J Chron Obstruct Pulmon Dis. 2016;11:649–55.
47. Malerba M, Ragnoli B, Salameh M, Sennino G, Sorlini ML, Radaeli A, Clini E. Sub-clinical left ventricular diastolic dysfunction in early stage of chronic obstructive pulmonary disease. J Biol Regul Homeost Agents. 2011;25:443–51.
48. Sabit R, Bolton CE, Fraser AG, Edwards JM, Edwards PH, Ionescu AA, Cockcroft JR, Shale DJ. Sub-clinical left and right ventricular dysfunction in patients with COPD. Respir Med. 2010;104:1171–8.
49. Funk GC, Lang I, Schenk P, Valipour A, Hartl S, Burghuber OC. Left ventricular diastolic dysfunction in patients with COPD in the presence and absence of elevated pulmonary arterial pressure. Chest. 2008;133:1354–9.
50. Schena M, Clini E, Errera D, Quadri A. Echo-Doppler evaluation of left ventricular impairment in chronic cor pulmonale. Chest. 1996;109:1446–51.
51. Freixa X, Portillo K, Pare C, Garcia-Aymerich J, Gomez FP, Benet M, Roca J, Farrero E, Ferrer J, Fernandez-Palomeque C, Antó JM, Barbera JA, PAC-COPD Study Investigators. Echocardiographic abnormalities in patients with copd at their first hospital admission. Eur Respir J. 2013;41(4):784–91.
52. Barr RG, Bluemke DA, Ahmed FS, Carr JJ, Enright PL, Hoffman EA, Jiang R, Kawut SM, Kronmal RA, Lima JA, Shahar E, Smith LJ, Watson KE. Percent emphysema, airflow obstruction, and impaired left ventricular filling. N Engl J Med. 2010;362:217–27.
53. McCord J, Borzak S. Multifocal atrial tachycardia. Chest. 1998;113:203–9.
54. Levine JH, Michael JR, Guarnieri T. Multifocal atrial tachycardia: a toxic effect of theophylline. Lancet. 1985;1:12–4.
55. Shih HT, Webb CR, Conway WA, Peterson E, Tilley B, Goldstein S. Frequency and significance of cardiac arrhythmias in chronic obstructive lung disease. Chest. 1988;94:44–8.
56. Buch P, Friberg J, Scharling H, Lange P, Prescott E. Reduced lung function and risk of atrial fibrillation in the Copenhagen City Heart Study. Eur Respir J. 2003;21:1012–6.
57. Li J, Agarwal SK, Alonso A, Blecker S, Chamberlain AM, London SJ, Loehr LR, McNeill AM, Poole C, Soliman EZ, Heiss G. Airflow obstruction, lung function, and incidence of atrial fibrillation: the Atherosclerosis Risk in Communities (ARIC) study. Circulation. 2014;129:971–80.
58. Konecny T, Park JY, Somers KR, Konecny D, Orban M, Soucek F, Parker KO, Scanlon PD, Asirvatham SJ, Brady PA, Rihal CS. Relation of chronic obstructive pulmonary disease to atrial and ventricular arrhythmias. Am J Cardiol. 2014;114:272–7.
59. Tukek T, Yildiz P, Akkaya V, Karan MA, Atilgan D, Yilmaz V, Korkut F. Factors associated with the development of atrial fibrillation in COPD patients: the role of P-wave dispersion. Ann Noninvasive Electrocardiol. 2002;7:222–7.
60. Bhatt SP, Nanda S, Kintzer JS. Arrhythmias as trigger for acute exacerbations of chronic obstructive pulmonary disease. Respir Med. 2012;106:1134–8.
61. Sarubbi B, Esposito V, Ducceschi V, Meoli I, Grella E, Santangelo L, Iacano A, Caputi M. Effect of blood gas derangement on QTc dispersion in severe chronic obstructive pulmonary disease: evidence of an electropathy? Int J Cardiol. 1997;58:287–92.
62. Warnier MJ, Blom MT, Bardai A, Berdowksi J, Souverein PC, Hoes AW, Rutten FH, de Boer A, Koster RW, De Bruin ML, Tan HL. Increased risk of sudden cardiac arrest in obstructive pulmonary disease: a case-control study. PLoS One. 2013;8:e65638.

63. Lahousse L, Niemeijer MN, van den Berg ME, Rijnbeek PR, Joos GF, Hofman A, Franco OH, Deckers JW, Eijgelsheim M, Stricker BH, Brusselle GG. Chronic obstructive pulmonary disease and sudden cardiac death: the Rotterdam study. Eur Heart J. 2015;36:1754–61.

64. van den Berg ME, Stricker BH, Brusselle GG, Lahousse L. Chronic obstructive pulmonary disease and sudden cardiac death: a systematic review. Trends Cardiovasc Med. 2016;26:606–13.

65. Iribarren C, Round AD, Peng JA, Lu M, Klatsky AL, Zaroff JG, Holve TJ, Prasad A, Stang P. Short QT in a cohort of 1.7 million persons: prevalence, correlates, and prognosis. Ann Noninvasive Electrocardiol. 2014;19:490–500.

66. Tukek T, Yildiz P, Atilgan D, Tuzcu V, Eren M, Erk O, Demirel S, Akkaya V, Dilmener M, Korkut F. Effect of diurnal variability of heart rate on development of arrhythmia in patients with chronic obstructive pulmonary disease. Int J Cardiol. 2003;88:199–206.

67. Hawkins NM, Petrie MC, Jhund PS, Chalmers GW, Dunn FG, McMurray JJ. Heart failure and chronic obstructive pulmonary disease: diagnostic pitfalls and epidemiology. Eur J Heart Fail. 2009;11:130–9.

68. Le Jemtel TH, Padeletti M, Jelic S. Diagnostic and therapeutic challenges in patients with coexistent chronic obstructive pulmonary disease and chronic heart failure. J Am Coll Cardiol. 2007;49:171–80.

69. Naum CC, Sciurba FC, Rogers RM. Pulmonary function abnormalities in chronic severe cardiomyopathy preceding cardiac transplantation. Am Rev Respir Dis. 1992;145:1334–8.

70. Light RW, George RB. Serial pulmonary function in patients with acute heart failure. Arch Intern Med. 1983;143:429–33.

71. Guder G, Rutten FH, Brenner S, Angermann CE, Berliner D, Ertl G, Jany B, Lammers JW, Hoes AW, Stork S. The impact of heart failure on the classification of COPD severity. J Card Fail. 2012;18:637–44.

72. Thomason JW, Ely EW, Chiles C, Ferretti G, Freimanis RI, Haponik EF. Appraising pulmonary edema using supine chest roentgenograms in ventilated patients. Am J Respir Crit Care Med. 1998;157:1600–8.

73. Martin GS, Ely EW, Carroll FE, Bernard GR. Findings on the portable chest radiograph correlate with fluid balance in critically ill patients. Chest. 2002;122:2087–95.

74. Lichtenstein DA, Meziere GA. Relevance of lung ultrasound in the diagnosis of acute respiratory failure: the BLUE protocol. Chest. 2008;134:117–25.

75. Picano E, Frassi F, Agricola E, Gligorova S, Gargani L, Mottola G. Ultrasound lung comets: a clinically useful sign of extravascular lung water. J Am Soc Echocardiogr. 2006;19:356–63.

76. Mayo PH, Copetti R, Feller-Kopman D, Mathis G, Maury E, Mongodi S, Mojoli F, Volpicelli G, Zanobetti M. Thoracic ultrasonography: a narrative review. Intensive Care Med. 2019;45:1200–11.

77. Gerges C, Gerges M, Lang MB, Zhang Y, Jakowitsch J, Probst P, Maurer G, Lang IM. Diastolic pulmonary vascular pressure gradient: a predictor of prognosis in "out-of-proportion" pulmonary hypertension. Chest. 2013;143:758–66.

Chapter 2
Origins of Cardiopulmonary Disease in Early Life

Michael J. Cuttica and Ravi Kalhan

> **Pearls**
> - Approaching the concept of lung health by focusing on the identification of early-life risk factors that drive the evolution of disease states later in life rather than defining disease and health by a dichotomized spirometric value will allow for more robust preventative health strategies targeted at lung disease.
> - Understanding heart-lung interactions early in life and the pathophysiologic mechanisms underlying them will allow a better understanding of the co-evolution of cardiopulmonary disease.

Lung Disease and Cardiovascular Disease

The association between lung disease and cardiovascular disease later in life has been well described. Both obstructive and restrictive lung physiology as measured with spirometry have been associated with cardiovascular disease and poor health outcomes [1–8]. In an aging population, it is not surprising that there would be overlaps between common lung diseases like COPD and common cardiovascular diseases like coronary artery disease especially considering that many of these diseases share common risk factors like tobacco use and aging. It is these common risk factors that give rise to the hypothesis that lung disease and heart disease are separate entities that evolve in parallel with the idea that environmental exposures such as tobacco smoke through direct injury to the lung and activation of inflammatory pathways lead to decline in lung function and eventually to COPD, while at the same time the activated inflammatory pathways also activate atherosclerotic pathways and

M. J. Cuttica · R. Kalhan (✉)
Northwestern University, Feinberg School of Medicine,
Division of Pulmonary and Critical Care Medicine, Chicago, IL, USA
e-mail: micuttic@nm.org; r-kalhan@northwestern.edu

© Springer Nature Switzerland AG 2020
S. P. Bhatt (ed.), *Cardiac Considerations in Chronic Lung Disease*,
Respiratory Medicine, https://doi.org/10.1007/978-3-030-43435-9_2

eventually lead to coronary artery disease. However, there is growing data that suggests that the association between diseases like COPD and cardiovascular disease occurs independent of these common risk factors [5]. As we see more evidence that lung and heart disease occur in individuals later in life, it raises an important question: are the processes that affect lung and heart function through life intertwined in such a way that they are actually causally linked in the development of shared disease states? Perhaps, instead of parallel development of lung disease and cardiac disease as individuals' age, these processes co-evolve into shared cardiopulmonary disease. If this is the case, then it becomes imperative that we look to the origins of this co-evolution early in life before disease is established to determine if we can intervene to delay or prevent these cardiopulmonary disease processes.

The Paradigm: Identification of Pre-cardiovascular Disease

No field in medicine has done a better job in the past than cardiovascular medicine in realizing the importance of identifying risk factors early in life that both predict the development of future disease and can be treated to modify and prevent development of disease. The paradigm in the cardiovascular community has been to conceptualize "ideal cardiovascular health" to include a set of factors, several situated directly along the causal pathway of transitions from health to disease, which protect against the development of cardiac disease. Considering cardiovascular health along such a continuum has facilitated identification of risk factors for loss of health, delineated intermediate endotypes which are deployed in clinical practice as screening tools, and, historically, has led to increasingly effective preventive health measures. Although a full review of the broad literature base related to cardiovascular disease prevention is beyond the focus of this chapter, one example to highlight the importance of approaching cardiovascular health along a continuum from health to disease is worth exploring. Probably one of the best examples of this are the guidelines on lipid management for the reduction of atherosclerotic cardiovascular disease events. The INTERHEART study, a large international case-control study, identified abnormal lipid levels as being associated with the highest population attributable risk for the occurrence of acute myocardial infarction compared to other modifiable risk factors [9]. This highlights one of many studies which identified cholesterol as not only an important risk factor in the development of coronary artery disease but via reduction of cholesterol levels through lifestyle and pharmacologic means as a major modifiable risk factor to prevent disease [10–13]. These epidemiologic studies looking at population-based effects of cholesterol on heart health along with multiple interventional studies exploring the direct effect of lipid-lowering interventions have allowed for the development of guidelines targeted at very specific patient groups [14–17]. For example, guidelines recommend statin therapy for individuals without atherosclerotic cardiovascular disease but with low density lipoprotein (LDL) cholesterol levels >190 mg/dL and for individuals aged 40–75 years old again without atherosclerotic cardiovascular disease but who have diabetes and LDL cholesterol levels in the range of 70–189 mg/dL [18]. Again, this does not mean to serve as a primary review of cholesterol based preventive health strategies for cardiovascular disease. Rather, it is as an excellent example of an approach where the focus lies on identifying and intervening on a continuum of health rather than awaiting intervention after the disease state has presented.

The Paradigm Shift: Loss of Lung Health and Identification of Pre-lung Disease

Although significant attention has been paid to the clinical manifestations of chronic lung disease, less is known about the evolution of respiratory conditions across the lifespan. Pulmonary physicians and respiratory researchers have traditionally defined lung health exclusively as the absence of lung disease. This simplistic definition has limited the development of a robust approach to lung disease prevention. Contrary to the experience of our cardiovascular colleagues who as outlined above have focused on the defining and intervening on the continuum of cardiovascular health as people age, there has been a distinct absence of life-course studies focused primarily on understanding the evolution of lung health as we age. As a result of this, it is a challenge to conceptualize how an individual might progress from ideal lung health to an intermediate phenotype of impaired respiratory health to chronic lung disease [19]. In the current paradigm, simple spirometry thresholds singularly delineate respiratory health from lung disease [20]. This simplistic approach does not acknowledge that the transition from health to chronic lung disease develops over years, a period of time when disease interception may be most efficacious. As a consequence, there are limited primary prevention strategies for chronic lung disease that are analogous to those implemented for cardiovascular conditions.

In recent years, there has been better identification of this gap in our knowledge base and the beginning of an increased focus on understanding the evolution of lung health. For instance, in an analysis of three independent primarily cardiovascular disease-focused cohorts in both the United States and Europe (the Framingham Offspring Cohort, the Copenhagen City Heart Study, and the Lovelace Smokers Cohort), participants with lower lung function (defined as an FEV_1 less than 80% of predicted) at cohort inception were at greater risk of chronic obstructive pulmonary disease (COPD) after 22 years of observation than those who had normal lung function at baseline [21]. This is an important study which shows that factors that impact an individual's peak lung function early in life have important implications for an individual's risk of developing obstructive lung disease as they age. This means lung function in early adulthood is an important risk factor for the development of lung disease later in life. One limitation of this study was that the mean age at cohort inception was about 40 years, ranging from 21 to 75 years across all three cohorts. This mean age is well beyond when most people attain peak lung function and presumably results in capturing people who have already accumulated environmental exposures that impact the risk of developing lung disease. However, these findings actually reinforced a prior report from the Coronary Artery Risk Development in Young Adults (CARDIA) cohort, which revealed that low baselineFEV$_1$ and FEV$_1$/forced vital capacity (FVC) between 18 and 30 years of age predicted airflow obstruction 20 years later independent of smoking status [22]. Of even more interest, most of the individuals in the CARDIA study with lower baseline lung function still had lung function values that would be considered in the "normal" range (i.e., FEV$_1$ greater than 80% of predicted and FEV$_1$/FVC greater than the lower limit of normal), did not report a diagnosis of any underlying lung disease, and typically would not have undergone spirometric testing in the context of routine clinical care. These again highlight the importance of approaching the idea of lung health as a continuum that evolves as we age rather than the traditional hard cut-off lung function value that separates "healthy" from "disease."

Our group has investigated the predictors and consequences of lung function decline in the CARDIA study [23], a longitudinal cohort aged 18–30 years at inception in 1985. We have identified features of impaired respiratory health that precede the development of chronic lung disease. These include: lower peak lung function in young adulthood [22], accelerated age-related decline in lung function, elevations in systemic inflammatory biomarkers [24], and the presence of respiratory symptoms [25]. We have shown the clinical relevance of impaired respiratory health [22, 25, 26], but our work to date does not provide a set of targets for the interception of chronic lung disease.

Co-evolution of Lung and Heart Disease: The Birth of Cardiopulmonary Disease

As more attention seems to be focused on trying to better define lung health, and where loss of lung health is on the path to the development of lung disease, there is an opportunity to explore how heart and lung disease coevolve as we age. It has long been recognized that measures of lung function are associated with cardiovascular outcomes. In the Framingham Heart Study, FVC measured at a mean age of 40–45 years was noted to be associated with risk of subsequent cardiovascular disease [27]. This finding reproduced similar associations noted in several older studies between lung function and cardiovascular outcomes but like its predecessors also failed to define a strong theory on the mechanism underlying the association [28–30]. As with the transgenerational cohort analysis discussed above [21], one limitation to the Framingham study is that the age range captured at the time of lung function testing (40–45 years old) is older than when most people attain peak lung function (typically around age 25–35 years) [31] and at an age when lung disease starts to become clinically apparent [21, 32, 33]. Occult coronary disease, smoking impacts on health, and hypoxic effects are presented as potential mechanisms driving the association even as the authors note that the associations in the statistical models are independent of these general risk factors [27]. This highlights the importance of being able to evaluate this association starting even earlier in life before the onset of disease and before common risk factors start to accumulate.

The CARDIA study again through its ability to look at measurements of lung function in early adulthood (ages 18–30 years) and link it to a robust cardiovascular outcomes database has provided a unique insight into the coevolution of heart and lung disease. Like the Framingham study before it, the CARDIA study was able to show an association independent of sex, race, smoking, BMI, total cholesterol, blood pressure, and diabetes between baseline lung function measured at mean age of 25 years and cardiovascular disease events over 29 years of follow-up. Unlike the Framingham study though, CARDIA captures an association occurring at a time when tobacco smoke exposure is low, lung function is at or near its peak, and, in almost all participants, the measurements of lung function are in the "normal" range [34]. The obvious implication of these findings is that lung function testing in early adulthood may provide an early window into cardiovascular health at a time when the evolution of potential heart and lung disease are in their initial stages.

These findings of links between peak lung function measurements in early adulthood and cardiovascular outcomes do not answer the questions related to the mechanisms that drive this association. It is intriguing that this study from CARDIA also showed that lung function was associated specifically with heart failure and cerebrovascular events and not coronary artery disease events like myocardial infarction or with indicators of atherosclerotic disease like coronary calcium scores. This is particularly interesting given the known association between lung disease like COPD and coronary artery disease events later in life [4, 35] and perhaps gives a window into different mechanistic pathways that may be present early in life versus pathways that develop through environmental exposure as we age. These early-life mechanistic pathways may lie more with metabolic changes linked to lung and cardiovascular function that impact overall vascular health. One example pointing toward this would be the evidence of associations between lung function and risk of diabetes, a disease with clear negative effects on both cardiac and vascular health outcomes [36–38]. How lung function is linked with diabetes risk is unclear, and exploring the roles of the interplay of physical fitness and common inflammatory pathways may lead to insights into the development of cardiopulmonary disease. It has also been shown in CARDIA that there is an association between FVC decline and incident hypertension. Although the mechanisms underlying this link remain to be understood, this association may provide a common pathway linking lung function to cardiovascular outcomes [39]. To help better understand this relationship, we further evaluated patterns of decline in lung health from peak lung function in young adulthood and their associations with heart structure and function in middle age. We found that patterns of loss of lung health are associated with distinct echocardiographic phenotypes in middle age such that a decline in the FEV_1/FVC ratio is associated with a decrease in left heart chamber size and lower cardiac output, whereas, a decline in the FVC but with a preserved FEV_1/FVC ratio is associated with left heart hypertrophy, increased cardiac output, and early diastolic dysfunction [26]. It is reasonable to hypothesize that as these divergent patterns of loss of lung health develop into distinct heart-lung phenotypes in middle age, the

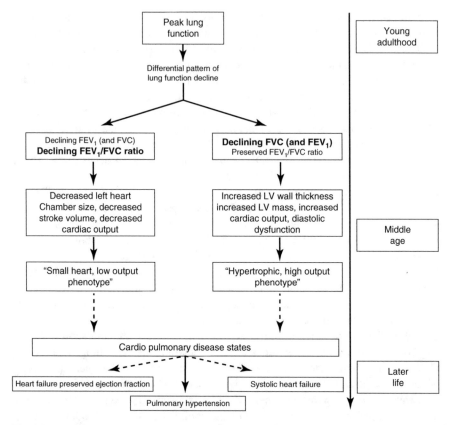

Fig. 2.1 Divergent patterns of loss of lung health and development of disease. Reproduced from Cuttica et al. [26])

groundwork is being laid for the eventual development of distinct heart failure syndromes seen later in life (Fig. 2.1).

Conclusion

All of these findings highlight the complexity of the early-life origins of the heart-lung interactions that evolve as we age to lead to the development of shared cardiopulmonary disease states. Almost all the data available evaluating this come from observational epidemiology studies which although providing interesting and important insights into the links between heart and lung disease are limited in their ability to explore mechanisms that drive this. Many intriguing findings have been reported raising many interesting questions regarding the origins of cardiopulmonary disease. Perhaps the next area of focus needs to be on interventional studies allowing for the delineation of the pathways that link the co-evolution heart and lung interactions. As our cardiovascular colleagues have shown, understanding these pathways will eventually allow us to modify and prevent the development of cardiopulmonary disease.

References

1. Mannino DM, Holguin F, Pavlin BI, Ferdinands JM. Risk factors for prevalence of and mortality related to restriction on spirometry: findings from the First National Health and Nutrition Examination Survey and follow-up. Int J Tuberc Lung Dis. 2005;9:613–21.
2. Duprez DA, Hearst MO, Lutsey PL, et al. Associations among lung function, arterial elasticity, and circulating endothelial and inflammation markers: the multiethnic study of atherosclerosis. Hypertension. 2013;61:542–8.
3. Ford ES, Wheaton AG, Mannino DM, Presley-Cantrell L, Li C, Croft JB. Elevated cardiovascular risk among adults with obstructive and restrictive airway functioning in the United States: a cross-sectional study of the National Health and Nutrition Examination Survey from 2007-2010. Respir Res. 2012;13:115.
4. Curkendall SM, DeLuise C, Jones JK, et al. Cardiovascular disease in patients with chronic obstructive pulmonary disease, Saskatchewan Canada cardiovascular disease in COPD patients. Ann Epidemiol. 2006;16:63–70.
5. Sin DD, Wu L, Man SF. The relationship between reduced lung function and cardiovascular mortality: a population-based study and a systematic review of the literature. Chest. 2005;127:1952–9.
6. Hole DJ, Watt GC, Davey-Smith G, Hart CL, Gillis CR, Hawthorne VM. Impaired lung function and mortality risk in men and women: findings from the Renfrew and Paisley prospective population study. BMJ. 1996;313:711–5; discussion 5–6.
7. Schunemann HJ, Dorn J, Grant BJ, Winkelstein W Jr, Trevisan M. Pulmonary function is a long-term predictor of mortality in the general population: 29-year follow-up of the Buffalo Health Study. Chest. 2000;118:656–64.
8. McGarvey LP, John M, Anderson JA, Zvarich M, Wise RA. Ascertainment of cause-specific mortality in COPD: operations of the TORCH Clinical Endpoint Committee. Thorax. 2007;62:411–5.
9. Yusuf S, Hawken S, Ounpuu S, et al. Effect of potentially modifiable risk factors associated with myocardial infarction in 52 countries (the INTERHEART study): case-control study. Lancet. 2004;364:937–52.
10. Bandosz P, O'Flaherty M, Drygas W, et al. Decline in mortality from coronary heart disease in Poland after socioeconomic transformation: modelling study. BMJ. 2012;344:d8136.
11. Bjorck L, Rosengren A, Bennett K, Lappas G, Capewell S. Modelling the decreasing coronary heart disease mortality in Sweden between 1986 and 2002. Eur Heart J. 2009;30:1046–56.
12. Wijeysundera HC, Machado M, Farahati F, et al. Association of temporal trends in risk factors and treatment uptake with coronary heart disease mortality, 1994-2005. JAMA. 2010;303:1841–7.
13. Ford ES, Ajani UA, Croft JB, et al. Explaining the decrease in U.S. deaths from coronary disease, 1980-2000. N Engl J Med. 2007;356:2388–98.
14. Downs JR, Clearfield M, Weis S, et al. Primary prevention of acute coronary events with lovastatin in men and women with average cholesterol levels: results of AFCAPS/TexCAPS. Air Force/Texas Coronary Atherosclerosis Prevention Study. JAMA. 1998;279:1615–22.
15. Nakamura H, Arakawa K, Itakura H, et al. Primary prevention of cardiovascular disease with pravastatin in Japan (MEGA Study): a prospective randomised controlled trial. Lancet. 2006;368:1155–63.
16. Ridker PM, Danielson E, Fonseca FA, et al. Rosuvastatin to prevent vascular events in men and women with elevated C-reactive protein. N Engl J Med. 2008;359:2195–207.

17. Cholesterol Treatment Trialists' (CTT) Collaboration, Baigent C, Blackwell L, et al. Efficacy and safety of more intensive lowering of LDL cholesterol: a meta-analysis of data from 170,000 participants in 26 randomised trials. Lancet. 2010;376:1670–81.
18. Stone NJ, Robinson JG, Lichtenstein AH, et al. 2013 ACC/AHA guideline on the treatment of blood cholesterol to reduce atherosclerotic cardiovascular risk in adults: a report of the American College of Cardiology/American Heart Association Task Force on Practice Guidelines. J Am Coll Cardiol. 2014;63:2889–934.
19. Reyfman PA, Washko GR, Dransfield MT, Spira A, Han MK, Kalhan R. Defining impaired respiratory health: a paradigm shift for pulmonary medicine. Am J Respir Crit Care Med. 2018;198(4):440–6.
20. Martinez FJ, Han MK, Allinson JP, et al. At the root: defining and halting progression of early chronic obstructive pulmonary disease. Am J Respir Crit Care Med. 2018;197:1540–51.
21. Agusti A, Noell G, Brugada J, Faner R. Lung function in early adulthood and health in later life: a transgenerational cohort analysis. Lancet Respir Med. 2017;5:935.
22. Kalhan R, Arynchyn A, Colangelo LA, Dransfield MT, Gerald LB, Smith LJ. Lung function in young adults predicts airflow obstruction 20 years later. Am J Med. 2010;123:468.e1–7.
23. Hughes GH, Cutter G, Donahue R, et al. Recruitment in the coronary artery disease risk development in young adults (Cardia) study. Control Clin Trials. 1987;8:68S–73S.
24. Kalhan R, Tran BT, Colangelo LA, et al. Systemic inflammation in young adults is associated with abnormal lung function in middle age. PLoS One. 2010;5:e11431.
25. Kalhan R, Dransfield MT, Colangelo LA, et al. Respiratory symptoms in young adults and future lung disease: the CARDIA lung study. Am J Respir Crit Care Med. 2018;197:1616–24.
26. Cuttica MJ, Colangelo LA, Shah S, et al. Loss of lung health from young adulthood and cardiac phenotypes in middle age. Am J Respir Crit Care Med. 2015;192:76–85.
27. Kannel WB, Hubert H, Lew EA. Vital capacity as a predictor of cardiovascular disease: the Framingham study. Am Heart J. 1983;105:311–5.
28. Keys A, Aravanis C, Blackburn H, et al. Lung function as a risk factor for coronary heart disease. Am J Public Health. 1972;62:1506–11.
29. Friedman GD, Klatsky AL, Siegelaub AB. Lung function and risk of myocardial infarction and sudden cardiac death. N Engl J Med. 1976;294:1071–5.
30. Higgins MW, Keller JB. Predictors of mortality in the adult population of Tecumseh. Arch Environ Health. 1970;21:418–24.
31. Beck GJ, Doyle CA, Schachter EN. A longitudinal study of respiratory health in a rural community. Am Rev Respir Dis. 1982;125:375–81.
32. Mannino DM, Gagnon RC, Petty TL, Lydick E. Obstructive lung disease and low lung function in adults in the United States: data from the National Health and Nutrition Examination Survey, 1988-1994. Arch Intern Med. 2000;160:1683–9.
33. Mannino DM, Homa DM, Akinbami LJ, Ford ES, Redd SC. Chronic obstructive pulmonary disease surveillance – United States, 1971-2000. Respir Care. 2002;47:1184–99.
34. Cuttica MJ, Colangelo L, Washko G, et al. Lung health and the association with cardiovascular disease outcomes: the CARDIA study. Am J Respir Crit Care Med. 2017;195:A1011.
35. Sidney S, Sorel M, Quesenberry CP Jr, DeLuise C, Lanes S, Eisner MD. COPD and incident cardiovascular disease hospitalizations and mortality: Kaiser Permanente Medical Care Program. Chest. 2005;128:2068–75.
36. Zaigham S, Nilsson PM, Wollmer P, Engstrom G. The temporal relationship between poor lung function and the risk of diabetes. BMC Pulm Med. 2016;16:75.
37. Lazarus R, Sparrow D, Weiss ST. Baseline ventilatory function predicts the development of higher levels of fasting insulin and fasting insulin resistance index: the Normative Aging Study. Eur Respir J. 1998;12:641–5.
38. Engstrom G, Hedblad B, Nilsson P, Wollmer P, Berglund G, Janzon L. Lung function, insulin resistance and incidence of cardiovascular disease: a longitudinal cohort study. J Intern Med. 2003;253:574–81.
39. Jacobs DR Jr, Yatsuya H, Hearst MO, et al. Rate of decline of forced vital capacity predicts future arterial hypertension: the Coronary Artery Risk Development in Young Adults Study. Hypertension. 2012;59:219–25.

Chapter 3
Cardiovascular Comorbidity in Chronic Lung Disease: Gender Differences

Christine Jenkins

Pearls
1. Asthma is associated with a higher probability of cardiovascular disease (CVD). The association is stronger in women than in men, for both morbidity and mortality.
2. Adult-onset asthma in women has the highest association with CVD, and women with asthma and CVD receive fewer interventions when they are admitted with myocardial infarction.
3. There are likely to be markedly different prevalence rates and clinical presentations between men and women with airway disease and CVD, depending on the country and the causes of obstructive lung disease.
4. CVD in men and women with asthma and COPD is under-recognized and treated differently, women tending to seek more healthcare interactions but receive fewer medications and interventions.
5. Sex- and gender-based differences in chronic lung disease with CVD urgently need further research to understand impact and to tailor better management.

There are substantial gender differences in chronic respiratory diseases as well as cardiovascular disease. In this chapter, gender differences in comorbid chronic lung disease (CLD) and cardiovascular disease (CVD) will be examined. Data on this

C. Jenkins (✉)
Concord Hospital Sydney, Concord, NSW, Australia

The George Institute for Global Health, Sydney, NSW, Australia

Faculty of Medicine, UNSW Sydney, Sydney, NSW, Australia

University of Sydney, Sydney, NSW, Australia
e-mail: christine.jenkins@sydney.edu.au

© Springer Nature Switzerland AG 2020
S. P. Bhatt (ed.), *Cardiac Considerations in Chronic Lung Disease*,
Respiratory Medicine, https://doi.org/10.1007/978-3-030-43435-9_3

intersection are limited and are found mostly in literature focused on asthma and chronic obstructive pulmonary disease (COPD). Interstitial lung disease (ILD) will not be included in this chapter as there are too few studies to allow meaningful conclusions to be drawn.

What Do We Mean by Sex and Gender?

Throughout the chapter, the Institute of Medicine definitions of sex as the classification of living things, generally as male or female according to their reproductive organs and functions assigned by chromosomal complement, will be used. Gender is a person's self-representation as male or female, or how that person is responded to by social institutions, on the basis of the individual's gender presentation [1].

Asthma, Cardiovascular Disease, and Sex Differences

The sex-specific aspects of asthma that are well recognized include a higher prevalence of asthma among boys in childhood and higher occurrence of new cases among girls, commencing around puberty and persisting through the life span. It is well known that young adult females may suffer from menstrual cycle-related asthma flare-ups, worsening asthma during pregnancy, and a higher risk of hospital admissions. Later in life, women with asthma also outnumber men, in both prevalence and mortality [2].

Asthma has been associated with increased cardiovascular disease (CVD) morbidity and mortality in multiple studies [3]. However, CVD is not a highly recognized comorbidity of asthma, and there are some conflicting results from different studies and populations. Very little is known about the impact of gender on CVD comorbidity in asthma.

What Can We Learn from General Population Studies?

In a large population-based cohort of men and women in Northern California, with a median follow-up 27 years [4], Iribarren et al. examined the sex-specific association between asthma and non-fatal and fatal coronary artery disease (CAD). After adjusting for age, ethnicity, education, occupational exposures, and several other risk factors, a history of asthma was associated with a 1.22-fold (95% CI: 1.14, 1.31) increased hazard of CAD among women compared to men. This was observed in never-smoking and ever-smoking women and in younger and older women. By contrast, asthma was not associated with CAD among men (adjusted hazard ratio = 0.99; 95% CI: 0.93, 1.05).

The Atherosclerosis Risk in Communities (ARIC) Study in four US communities included 15,792 men and women aged 45–64, followed for 14 years for incidence of CAD and stroke events to 2001 [5]. Compared with never having asthma, the adjusted hazard ratio (HR) of stroke was 1.50 (95% CI 1.04–2.15) for those reporting ever having asthma (prevalence 5.2%) and 1.55 (95% CI 0.95–2.52) for current asthma (prevalence 2.7%). Those reporting wheeze attacks with shortness of breath also had greater risk for stroke (HR = 1.56, 95% CI 1.18–2.06) than participants without these symptoms.

In the same study population, women with adult-onset asthma (but not those with child-onset asthma) experienced a twofold increase in incident CAD and stroke which was independent of other known risk factors, and this increase persisted when the analysis was restricted to never-smokers [6]. No significant association was found among women with childhood-onset asthma or among men. The authors concluded that adult-onset asthma may be a significant risk factor for CAD and stroke among women but not men. Subsequently they found carotid artery intimal-medial wall thickness (IMT) to be slightly greater for women with history of adult-onset asthma than that of women without asthma, but mean IMT did not differ significantly according to asthma history among men. The interaction between adult-onset asthma and gender was significant, even after adjusting for age, race, body mass index, smoking status, smoking pack-years, diabetes, hypertension, physical activity, education level, and high- and low-density lipoprotein levels. They concluded that adult-onset asthma is associated with increased carotid atherosclerosis among women but not among men, an observation that provides one possible contributory mechanism for the higher probability of stroke and CAD in women.

By contrast, in the Canadian Community Health Survey [7], there was no clear relationship between age of onset of asthma and CVD risk. Asthmatics were 43% (odds ratio, OR = 1.43, 95% CI 1.19–1.72) more likely to have heart disease and 36% (OR = 1.36, 95% CI 1.21–1.53) more likely to have high blood pressure than non-asthmatics. Males with adult-onset asthma (>20 years old) were 63% more likely to have high blood pressure than males with early-onset asthma, but otherwise there were no significant differences between males and females.

In a large Italian database, a diagnosis of asthma was modestly associated with the diagnosis of different cardiovascular comorbidities although significantly less strongly than for COPD [8]. In the whole population, cardiovascular comorbidities affected minimally more women than men (male:female = 0.98). Among patients with diagnosed asthma, the OR for angina and coronary disease was higher in women compared to men, but no difference was seen for association with all cardiovascular diseases.

Asthma and CVD in Case-Control Studies

In a US cohort of 203,595 adults with asthma and a parallel asthma-free cohort matched for age, sex, and ethnicity, asthma was associated with a 1.40-fold increased hazard of CAD, a 1.20-fold hazard of cerebrovascular disease, a 2.14-fold hazard of heart failure, and a 3.28-fold hazard of all-cause mortality after adjustment for multiple risk factors [4]. Stronger associations were noted among women. However, only those using asthma medications (particularly those on oral corticosteroids alone or in combination) were at enhanced risk of CVD. These data suggest that severity of asthma is a determinant of CVD morbidity, and sex is a cofactor modifying this.

Further exploring this, among 100 asthmatic patients and 129 COPD patients consecutively recruited from an Italian university outpatient clinic, a high prevalence of CVD was found. On the basis of history, clinical, and echocardiographic data, CVD was found in 81% of this population, 51% of these having COPD and 30% having asthma [9]. CVD was associated with older age and more severe airflow obstruction both in asthma and COPD. Distributions of pressure and volume overload showed a clear increase with increasing severity of asthma, in contrast to COPD where the prevalence of each type of CVD was similar across GOLD stages.

In a Danish study comparing mortality rates in asthma and COPD patients to the general population over a mean follow-up of 13 years, and after adjustment for predictors of survival (age, $FEV_1\%$ predicted, body mass index, smoking status, oral prednisolone, CAD, and cor pulmonale), the relative risk of death was 1.21 and 0.98 in females compared with males in asthma and COPD, respectively [10]. When standardized mortality rates were used, the relationship was stronger with a rate ratio of 1.24 (95% CI 0.82–1.84) in asthma. However, females and males with the same level of obstructive lung disease appeared to have similar mortality rates.

Gender Effects on Outcomes in Asthma with CVD Comorbidity

A recent meta-analysis examined the relationship between asthma and CVD or all-cause mortality in prospective and retrospective cohort studies, containing over 400,000 participants [11]. The summary relative risk for all-cause mortality in patients with asthma and CVD was 1.33 (95% CI 1.15–1.53). For asthma and CVD in women, the relative risk for mortality was 1.55 (95% CI 1.20–2.00), 1.20 (95% CI 0.92–1.56) in men, and 1.36 (95% CI 1.01–1.83) for all-cause mortality in both genders. Women with asthma experienced a higher risk of CVD than men with asthma, these findings remaining consistent after sensitivity analysis.

In a study of myocardial infarction (MI) and post-MI outcomes in people with asthma (who constituted 3% of the total database) compared to the general population in the United Kingdom, analysis of over 300,000 people showed that people with asthma were more likely to have adverse outcomes [12]. These included a delay in their MI diagnosis following an ST-segment elevation myocardial infarction (STEMI), OR 1.38, and 95% CI 1.06–1.79, but not a non-STEMI, OR 1.04, and 95% CI 0.92–1.17, compared to people without asthma. They also experienced a delay in reperfusion (OR 1.19, 95% CI 1.09–1.30) following a STEMI. People with asthma were much less likely to be discharged on a beta-blocker following a myocardial infarction (STEMI or non-STEMI), OR 0.24, 95% CI 0.21–0.28 and OR 0.27, 95% CI 0.24–0.30. While this is not surprising, withholding highly efficacious medications such as beta-blockers which reduce post-MI mortality could be one mechanism by which mortality from MI is increased in people with asthma.

On presentation with an MI, people with asthma were older than those without (mean age 72.8 vs. 67.3) and more likely to be female (54.4% vs. 32.5%). Although there was a higher prevalence of comorbid conditions such as chronic kidney disease, diabetes, and congestive cardiac failure among people with asthma, after controlling for age, sex, smoking status, and comorbidities, there was no difference in in-hospital mortality between people with and without asthma.

In another UK study of asthma deaths in hospital, ascertained through anonymized National Health Service (NHS) data from 2000 to 2005, respiratory infection was the single most common comorbidity (25%), but CVD diagnoses (atrial fibrillation and flutter, hypertension, left ventricular failure, and CAD) accounted for 54% of all listed comorbidities [13]. Females and those over 45 years were at the highest risk of death after a hospitalization for asthma. Conceivably, infection interacts with other comorbidities such as heart disease to increase risk of admission or death, such as is now known for pneumococcal infection.

Gender-Related Factors Affect the Presentation and Management of Asthma with CVD

In relation to the impact of CVD in asthma, an analysis of sex differences in health service and medication use in the German statutory health insurance database of over 26 million people [14] showed that men had on average 17.1% (95% CI 14.1–20.2) higher costs for inpatient care after adjusting for age and comorbidity. On average women received more prescriptions than men, but costs per medication for men were higher per prescription. Men and women received about the same percentage of prescriptions for beta-2 agonists and inhaled steroids. While not directly informing us about the impact of gender on the association between CVD and asthma, this analysis indicates that in this population, men and women received different treatments for similar diseases. This may result from different presentation patterns and physician contacts as well as different prescribing behaviors.

Other studies confirm the different prescribing patterns for men and women with asthma. In an analysis of over 11 million ambulatory visits in COPD patients in the United States [15], there was a significantly lower bronchodilator treatment rate among patients with comorbid CVD (32.3%) than among patients without CVD (57.6%). There were significant interactions between CVD and gender, concomitant beta-blocker drugs, and concomitant asthma. The presence of CVD diagnosis significantly decreased the likelihood of bronchodilator prescribing by 97% for females with asthma who were not taking beta-blockers and by 83% in males with similar characteristics. De-prescribing was more pronounced for females than males, and bronchodilator prescribing in females with CVD taking beta-blockers with coexisting asthma was 79% less than those without CVD (OR = 0.21, 95% CI 0.14–0.30). In females who had asthma and did not use beta-blockers, there was only a 3% chance of taking bronchodilators compared with the non-comorbid CVD group. In males with no asthma and no beta-blocker use, there was a higher bronchodilator prescribing rate of 68% (OR = 0.32, 95% CI 0.25–0.40). CVD did not affect the prescribing outcome in male beta-blocker users, regardless of asthma status. The authors commented that the lower utilization rates in females suggest more conservative prescribing practices for females than for males.

In many countries the female:male ratio for deaths in severe asthma is still very high, even allowing for the fact that there is a greater proportion of females with asthma. Since more older women than men die from asthma, and the majority of deaths from asthma in older adults are associated with cardiac events [13], on the basis of these data, the coexistence of CVD in asthma in women is a warning flag for increased mortality risk from asthma.

Mechanisms for the Increased Prevalence of CVD in Asthma

There are several possible reasons for an increased risk of CVD among people with asthma, but these mostly remain theoretical and unproven. Several investigators propose that tobacco smoking is the main explanation of poor CV prognosis in some individuals with asthma. This is based on studies such as the Copenhagen Heart Study [16], which found that the increased CVD risk in patients with asthma was restricted to former and current smokers, and no difference in CVD risk existed between never-smokers with asthma and never-smokers without asthma.

This contrasts however with other studies suggesting that the higher risk of CVD in patients with asthma is the result of a causal or contributory effect of asthma on CVD, potentially mediated by common inflammatory pathways, asthma medication, cardiopulmonary interactions, or other mechanisms and related in some studies to asthma severity. When the analysis is restricted to never-smokers and after an adjustment for potential confounders, some studies have found no association between asthma and CVD [16].

Although inflammation has been proposed as the common pathway in asthma and CVD [17], this common mechanistic pathway has not been proven. Inflammation in CVD and asthma may be driven by different etiologic factors, such as allergen exposure or dietary fat intake, as well as some very similar factors, such as air pollution, which significantly increases all-cause mortality and cardiorespiratory mortality. Although these effects could be additive, this has yet to be demonstrated and would be challenging.

Several studies have shown an association between allergic features (history or high IgE) and risk of atherosclerosis [18, 19], although a sex difference has not been shown. A positive skin prick test was associated with a 1.7 times (1.4–2.2) increased risk of CVD mortality in one study [17], and others have shown a significant association (OR = 3.8, 95% CI 1.4–10.2) between allergic disorders, such as asthma and allergic rhinitis, with atherosclerosis [19].

In a study of Hutterites, sex was a significant predictor trait value in a linear regression model for 16 of 19 phenotypes characterizing different aspects of CVD, DM, OA, and asthma [20]. For asthma, these included FEV_1, the ratio of FEV_1/FVC, eosinophil count, and total immunoglobulin E (IgE) as well as more systemic features such as body mass index and fat free mass. These could potentially interact with CVD-associated traits such as HDL-cholesterol, lipoprotein A, triglycerides, and diastolic and systolic blood pressure, with a female bias.

Are There Sex Differences in the Mechanisms Underlying the Association Between CVD and Asthma?

The observation that the association between asthma and cardiovascular disease only occurs in women in most studies, and most strongly in those with adult-onset asthma, leads to a consideration of hormonal influences as major contributors. Estrogen levels increase at puberty, exactly the time when the higher male:female ratio of prevalence switches, and over the life span, asthma is not only more prevalent in women but also more severe. In vitro, estrogen modulates the release of pro-inflammatory cytokines from activated monocytes, macrophages, and vascular cells and also regulates the production of leukotrienes from mast cells. It is speculated that women who develop asthma after puberty may be particularly susceptible to estrogen-modulated alterations in inflammatory cytokine and leukotriene regulation [21].

The effects of estrogen on CVD however may be quite different [22]. The heart contains receptors for sex hormones, including estrogen, and in animal models, estrogen has been shown to improve cardiac function and reduce the severity of ischemic injury. Estrogen can also act as an anti-oxidant [23]. Post menopause, however, when estrogen levels drop markedly, the cardioprotective effects are lost, and the prevalence of CVD in women increases dramatically. When combined with the increased prevalence of asthma in women, this effect may be additive or synergistic, helping to explain the significant risk of CVD in women, particularly those with adult-onset asthma. Other comorbidities may play some role in this also [24]. Diabetes is increased in asthma, and of the many CVD risk factors, diabetes, high-density lipoprotein levels, and triglyceride levels have a greater impact on CVD in women than men. Diabetic men have a two- to threefold increased risk of CVD, whereas women have a three- to sevenfold increased risk. It could be postulated that the risks of CVD in asthma is magnified, when all three are combined in women – asthma, CVD, and diabetes. Given the high prevalence of all these chronic diseases in the adult population, this requires further research.

Sex Differences in Chronic Obstructive Pulmonary Disease (COPD) with Comorbid CVD

COPD is now the third most frequent cause of death in the world, behind ischemic heart disease and stroke, the two major causes of death from CVD. Given the common risk factors of tobacco smoking, air pollution, deprivation, and early-life determinants of CVD and lung health, it is not surprising that these two diseases occur together and may interact in a significant proportion of cases [25]. Large population-based studies suggest that patients with COPD are two to three times more at risk for cardiovascular mortality, and COPD-related and CVD-related deaths account for around 50% of total number of deaths [26]. All-cause mortality is related to the presence of airflow obstruction, whether diagnosed or not, symptomatic or not [25].

Symptoms alone contribute to all-cause and CVD mortality risk in COPD. In NHANES, having symptoms of chronic bronchitis alone increased the risk of coronary death by 50% [27], and in two Scandinavian studies, having a mucus hypersecretion-chronic bronchitic phenotype had a similar impact [28]. In some older studies, poor lung function was as powerful a predictor of cardiac mortality as established risk factors such as total serum cholesterol [29]. Although the availability of statins and other effective lipid-lowering medications has significantly ameliorated the consequences of hypercholesterolemia, the impact of FEV_1 on CVD and all-cause mortality may change very slowly. This is because of the combined effect of the increasing global burden of COPD; the continuing exposure to smoke, dusts, and fumes of many millions around the world; the lack of effective detection of early COPD; and the inability of currently available treatments to slow the rate of FEV_1 decline.

Sex Differences in COPD Prevalence and Impact

It is becoming clear that COPD affects men and women differently, develops in response to different exposures and doses, and presents differently clinically [30]. The prevalence of COPD in women is rapidly rising, and in some countries, mortality is equal to that in men. Women are therefore increasingly likely to be affected by COPD comorbidities, but the sex differences of COPD comorbidities are a poorly studied area, and little is known about their frequency and impact [31]. Patients with COPD are frequently excluded from clinical trials of drugs which reduce cardiac morbidity and mortality, and many studies show that CVD in COPD patients is under-recognized and under-treated. Given the relative over-representation of men in randomized controlled trials of COPD, and the exclusion of COPD patients from CVD trials, where COPD and CVD coexist, it may be some time before the gender differences in treatment outcomes are known.

In some contrast to COPD, increasingly important sex differences are known to affect CVD pathophysiology [32], presentation, management, and outcomes

[33], even though women are also under-represented in CVD trials [34]. In relation to CVD in COPD, much of what is known pertains to tobacco-related COPD and treatment effects derived from trials with a predominantly male population. Although the interaction between CVD and COPD could have different manifestations in men and women, there is a dearth of research addressing this specifically, although much can be gleaned from database studies and randomized clinical trials.

Risk of Developing COPD Differs by Dose and Type of Exposure

There is increasing evidence that women are more susceptible to the effects of cigarette smoke than men [35, 36], for a given number of cigarettes smoked per day and total intake. There are many possible mechanisms for this, including different molecular and metabolic responses to cigarette and biomass smoke, different airway geometry, patterns of inhalation, intensity and diversity of exposure, and cellular vulnerability [37–41].

Multiple studies from different regions of the world have suggested both increased risk and greater impact of COPD in women who smoke [42]. Two longitudinal Danish studies [43], the Copenhagen City Heart Study and the Glostrup Population Study combined, found that after adjusting for smoking, women had a 1.5 times greater probability of COPD-related hospitalizations than men, which could not be accounted for by higher rates of hospitalization in women in general. For each pack-year of smoking, women had greater excess loss of FEV_1 in ml per year. In another study, women were disproportionately represented in the subset of patients with COPD with severe disease despite minimal tobacco smoke exposure (defined as <20 pack-years) [44]. Women were also more likely to present with COPD before the age of 60 years.

In a study from Nanjing China exploring the relationship between cigarette smoking and COPD among urban and rural adults >35 years old, the overall prevalence of diagnosed COPD was significantly higher among men than in women [45]. However the relationship between prevalence of COPD and total cigarette smoking was dose dependent in women, while only men with the highest cigarette smoking rates were more likely to have COPD. This finding is similar to a Finnish analysis of medical records of 844 COPD patients in which women reported significantly fewer pack-years than men [46]. Compared to the men, women had less advanced airflow obstruction but more severe gas transfer impairment. This cohort showed several significant gender dependent differences in their clinical presentation including women having a lower body mass index, and more psychiatric conditions, especially depression, and men being more likely to have cardiovascular diseases, diabetes, and alcoholism.

Increased Susceptibility of Women to Tobacco and Biomass Smoke Inhalation

The recently published study from the UK Biobank confirms the increased susceptibility of women to cigarette smoke. In a very large database of approximately 500,000 subjects aged 40–69 years, the association of airflow obstruction and smoking was stronger in women than in men [35]. There was a greater probability of having airflow obstruction with a lower self-reported cigarette smoke exposure among women, and women were at increased risk of airflow obstruction after only 15 years of smoking and five cigarettes per day.

In the BOLD study, the prevalence of stage II or higher COPD was 10.1% overall, 11.8% for men, and 8.5% for women. Even allowing for a greater susceptibility to tobacco-related lung damage, and lower smoking rates than men, this difference is not as great as might be expected. In countries where women have much less tobacco exposure, factors other than cigarette smoking contribute to COPD prevalence. The prevalence of airway hyperresponsiveness in women with COPD is greater than in men; hyperresponsiveness is an important predictor of decline in lung function, which may, at least partially, account for some of the variability between genders in symptoms such as dyspnea, and possibly FEV_1, although further studies are required. Airway reactivity was more strongly related to rates of FEV_1 decline in women than in men in the Lung Health Study [47].

In low- to middle-income countries, early-life nutritional deficiencies may contribute to both CVD risk and poor lung growth, subsequently increasing COPD risk. Women and men experience different domestic air pollution exposures, accounting for the more equal prevalence of COPD despite the fact that women are usually not tobacco smokers [48]. However, there is a strong cardiovascular risk associated with secondhand smoke exposure, and studies demonstrate a consistent 25–30% increased risk for coronary disease associated with secondhand smoke [49, 50]. The best established mechanisms underlying this effect include endothelial dysfunction and a prothrombotic effect.

Little is known about the sex differences in risk of CVD in settings where COPD is not tobacco smoke related, such as biomass-related COPD [51]. A few studies have shown increased risk of CVD in non-tobacco-related COPD [52, 53], but a link between biomass or solid fuel exposure, COPD, and CVD has not been demonstrated yet. Men and women may not only have different susceptibility but also markedly different combined exposures, women usually not smoking but working in unskilled jobs or cottage industries where smoke and dust exposure are very high and men smoking and working unprotected in very dusty jobs. Early-life exposures combined with nutritional deficiencies may combine to compound vulnerability.

Different Symptom Profile and Burden in Men and Women with COPD

Some studies have shown similar COPD symptoms between men and women [54, 55], but others report higher levels of dyspnea in women compared with men, higher exacerbation rates and hospital admissions but lower mortality rates [56–58]. This could conceivably relate to a lower risk of acute MI and CVD complications post exacerbation. In a study detailing the under-diagnosis of acute MI in COPD, men had slightly higher cardiac injury scores, but women and younger age groups were less likely to have an established MI diagnosis despite electrocardiographic evidence of a previous infarction [59].

The higher rate of exacerbations in women versus men with COPD, identified in some studies, may contribute to the overall higher death rate in women in some countries, such as the United States [57, 60]. In the Evaluation of COPD Longitudinally to Identify Predictive Surrogate End-points (ECLIPSE) cohort ($n = 2164$), the rate of exacerbations was found to be significantly higher in women than men at each GOLD stage [56]. Similarly, in a post hoc analysis from the Prevention of Exacerbations with Tiotropium in COPD (POET-COPD) trial, the risk of first exacerbation was higher for women compared with men (HR 1.31, 95% CI 1.19–1.43) [61]. Data from the TOwards a Revolution in COPD Health (TORCH) study also showed that the time to first exacerbation was shorter and the rate of exacerbations was 25% higher in women than in men (95% CI 16–34%; $P < 0.001$), although the number of hospital admissions caused by exacerbations was similar in both sexes [57].

Although several studies show that women are more likely to be admitted to hospital for an exacerbation [43], they appear less likely to die in hospital [62]. In a population of >40,000 participants in the Quebec Insurance databases, males had a significantly increased risk of death (adjusted HR 1.45, 95% CI 1.42–1.49) and re-hospitalization for COPD (adjusted HR 1.12, 95% CI 1.09–1.15) [63].

Men and women appear to experience a different spectrum and severity of symptoms for a given severity of spirometric abnormality [64]. In a Spanish study, women were younger, smoked less, had better PaO2 and lower PaCO but more exacerbations in the last year and fewer comorbidities. However they performed less well than men in walking distance, had worse St. George Respiratory Questionnaire (SGRQ) total, symptoms and activity scores, and had a higher degree of dyspnea [65]. Several studies have shown a greater predominance of anxiety, depression, osteoporosis, and sleep disturbance but a lower prevalence of cardiovascular diagnoses among women [66, 67]. In combination, differences in dyspnea and exercise capacity contribute to poorer prognostic scores such as the BODE (Body mass index, airflow Obstruction, Dyspnea, and Exercise capacity) score in women compared with men who are matched for lung function and age [58].

Different Responses of Clinicians to Men and Women with COPD

Finally, it is well recognized that the responses of clinicians may also differ to men and women, and this can markedly affect the rapidity of diagnosis. Women with COPD are likely to have more frequent interactions with healthcare providers and use more healthcare resources than men [56, 62]. However, there is a higher rate of misdiagnosis or delayed diagnosis in women with COPD compared with men, potentially leading to suboptimal treatment [31, 68]. Although the gender bias in diagnosis is reduced by the use of spirometry, spirometry in general remains underused, particularly in women. COPD patients with concurrent CVD were less likely to be prescribed bronchodilators, with the exception of males who were also prescribed beta-blockers.

Potential Mechanisms for Sex Differences in Increased Risk of CVD and COPD

Gender differences are especially prevalent in cardiovascular disease. Males tend to suffer from myocardial infarctions earlier than females, and a woman's risk of cardiovascular disease increases after menopause reaching a similar prevalence to males in the sixth decade. Several studies indicate that there is an apparent association between gender and oxidative stress, where women seem to be less susceptible to oxidative stress but lose this protection after menopause.

Multiple factors contribute to the risk of CVD, as they do in COPD, apart from known environmental exposures such as tobacco smoking or hyperlipidemia. Many studies show a strong association between childhood adversity and CVD. A study of sex differences in vascular physiology and pathophysiology [22] in Canadians aged 18–49 years showed an OR of 2.14 (95% CI, 1.56–2.94) for 3+ childhood adversities. The association was stronger with increasing stressful events, and female patients with 3+ stressful events exhibited the highest risk of CVD (OR 4.40, 95% CI 1.98–9.75), indicating that the effect of childhood adverse events on CVD is heightened among women, particularly women with stressful adulthoods. This difference was not mediated by depression, smoking, or poor diet. Such differences however could interact with the increased vulnerability of women to smoking-related airflow limitation, increasing their probability of having both COPD and CVD.

COPD, CVD Clinical Manifestations, and Sex Differences

COPD patients carry an excessive risk of cardiac disease beyond what would be expected from a common initiating pathway such as cigarette smoking or atmospheric pollution. In large population databases, there is a strong association between COPD and vascular disease, which confers worse outcomes and is likely to contribute to the high mortality of COPD. CVD accounts for around 30% of deaths in COPD patients [69], and this is so even in younger patients and those with milder COPD. This risk is particularly increased in the weeks immediately following an acute exacerbation of COPD (AECOPD), although to date there is no strong evidence of a sex difference. This may be due to the relatively small numbers of patients in longitudinal COPD studies, and prospective studies will be needed to ascertain whether sex differences in COPD-cardiac comorbidity exist.

In a UK analysis of 18,342 subjects aged ≥40 years, COPD patients ($n = 958$) were at higher risk of having CAD, angina, myocardial infarction, stroke, congestive heart failure, poor lower limb circulation, and arrhythmia. Overall, the presence of COPD increased the odds of having CVD by a factor of 2.7 (95% CI 2.3–3.2). Older age, lower family income, underweight, smoking, drinking, diabetes, hypertension, and high cholesterol were significantly associated with increased risk of CVD. In gender-related differences, there was no significant difference between ORs for CVD or any CVD category except for CAD, which was significantly greater in females than in males.

In another UK study of >25,000 patients with COPD, there was a 2.27-fold (95% CI, 1.1–4.7) increased risk of MI 1–5 days after exacerbation. The increased risk diminished over time and was not significantly different from the baseline MI risk at times longer than 5 days post MI. There was a slight preponderance of men who experienced MI, a smaller difference than suggested by a recent analysis assessing the burden of CVD, where around three times as many men had a MI compared with women in the UK.

Large clinical trials, especially those with a longitudinal follow-up, have provided substantial information on CVD risk in COPD, but few have analyzed or commented on sex differences in treatment effects. The Lung Health Study recruited predominantly asymptomatic smokers aged 35–60 years old with mild, predominantly early GOLD stage II COPD patients [70]. Cardiovascular events accounted for 42% of the first hospitalizations and 48% of the second hospitalizations in the 13% of the cohort who experienced at least one hospitalization during the 5-year follow-up. Coronary artery disease accounted for approximately two-thirds of nonfatal CVD. Baseline FEV_1% predicted was inversely related to all-cause mortality and to deaths from coronary artery disease and CVD. Mortality did not differ significantly between groups by sex. Increased body mass index was a risk factor for respiratory illnesses, as was female sex.

In this same study, among participants who quit smoking in the first year, FEV_1% predicted increased more in women (3.7%) than in men (1.6%) [47]. The relationship between all-cause mortality, CVD mortality, and FEV_1 raises the possibility that women may gain more than men in reduced mortality from CVD when they give up smoking.

Clinically, there is frequent uncertainty in determining whether worsening dyspnea is due to AECOPD, heart failure, or acute ischemia. Differentiating between HF and AECOPD can be difficult, and both frequently coexist. CVD has been detected in up to 55% of patients admitted with AECOPD, suggesting that up to 20% of AECOPD could be due to cardiac events.

In the Understanding Potential Long-term Impacts on Function with Tiotropium (UPLIFT) trial, another large RCT of patients with GOLD stage II–IV disease, there were >900 deaths, with 11% deaths due to CVD and 4.4% due to sudden cardiac death. Interestingly, the panel and study investigators agreed closely on causes of death *except* in the case of a threefold greater rate attributed to "cardiac disorders" by study investigators compared to the adjudication panel. An analysis based on gender was not reported.

In the TORCH study, an independent adjudication committee determined that 23% of participants who died did so from CVD causes [71]. At baseline, 7% of patients reported a history of previous MI, 41% were taking CVD medications, and during the study 17–20% and 10–12% of patients had cardiac adverse events or severe adverse events, respectively. A history of MI doubled the probability of cardiovascular adverse events, but the likelihood of experiencing a cardiovascular adverse event was unaffected by gender and current smoking status.

A crucial question, given the high rate of cardiac comorbidity in COPD, is whether treating COPD with medications that reduce exacerbations also reduces cardiac comorbidity. In the Study to Understand Mortality and Morbidity in COPD (SUMMIT) study [72], combination ICS-LABA therapy had no effect on composite cardiovascular events, even though ICS and LABA alone or in combination reduced the rate of moderate and severe AECOPD. As so often in randomized trials in COPD, the statistical analysis model (in this case the Cox proportionate hazards model) "allowed" for the covariates of age and sex. Any approach to RCT analysis that makes adjustments for sex inevitably standardizes the treatment effect in men and women and so does not report on sex differences – and is unlikely to show differences.

Potential Mechanisms for Sex Differences Affecting the Increased Cardiovascular Risk Associated with COPD

The pathophysiologic mechanisms which contribute to the increased prevalence and impact of CVD in patients with COPD, and vice versa, will be fully explored in Chap. 6. Very briefly, these include but are not limited to increases in structural vascular changes such as carotid intima-media thickness, plaques, and arterial stiffness, which are more prevalent in patients with COPD compared to matched smokers without COPD. Key COPD events such as exacerbations are associated with increases in arterial stiffness, increased myocardial oxygen demand in a hypoxemic state, and increased pulmonary vascular pressures. Additional demand occurs through medications such as beta-2 agonists, frequently administered at very high doses.

Changes in inflammatory parameters, such as C-reactive protein, vascular adhesion molecules and fibrinogen levels, cytokines, and TNF-α, all contribute to the higher CVD mortality and morbidity observed in frequent exacerbators. Increases in BNP and troponin have been demonstrated in even moderate exacerbations of COPD [73], and retrospective analyses show that undiagnosed ischemic damage is common in hospitalized patients with AECOPD. Infection-related exacerbations are especially related to greater increases in arterial stiffness which is consistent with observations that lung infections are associated with increased acute and long term risk of cardiovascular disease.

Even in the stable state, COPD is a disease associated with increased markers of systemic inflammation, oxidative stress, physiological stress, and accelerated aging [74], which are known to occur differently in men and women. However, there are no robust data on the extent to which these inflammatory mechanisms operate similarly or differently in men and women when COPD and CVD coexist. The different impact of similar and dissimilar exposures, such as active and passive smoking, dusty work environments, and domestic biomass fuel exposures, is likely to add complexity to the interactions of inflammatory mechanisms, hormonal effects, and physiologic responses in the CVD-COPD interaction.

Summary: Cardiovascular Comorbidity in Airway Disease: Gender Differences

In summary, cardiovascular comorbidity in airway disease shows significant gender differences. In asthma, there is an increased risk of CVD as a comorbidity and an increased risk of CVD death in women, especially those with later-onset disease, and in those who have been smokers. There is evidence of different prescribing patterns for men and women, the latter receiving less medication targeted at both their lung and heart diseases. A different pattern of comorbidities exists in men and women with asthma that may further influence the risks of adverse outcomes for those with asthma and CVD.

In COPD, the increased risk of CVD as a comorbidity is common, frequently symptomatic but often undertreated, and appears to affect men and women equally but increases mortality risk compared to COPD alone. CVD is a major contributor to mortality in COPD, and research is needed to determine the optimal management of patients with both diseases, particularly urgent because of the rising prevalence of COPD globally. Although men and women present differently and receive different management, in both diseases there are very limited data on the gender differences in treatment outcomes, despite the many opportunities available through large randomized trials of asthma and COPD.

References

1. Clayton J, Tannenbaum C. Reporting sex, gender, or both in clinical research? JAMA. 2016;316(18):1863–4.
2. Tai A, Tran H, Roberts M, Clarke N, Gibson AM, Vidmar S, et al. Outcomes of childhood asthma to the age of 50 years. J Allergy Clin Immunol. 2014;133(6):1572–8.e3.
3. Tattersall MC, Barnet JH, Korcarz CE, Hagen EW, Peppard PE, Stein JH. Late-onset asthma predicts cardiovascular disease events: the Wisconsin sleep cohort. J Am Heart Assoc. 2016;5(9):24.
4. Iribarren C, Tolstykh IV, Miller MK, Sobel E, Eisner MD. Adult asthma and risk of coronary heart disease, cerebrovascular disease, and heart failure: a prospective study of 2 matched cohorts. Am J Epidemiol. 2012;176(11):1014–24.
5. Schanen JG, Iribarren C, Shahar E, Punjabi NM, Rich SS, Sorlie PD, et al. Asthma and incident cardiovascular disease: the Atherosclerosis Risk in Communities Study. Thorax. 2005;60(8):633–8.
6. Onufrak SJ, Abramson JL, Austin HD, Holguin F, McClellan WM, Vaccarino LV. Relation of adult-onset asthma to coronary heart disease and stroke. Am J Cardiol. 2008;101(9):1247–52.
7. Dogra S, Ardern CI, Baker J. The relationship between age of asthma onset and cardiovascular disease in Canadians. J Asthma. 2007;44(10):849–54.
8. Cazzola M, Calzetta L, Bettoncelli G, Cricelli C, Romeo F, Matera MG, et al. Cardiovascular disease in asthma and COPD: a population-based retrospective cross-sectional study. Respir Med. 2012;106(2):249–56.
9. Bellocchia M, Masoero M, Ciuffreda A, Croce S, Vaudano A, Torchio R, et al. Predictors of cardiovascular disease in asthma and chronic obstructive pulmonary disease. Multidiscip Respir Med. 2013;8(1):58.
10. Ringbaek T, Seersholm N, Viskum K. Standardised mortality rates in females and males with COPD and asthma. Eur Respir J. 2005;25(5):891–5.
11. Xu M, Xu J, Yang X. Asthma and risk of cardiovascular disease or all-cause mortality: a meta-analysis. Ann Saudi Med. 2017;37(2):99–105.
12. Pinto P, Rothnie KJ, Lui K, Timmis A, Smeeth L, Quint JK. Presentation, management and mortality after a first MI in people with and without asthma: a study using UK MINAP data. Chron Respir Dis. 2018;15(1):60–70.
13. Watson L, Turk F, James P, Holgate ST. Factors associated with mortality after an asthma admission: a national United Kingdom database analysis. Respir Med. 2007;101(8):1659–64.
14. Stock SA, Stollenwerk B, Redaelli M, Civello D, Lauterbach KW. Sex differences in treatment patterns of six chronic diseases: an analysis from the German statutory health insurance. J Womens Health. 2008;17(3):343–54.
15. Adesanoye DT, Willey CJ. Does cardiovascular comorbidity influence the prescribing of bronchodilators in chronic obstructive pulmonary disease? Ann Pharmacother. 2017;51(10):855–61.
16. Colak Y, Afzal S, Nordestgaard BG, Lange P. Characteristics and prognosis of never-smokers and smokers with asthma in the Copenhagen General Population Study. A prospective cohort study. Am J Respir Crit Care Med. 2015;192(2):172–81.
17. Ilmarinen P, Tuomisto LE, Kankaanranta H. Phenotypes, risk factors, and mechanisms of adult onset asthma. Mediat Inflamm. 2015;2015:514868.
18. Hospers JJ, Rijcken B, Schouten JP, Postma DS, Weiss ST. Eosinophilia and positive skin tests predict cardiovascular mortality in a general population sample followed for 30 years. Am J Epidemiol. 1999;150(5):482–91.
19. Knoflach M, Kiechl S, Mayr A, Willeit J, Poewe W, Wick G. Allergic rhinitis, asthma, and atherosclerosis in the Bruneck and ARMY studies. Arch Intern Med. 2005;165(21):2521–6.
20. Abney M, McPeek MS, Ober C. Broad and narrow heritabilities of quantitative traits in a founder population. Am J Hum Genet. 2001;68(5):1302–7.

21. Onufrak S, Abramson J, Vaccarino V. Adult-onset asthma is associated with increased carotid atherosclerosis among women in the Atherosclerosis Risk in Communities (ARIC) study. Atherosclerosis. 2007;195(1):129–37.
22. Boese AC, Kim SC, Yin KJ, Lee JP, Hamblin MH. Sex differences in vascular physiology and pathophysiology: estrogen and androgen signaling in health and disease. Am J Physiol Heart Circ Physiol. 2017;313(3):H524–H45.
23. Kander MC, Cui Y, Liu Z. Gender difference in oxidative stress: a new look at the mechanisms for cardiovascular diseases. J Cell Mol Med. 2017;21(5):1024–32.
24. Kauppi P, Linna M, Jantunen J, Martikainen JE, Haahtela T, Pelkonen A, et al. Chronic comorbidities contribute to the burden and costs of persistent asthma. Mediat Inflamm. 2015;2015:819194.
25. Maclay JD, MacNee W. Cardiovascular disease in COPD: mechanisms. Chest. 2013;143(3):798–807.
26. Sin DD, Man SFP. Chronic obstructive pulmonary disease as a risk factor for cardiovascular morbidity and mortality. Proc Am Thorac Soc. 2005;2(1):8–11.
27. Mannino DM. Lung function and mortality in the United States: data from the First National Health and Nutrition Examination Survey follow up study. Thorax. 2003;58(5):388–93.
28. Stavem K, Sandvik L, Erikssen J. Breathlessness, phlegm and mortality: 26 years of follow-up in healthy middle-aged Norwegian men. J Intern Med. 2006;260(4):332–42.
29. Hole DJ, Watt GCM, Davey-Smith G, Hart CL, Gillis CR, Hawthorne VM. Impaired lung function and mortality risk in men and women: findings from the Renfrew and Paisley prospective population study. BMJ. 1996;313(7059):711–5; discussion 715–6.
30. Jenkins CR, Chapman KR, Donohue JF, Roche N, Tsiligianni I, Han MK. Improving the management of COPD in women. Chest. 2017;151(3):686–96.
31. Han MK, Postma D, Mannino DM, Giardino ND, Buist S, Curtis JL, et al. Gender and chronic obstructive pulmonary disease: why it matters. Am J Respir Crit Care Med. 2007;176(12):1179–84.
32. Pedersen LR, Frestad D, Michelsen MM, Mygind ND, Rasmusen H, Suhrs HE, et al. Risk factors for myocardial infarction in women and men: a review of the current literature. Curr Pharm Des. 2016;22(25):3835–52.
33. Czubryt MP, Espira L, Lamoureux L, Abrenica B. The role of sex in cardiac function and disease. Can J Physiol Pharmacol. 2006;84(1):93–109.
34. Vitale C, Fini M, Spoletini I, Lainscak M, Seferovic P, Rosano GM. Under-representation of elderly and women in clinical trials. Int J Cardiol. 2017;232:216–21.
35. Amaral AFS, Strachan DP, Burney PGJ, Jarvis DL. Female smokers are at greater risk of airflow obstruction than male smokers. UK Biobank. Am J Respir Crit Care Med. 2017;195(9):1226–35.
36. Sansores R, Ramírez-Venegas A. COPD in women: susceptibility or vulnerability? Eur Respir J. 2016;47:19–22.
37. Ben-Zaken Cohen S, Pare PD, Man SF, Sin DD. The growing burden of chronic obstructive pulmonary disease and lung cancer in women: examining sex differences in cigarette smoke metabolism. Am J Respir Crit Care Med. 2007;176(2):113–20.
38. Becklake M, Kauffmann F. Gender differences in airway behaviour over the human lifespan. Thorax. 1999;54:1119–38.
39. Barnes P. Sex differences in chronic obstructive pulmonary disease mechanisms. Am J Respir Crit Care Med. 2016;193(8):813–4.
40. Tam A, Churg A, Wright JL, Zhou S, Kirby M, Coxson HO, et al. Sex differences in airway remodeling in a mouse model of chronic obstructive pulmonary disease. Am J Respir Crit Care Med. 2016;193(8):825–34.
41. Hardin M, Cho MH, Sharma S, Glass K, Castaldi PJ, McDonald ML, et al. Sex-based genetic association study identifies CELSR1 as a possible chronic obstructive pulmonary disease risk locus among women. Am J Respir Cell Mol Biol. 2017;56(3):332–41.

42. Gershon A, Hwee J, Victor JC, Wilton A, Wu R, Day A, et al. Mortality trends in women and men with COPD in Ontario, Canada, 1996-2012. Thorax. 2015;70(2):121–6.

43. Prescott E, Bjerg AM, Andersen PK, Lange P, Vestbo J. Gender difference in smoking effects on lung function and risk of hospitalization for COPD: results from a Danish longitudinal population study. Eur Respir J. 1997;10(4):822–7.

44. Martinez FJ, Curtis JL, Sciurba F, Mumford J, Giardino ND, Weinmann G, et al. Sex differences in severe pulmonary emphysema. Am J Respir Crit Care Med. 2007;176(3):243–52.

45. Xu F, Yin XM, Zhang M, Shen HB, Lu LG, Xu YC. Prevalence of physician-diagnosed COPD and its association with smoking among urban and rural residents in regional mainland China. Chest. 2005;128:2818–23.

46. Laitinen THU, Kupiainen H, Tammilehto L, Haahtela T, et al. Real-world clinical data identifies gender-related profiles in chronic obstructive pulmonary disease. J Chronic Obstr Pulm Dis. 2009;6:256–62.

47. Connett JE, Murray RP, Buist AS, Wise RA, Bailey WC, Lindgren PG, et al. Changes in smoking status affect women more than men: results of the Lung Health Study. Am J Epidemiol. 2003;157:973–9.

48. Zhou Y, Wang C, Yao W, Chen P, Kang J, Huang S, et al. COPD in Chinese nonsmokers. Eur Respir J. 2009;33(3):509–18.

49. Reed RM, Dransfield MT, Eberlein M, Miller M, Netzer G, Pavlovich M, et al. Gender differences in first and secondhand smoke exposure, spirometric lung function and cardiometabolic health in the old order Amish: a novel population without female smoking. PLoS One. 2017;12(3):e0174354.

50. He Y, Jiang B, Li LS, Li LS, Ko L, Wu L, et al. Secondhand smoke exposure predicted COPD and other tobacco-related mortality in a 17-year cohort study in China. Chest. 2012;142(4):909–18.

51. Lopez Varela MV, Montes de Oca M, Halbert R, Muino A, Talamo C, Perez-Padilla R, et al. Comorbidities and health status in individuals with and without COPD in five Latin American cities: the PLATINO study. Arch Bronconeumol. 2013;49(11):468–74.

52. Mortimer K, Gordon SB, Jindal SK, Accinelli RA, Balmes J, Martin WJ 2nd. Household air pollution is a major avoidable risk factor for cardiorespiratory disease. Chest. 2012;142(5):1308–15.

53. Samet JM, Bahrami H, Berhane K. Indoor air pollution and cardiovascular disease: new evidence from Iran. Circulation. 2016;133(24):2342–4.

54. Raherison C, Tillie-Leblond I, Prudhomme A, Taille C, Biron E, Nocent-Ejnaini C, et al. Clinical characteristics and quality of life in women with COPD: an observational study. BMC Womens Health. 2014;14(1):31.

55. Skumlien S, Haave E, Morland L, Bjortuft O, Ryg MS. Gender differences in the performance of activities of daily living among patients with chronic obstructive pulmonary disease. Chron Respir Dis. 2006;3(3):141–8.

56. Agusti A, Calverley PM, Celli B, Coxson HO, Edwards LD, Lomas DA, et al. Characterisation of COPD heterogeneity in the ECLIPSE cohort. Respir Res. 2010;11:122.

57. Celli B, Vestbo J, Jenkins CR, Jones PW, Ferguson GT, Calverley PM, et al. Sex differences in mortality and clinical expressions of patients with chronic obstructive pulmonary disease. The TORCH experience. Am J Respir Crit Care Med. 2011;183(3):317–22.

58. Roche N, Deslee G, Caillaud D, Brinchault G, Court-Fortune I, Nesme-Meyer P, et al. Impact of gender on COPD expression in a real-life cohort. Respir Res. 2014;15:20.

59. Brekke P, Omland T, Smith P, Søyseth V. Underdiagnosis of myocardial infarction in COPD: Cardiac Infarction Injury Score (CIIS) in patients hospitalised for COPD exacerbation. Respir Med. 2008;102:1243–7.

60. Han MK, Kazerooni EA, Lynch DA, Liu LX, Murray S, Curtis JL, et al. Chronic obstructive pulmonary disease exacerbations in the COPDGene study: associated radiologic phenotypes. Radiology. 2011;261(1):274–82.

61. Beeh KM, Glaab T, Stowasser S, Schmidt H, Fabbri LM, Rabe KF, et al. Characterisation of exacerbation risk and exacerbator phenotypes in the POET-COPD trial. Respir Res. 2013;14(1):116.
62. Ekstrom MP, Jogreus C, Strom KE. Comorbidity and sex-related differences in mortality in oxygen-dependent chronic obstructive pulmonary disease. PLoS One. 2012;7(4):e35806.
63. Gonzalez AV, Suissa S, Ernst P. Gender differences in survival following hospitalisation for COPD. Thorax. 2011;66(1):38–42.
64. Lamprecht B, Vanfleteren LE, Studnicka M, Allison M, McBurnie MA, Vollmer WM, et al. Sex-related differences in respiratory symptoms: results from the BOLD Study. Eur Respir J. 2013;42(3):858–60.
65. de Torres J, Casanova C, Hernández C, Abreu J, Aguirre-Jaime A, Celli BR. Gender and COPD in patients attending a pulmonary clinic. Chest. 2005;128:2012–6.
66. Martinez CH, Raparla S, Plauschinat CA, Giardino ND, Rogers B, Beresford J, et al. Gender differences in symptoms and care delivery for chronic obstructive pulmonary disease. J Womens Health (Larchmt). 2012;21(12):1267–74.
67. Watson L, Vestbo J, Postma DS, Decramer M, Rennard S, Kiri VA, et al. Gender differences in the management and experience of Chronic Obstructive Pulmonary Disease. Respir Med. 2004;98(12):1207–13.
68. Ancochea J, Miravitlles M, García-Río F, Muñoz L, Sánchez G, Sobradillo V, et al. Underdiagnosis of chronic obstructive pulmonary disease in women: quantification of the problem, determinants and proposed actions. Arch Bronconeumol. 2013;49(6):223–9.
69. McGarvey L, John M, Anderson J, Zvarich M, RA W. Ascertainment of cause-specific mortality in COPD: operations of the TORCH Clinical Endpoint Ascertainment of cause-specific mortality in COPD. Thorax. 2007;62:411–5.
70. Anthonisen NR, Connett JE, Enright PL, Manfreda J. Hospitalizations and mortality in the Lung Health Study. Am J Respir Crit Care Med. 2002;166:333–9.
71. Calverley PM, Anderson JA, Celli B, Ferguson GT, Jenkins C, Jones PW, et al. Cardiovascular events in patients with COPD: TORCH study results. Thorax. 2010;65(8):719–25.
72. Vestbo J, Anderson JA, Brook RD, Calverley PMA, Celli BR, Crim C, et al. Fluticasone furoate and vilanterol and survival in chronic obstructive pulmonary disease with heightened cardiovascular risk (SUMMIT): a double-blind randomised controlled trial. Lancet. 2016;387(10030):1817–26.
73. Patel AR, Kowlessar BS, Donaldson GC, Mackay AJ, Singh R, George SN, et al. Cardiovascular risk, myocardial injury, and exacerbations of chronic obstructive pulmonary disease. Am J Respir Crit Care Med. 2013;188(9):1091–9.
74. Stone IS, Barnes NC, Petersen SE. Chronic obstructive pulmonary disease: a modifiable risk factor for cardiovascular disease? Heart. 2012;98(14):1055–62.

Chapter 4
Pathophysiology of Cardiovascular Disease in Chronic Lung Disease

Trisha M. Parekh and Mark T. Dransfield

> **Pearls**
> - Chronic lung diseases and cardiovascular diseases share many risk factors and are common comorbid conditions.
> - Impairment of lung function is associated with an increased risk of cardiovascular events.
> - Arterial abnormalities, accelerated aging, systemic inflammation, and oxidative stress play a role in the development of cardiovascular disease in chronic lung diseases.

Introduction

Multiple factors contribute to the complex link between cardiovascular disease (CVD) and chronic lung diseases (CLD). Despite having numerous shared risk factors including smoking and socioeconomic status, there is now growing evidence to suggest potential causality between CLD and CVD rather than simple association. In this chapter, we will review the pathobiologic processes that may drive the development of CVD in patients with CLD. This chapter will focus primarily on the

T. M. Parekh
Lung Health Center, Division of Pulmonary, Allergy, and Critical Care, University of Alabama at Birmingham, Birmingham, AL, USA

M. T. Dransfield (✉)
Lung Health Center, Division of Pulmonary, Allergy, and Critical Care, University of Alabama at Birmingham, Birmingham, AL, USA

Birmingham VA Medical Center, Birmingham, AL, USA
e-mail: mdransfield@uabmc.edu

© Springer Nature Switzerland AG 2020   45
S. P. Bhatt (ed.), *Cardiac Considerations in Chronic Lung Disease*,
Respiratory Medicine, https://doi.org/10.1007/978-3-030-43435-9_4

relationship between chronic obstructive pulmonary disease (COPD) and coronary artery disease (CAD) but will also briefly examine the associations with congestive heart failure, peripheral arterial disease, and cerebral vascular disease as well as the relationship between other CLDs and CVD.

Epidemiology of COPD and CVD

COPD is the fourth leading cause of mortality worldwide [1]. The epidemiology of COPD and CVD overlaps, with the two diseases sharing many risk factors, and the presence of one worsens the prognosis and complicates the management of the other. CVD is a leading cause of death in COPD [2], and the presence of COPD predicts mortality in patients with heart disease [3]. COPD is associated with a significantly increased risk of incident and recurrent myocardial infarction [4], while a rise in troponin during a COPD exacerbation also predicts mortality [5]. The risk for cardiovascular events increase in the period after COPD exacerbations [6–8], with the risk highest in the first 30 days but lasting up to 1 year [9]. Patients with both COPD and CVD also incur significantly greater morbidity and healthcare costs with increased number of hospitalizations and prolonged exacerbations compared to patients who have COPD alone [10–12]. In order to decrease the burden of CVD in CLD patients, it is crucial to understand the mechanisms that underlie the relationship between CLD and CVD.

Relationship Between Lung Function and CVD

There is a clear association between impaired lung function and the risk of cardiovascular disease as low baseline forced expiratory volume (FEV_1), forced vital capacity (FVC), and declines in FEV_1 predict cardiovascular events independent of traditional cardiac risk factors [2, 10, 11, 13]. The association of impaired lung function and increased risk of cardiovascular events is evident across age groups, including the young and elderly populations [12, 13]. A population-based study found that individuals in the lowest FEV_1 quintile had a fivefold increased risk of cardiovascular mortality [14].

Pathobiologic Processes Underlying CVD Risk in COPD

Arterial Abnormalities

A number of vascular abnormalities have been described in patients with CVD including arterial thickening, impaired vasodilation, stiffness, and calcification, and these may be more prevalent or severe in patients with COPD.

Carotid intimal medial thickness (CIMT) is a surrogate indicator of atherosclerotic heart disease, with an increased thickness of the intima or media associated with an increased risk of CVD. In smokers with airflow obstruction compared to smokers without airflow obstruction as well as non-smokers, CIMT is increased and is independently associated with lower FEV_1 [14]. COPD patients with an increased CIMT also have a higher risk of mortality from CVD [15]. COPD is also an independent predictor of carotid plaque development [16], including vulnerable plaques [17].

Flow-mediated dilation (FMD) is another noninvasive tool used to assess endothelial function and early development of atherosclerosis [18]. FMD is determined by measuring the brachial artery diameter in response to hyperemia. FMD measurements have been shown to correlate inversely with CIMT [19] as well as predict future cardiovascular events [20]. After adjusting for cardiovascular risk factors and age, FMD was found to correlate with percent predicted FEV_1 [21], measurements of which are reproducible over time [22]. In patients with AECOPD requiring hospitalization, FMD was found to be lower during exacerbation and improved upon resolution of exacerbation 3 months later [23]. Evidence supports the presence of endothelial dysfunction in stable and exacerbating COPD patients and provides a possible explanation for the increased risk of CVD, especially during exacerbations.

Arterial stiffness occurs as a consequence of atherosclerosis and normal aging and can be measured by pulse wave velocity (PWV) [24]. Independent of smoking and prior myocardial infarction history, COPD patients are twice as likely to have increased arterial stiffness compared to non-smoking controls [25]. PWV is inversely related to FEV_1 and FVC [26] as well as emphysema severity [27]. Systemic inflammation may be a mechanism for this relationship [28]. Elastin degradation may be another mechanism for increased arterial stiffness in COPD. Skin elastin degradation is increased in COPD, and this is associated with airflow obstruction, emphysema severity, and PWV [29].

Arterial calcification is also a predictor for CVD and coronary artery calcification is increased in COPD patients and associated with mortality [30]. In the National Lung Screening Trial, CT emphysema was also associated with increased thoracic aortic calcification [31]. Some have suggested that individuals with COPD should be screened for arterial stiffness and calcification; however, this is not yet recommended by clinical guidelines [32].

Accelerated Aging

Both COPD and CVD are diseases that are associated with accelerated aging. Shortened telomere length, increased apoptosis, and reductions of anti-aging proteins are potential mediators of an increased CVD risk in COPD patients. Shortened telomeres and increased cell senescence occur naturally with aging. However in comparison to age-matched control smokers, telomere length was shortened in COPD patients [33]. Markers of cellular senescence (p16 and p21) are also increased in samples of lung tissue from patients with emphysema [34]. Evidence suggests that telomere shortening and senescent pulmonary vascular endothelial cells promote the release of inflammatory cells [35], further perpetuating the vicious cycle of inflammation and aging.

Accelerated aging may also contribute to the development of emphysema through increased apoptosis. Cellular senescence and reduced levels of vascular endothelial growth factor receptor-2 increase apoptosis in endothelial and epithelial cells as a protective response to harmful exposures like smoke [36]. In the lung, this can prevent regeneration of lung parenchyma, leading to loss of cells in the alveolar walls causing emphysema [37].

Decreased levels of proteins including sirtuin-1 and Werner's syndrome protein may also contribute to accelerated aging in COPD patients. Sirtuin-1, an anti-aging protein, plays a major role in cellular stress management, and, compared to non-smoking controls, levels of sirtuin-1 were shown to be reduced in lung samples of COPD patients [38]. Animal studies have shown that sirtuin-1 overexpression suppresses markers associated with aging (p21, p16, p53). A reduction in sirtuin-1 also predated the development of emphysema in mice models [39]. Reductions of sirtuin-1 may be the result of increased levels of oxidative stress and inflammation, both of which are prominent in COPD patients [40]. Suppression of Werner's syndrome protein, which is associated with increased cell senescence in fibroblasts isolated from patients with emphysema, has also been proposed as a mechanism of accelerated aging in COPD patients [41].

Cellular senescence has an established association with CVD. Shortened telomere length is associated with arterial stiffness [42] and is a predictor of future cardiovascular events [43]. Senescent endothelial cells are found on plaque surfaces and may be involved in the development of CVD [44].

Systemic Inflammation

Inflammation plays a major role in the pathophysiology of most CLD, including COPD, ILD, and asthma. Inflammatory molecules, including C-reactive protein, tumor necrosis factor alpha, fibrinogen, IL-6, and IL-8, are known to be elevated in COPD [45, 46] and have all been evaluated as possible disease-related biomarkers. Nuclear studies have also documented greater inflammation seen in the aorta of COPD patients compared to ex-smoking controls [47]. The systemic effects of inflammation in COPD also play a role in the development of comorbidities, including diabetes, hypertension, and CVD [48]. Coronary artery disease is accepted as a disease of inflammation [49, 50]. CRP, IL-6, and fibrinogen are involved in the formation of plaque [51] and progression of atherosclerosis [52]. Elevated CRP in the presence of airflow obstruction has been associated with increased risk of cardiac injury [53]. CT findings of coronary artery calcification, presence of metabolic syndrome, and elevated CRP were also associated with lower FEV_1 [54]. Levels of inflammatory markers are higher during AECOPD [55], a time when CV events are known to occur [6]. This may be due to dysfunctional endothelial progenitor cells that alter the vascular endothelium during AECOPD [56]. Systemic inflammation, oxidative stress, and endothelial dysfunction are common in both COPD and CVD, and their interrelationship mechanisms are complex.

Oxidative Stress

An imbalance between reactive oxygen species and antioxidants can produce a state of oxidative stress which can lead to tissue damage in the lungs and systemic vessels. Cigarette smoking and frequent exacerbations perpetuate the imbalance of free radicals in COPD [57] which can lead to increased mucous secretion, direct injury to lung cells, and protease/antiprotease imbalance [58]. Reactive oxygen species can also upregulate pro-inflammatory cytokines in COPD [59] contributing to the negative effects caused by chronic inflammation. Oxidative stress increases lipid peroxidation, a mechanism that promotes atherosclerosis, specifically during AECOPD [60], and levels of oxidized low-density lipoproteins are elevated in COPD patients [61]. End products of lipid peroxidation induce apoptosis in multiple cell lines. This can be combated by antioxidant enzymes like glutathione s-transferase [62]. Evidence also points to increased prevalence of glutathione s-transferase polymorphisms in COPD patients [63] which predisposes the individual to increased damage from reactive oxygen species, including upregulation of inflammation and development of atherosclerosis.

Protease/Antiprotease Imbalance

Proteases are enzymes that digest proteins in the connective tissues. They are the primary culprit in the development of emphysema. Elevated neutrophil elastase, matrix metalloproteases (MMP), and cathepsins are mechanisms that may contribute to both CLD and CVD. Unregulated neutrophil elastase promotes the development of emphysema [64]. Elevated levels are also found in unstable angina and myocardial infarction patients [65] as well as on the surface of fibrous and atherosclerotic plaques [66]. MMPs, specifically MMP-1, MMP-2, MMP-7, MMP-9, and MMP-12, are involved in the degradation of various components of the matrix framework, and their imbalance plays a key role in the development of COPD, ILD, and asthma [67]. MMPs have also been involved in the development of CVD. MMP-9 is associated with aortic stiffness in patients with systolic hypertension and in healthy individuals [68]. Polymorphisms of MMP-3 have also been associated with plaque rupture and acute myocardial infarction [69]. Cathepsin K is an enzyme primarily involved in bone resorption but also has implications for the development of emphysema and atherosclerosis. Levels of cathepsin K have been shown to be elevated in humans with emphysema and in animal models [70]. Cathepsin K levels are also elevated in patients with coronary artery disease [71]. In animal models, the knockout of cathepsin K is associated with a reduction in atherosclerosis [72] as well as age-related cardiac dysfunction [73].

Renin-Angiotensin System

The renin-angiotensin system (RAS) functions to regulate the body's systemic blood pressure and electrolyte and fluid balance. The RAS also plays a role in the development of CLD, including COPD and interstitial lung diseases. During periods of hypoxia, as is frequently seen in CLD patients, the RAS is activated [74], and this has pro-inflammatory and pro-fibrotic effects that contribute to the development of systemic inflammation and fibrosis in CLD [75]. Upregulation of the RAS is also involved in the development of atherosclerosis through vascular inflammation, plaque development, and cardiac remodeling [76, 77]. Animal models show that instillation of angiotensin-II, a main effector molecule of the RAS, is associated with increased plaque vulnerability [78]. The chronic hypoxia seen in CLD patients can upregulate the RAS causing increased production of angiotensin II and increased risk of a cardiovascular event.

Hypercoagulability

Abnormal blood clotting increases the body's susceptibility to vascular events. Fibrinogen is a protein that functions mainly to promote hemostasis but in excess can cause infarctions in the heart, brain, and extremities. COPD patients have higher levels of coagulation markers, including thrombin-antithrombin complex [79] and fibrinogen [80], which are also associated with the development of acute coronary syndrome [81]. COPD patients undergoing percutaneous stent placement are at higher risk of major adverse cardiac events, stent thrombosis, and myocardial infarction compared to patients without COPD [82]. Specific mechanisms underlying the cause of hypercoagulability in COPD patients remain undetermined, and this may be in part due to thrombocytosis [83].

Hypoxia and Sympathetic Nervous System Activation

Patients with severe CLD experience episodes of hypoxia frequently. Chronic hypoxia has been associated with increased levels of inflammation, platelet activation, cell apoptosis, RAS activation, and oxidative stress [84–88], the CVD-related mechanisms of which are discussed above. Hypoxia can also cause significant hemodynamic changes through activation of the sympathetic nervous system [89]. In a study of healthy men, heart rate increased and systemic vascular resistance decreased after 1 hour of hypoxia [90]. Muscle sympathetic nerve activity increase in response to hypoxia and hypercapnia can persist up to 20 minutes after return to room air breathing [91]. As a result, COPD patients frequently have an elevated resting heart rate [92]. Autonomic dysregulation and tachycardia are both risk factors for cardiovascular mortality [93, 94].

Heart Failure

COPD patients have a 4.5-fold higher risk of developing heart failure (HF) compared to age-matched controls without COPD [95], and patients with both conditions have worse outcomes [96]. Through mechanisms discussed earlier, COPD increases the risk of ischemic coronary events, which predisposes patients to the development of systolic heart failure. With a prevalence of 90% in one study of stable severe COPD patients [97], diastolic heart failure can also develop in CLD and occurs primarily from lung hyperinflation causing a reduction in left ventricular preload [98, 99]. In a cohort of 615 COPD participants, lung hyperinflation and lower FEV_1 were associated with echocardiographic markers of diastolic dysfunction [100]. These data also suggest that a reduction in hyperinflation could improve diastolic filling, a hypothesis supported by several randomized trials of inhaled treatments. Hohlfeld et al. found that use of dual bronchodilator therapy with a long-acting muscarinic antagonist and long-acting beta-agonist over 14 days was associated with a 10% increase in left ventricular end diastolic volume in the treatment group compared to placebo group as well as a reduction in lung hyperinflation [101]. Similar improvements in left as well as right ventricular end diastolic volume was also reported after 14 days of treatment with an inhaled steroid and long acting beta-agonist combination as compared to placebo [102]. It is also possible that the improvement in ventricular filling after lung deflation could improve cardiac performance as supported by the study by Come et al., who found improvements in oxygen pulse in patients in the National Emphysema Treatment Trial who achieved significant reductions in hyperinflation with lung volume reduction surgery [103].

Right heart failure occurs secondary to the development of pulmonary hypertension in patients with COPD. Mechanisms leading to the development of pulmonary hypertension in COPD patients include hyperinflation, systemic inflammation, and hypoxic vasoconstriction [104]. This topic is discussed separately in Chap. 7.

Cerebrovascular and Peripheral Artery Disease

The evidence supporting a causal relationship between COPD and cerebrovascular diseases is less compelling. Population-based studies have found COPD patients have an up to 20% higher risk of stroke; however, the association is significantly weaker after accounting for smoking status [7], indicating that this and perhaps other shared risk factors may largely account for the risk. Peripheral artery disease (PAD) also occurs in COPD patients and can have a significant impact on functional capacity and quality of life. Similar to stroke and CAD, PAD risk is inversely associated with FEV_1 (% predicted) [105]. Proposed mechanisms for development of stroke and PAD in COPD patients are similar to the mechanisms involved in the pathogenesis of CAD.

Idiopathic Pulmonary Fibrosis and Asthma

Other chronic lung diseases including idiopathic pulmonary fibrosis (IPF) and asthma are also associated with the development of cardiovascular diseases; however, they are much less researched. Similar to COPD, IPF patients have an increased risk of cardiovascular disease that is not fully explained by shared risk factors [106, 107]. In a cohort of patients undergoing transplant evaluation, IPF patients had a significantly increased prevalence of CAD compared to COPD patients as well as worse survival outcomes [108]. In the Multiethnic Study of Atherosclerosis, persistent asthmatic patients had a 1.6-fold increased risk of cardiovascular events compared to age- and risk-matched non-asthmatic controls [109]. Many of the mechanisms discussed previously that explain the relationship between COPD and CVD, including systemic inflammation, hypoxia, and sympathetic activation, may also underlie the relationship between other CLDs and CVD.

Conclusion

CVD is a common comorbidity in COPD independent of shared risk factors. A variety of altered pathobiologic pathways have been described in patients with COPD including increased systemic inflammation, accelerated aging, vascular abnormalities, oxidative stress, hypoxia, sympathetic nervous system activation, hypercoagulability, and protease/anti-protease imbalance, and these likely underlie the increased risk for CVD. Though a definitive cause and effect pathway has not been established and there is no COPD-specific marker of CVD risk, the presence of COPD should raise suspicion for the presence of clinically overt and subclinical CVD. More research is needed to further define the exact pathobiologic relationship between COPD and CVD and to explore potential therapies for both. The mechanisms underlying CVD development in other CLD including IPF and asthma also warrant further studies.

References

1. WHO. The top 10 causes of death [Internet]. WHO. 2018 [cited 2018 Apr 2]. Available from: http://www.who.int/mediacentre/factsheets/fs310/en/.
2. Anthonisen NR, Connett JE, Enright PL, Manfreda J, Lung Health Study Research Group. Hospitalizations and mortality in the Lung Health Study. Am J Respir Crit Care Med. 2002;166(3):333–9.
3. Komajda M, Kerneis M, Tavazzi L, Balanescu S, Cosentino F, Cremonesi A, et al. The chronic ischaemic cardiovascular disease ESC Pilot Registry: results of the six-month follow-up. Eur J Prev Cardiol. 2018;25(4):377–87.
4. Yin L, Lensmar C, Ingelsson E, Bäck M. Differential association of chronic obstructive pulmonary disease with myocardial infarction and ischemic stroke in a nation-wide cohort. Int J Cardiol. 2014;173(3):601–3.
5. Chang CL, Robinson SC, Mills GD, Sullivan GD, Karalus NC, McLachlan JD, et al. Biochemical markers of cardiac dysfunction predict mortality in acute exacerbations of COPD. Thorax. 2011;66(9):764–8.
6. Donaldson GC, Hurst JR, Smith CJ, Hubbard RB, Wedzicha JA. Increased risk of myocardial infarction and stroke following exacerbation of COPD. Chest. 2010;137(5):1091–7.
7. Portegies MLP, Lahousse L, Joos GF, Hofman A, Koudstaal PJ, Stricker BH, et al. Chronic obstructive pulmonary disease and the risk of stroke. The Rotterdam Study. Am J Respir Crit Care Med. 2016;193(3):251–8.
8. McAllister DA, Maclay JD, Mills NL, Leitch A, Reid P, Carruthers R, et al. Diagnosis of myocardial infarction following hospitalisation for exacerbation of COPD. Eur Respir J. 2012;39(5):1097–103.
9. Kunisaki KM, Dransfield MT, Anderson JA, Brook RD, Calverley PMA, Celli BR, et al. Exacerbations of chronic obstructive pulmonary disease and cardiac events: a cohort analysis. Am J Respir Crit Care Med. 2018;198(1):51–7.
10. Dalal AA, Shah M, Lunacsek O, Hanania NA. Clinical and economic burden of patients diagnosed with COPD with comorbid cardiovascular disease. Respir Med. 2011;105(10):1516–22.
11. Patel ARC, Donaldson GC, Mackay AJ, Wedzicha JA, Hurst JR. The impact of ischemic heart disease on symptoms, health status, and exacerbations in patients with COPD. Chest. 2012;141(4):851–7.
12. Sidney S, Sorel M, Quesenberry CP, DeLuise C, Lanes S, Eisner MD. COPD and incident cardiovascular disease hospitalizations and mortality: Kaiser Permanente Medical Care Program. Chest. 2005;128(4):2068–75.
13. Lee HM, Le H, Lee BT, Lopez VA, Wong ND. Forced vital capacity paired with Framingham Risk Score for prediction of all-cause mortality. Eur Respir J. 2010;36(5):1002–6.
14. Iwamoto H, Yokoyama A, Kitahara Y, Ishikawa N, Haruta Y, Yamane K, et al. Airflow limitation in smokers is associated with subclinical atherosclerosis. Am J Respir Crit Care Med. 2009;179(1):35–40.
15. van Gestel YRBM, Flu W-J, van Kuijk J-P, Hoeks SE, Bax JJ, Sin DD, et al. Association of COPD with carotid wall intima-media thickness in vascular surgery patients. Respir Med. 2010;104(5):712–6.
16. Chindhi S, Thakur S, Sarkar M, Negi PC. Subclinical atherosclerotic vascular disease in chronic obstructive pulmonary disease: prospective hospital-based case control study. Lung India. 2015;32(2):137–41.
17. Lahousse L, van den Bouwhuijsen QJA, Loth DW, Joos GF, Hofman A, Witteman JCM, et al. Chronic obstructive pulmonary disease and lipid core carotid artery plaques in the elderly: the Rotterdam Study. Am J Respir Crit Care Med. 2013;187(1):58–64.
18. Charakida M, Masi S, Lüscher TF, Kastelein JJP, Deanfield JE. Assessment of atherosclerosis: the role of flow-mediated dilatation. Eur Heart J. 2010;31(23):2854–61.
19. Juonala M, Viikari JSA, Laitinen T, Marniemi J, Helenius H, Rönnemaa T, et al. Interrelations between brachial endothelial function and carotid intima-media thickness in young adults: the cardiovascular risk in young Finns study. Circulation. 2004;110(18):2918–23.

20. Thijssen DHJ, Black MA, Pyke KE, Padilla J, Atkinson G, Harris RA, et al. Assessment of flow-mediated dilation in humans: a methodological and physiological guideline. Am J Physiol Heart Circ Physiol. 2010;300(1):H2–12.
21. Clarenbach CF, Senn O, Sievi NA, Camen G, van Gestel AJR, Rossi VA, et al. Determinants of endothelial function in patients with COPD. Eur Respir J. 2013;42(5):1194–204.
22. Rodriguez-Miguelez P, Seigler N, Bass L, Dillard TA, Harris RA. Assessments of endothelial function and arterial stiffness are reproducible in patients with COPD. Int J Chron Obstruct Pulmon Dis. 2015;10:1977–86.
23. Marchetti N, Ciccolella DE, Jacobs MR, Crookshank A, Gaughan JP, Kashem MA, et al. Hospitalized acute exacerbation of COPD impairs flow and nitroglycerin-mediated peripheral vascular dilation. COPD. 2011;8(2):60–5.
24. Vivodtzev I, Minet C, Tamisier R, Arbib F, Borel J-C, Baguet J-P, et al. Arterial stiffness by pulse wave velocity in COPD: reliability and reproducibility. Eur Respir J. 2013;42(4):1140–2.
25. Fisk M, McEniery CM, Gale N, Mäki-Petäjä K, Forman JR, Munnery M, et al. Surrogate markers of cardiovascular risk and chronic obstructive pulmonary disease: a large case-controlled study. Hypertensions. 2018;71(3):499–506.
26. Zureik M, Benetos A, Neukirch C, Courbon D, Bean K, Thomas F, et al. Reduced pulmonary function is associated with central arterial stiffness in men. Am J Respir Crit Care Med. 2001;164(12):2181–5.
27. McAllister DA, Maclay JD, Mills NL, Mair G, Miller J, Anderson D, et al. Arterial stiffness is independently associated with emphysema severity in patients with chronic obstructive pulmonary disease. Am J Respir Crit Care Med. 2007;176(12):1208–14.
28. Vivodtzev I, Tamisier R, Baguet JP, Borel JC, Levy P, Pépin JL. Arterial stiffness in COPD. Chest. 2014;145(4):861–75.
29. Maclay JD, McAllister DA, Rabinovich R, Haq I, Maxwell S, Hartland S, et al. Systemic elastin degradation in chronic obstructive pulmonary disease. Thorax. 2012;67(7):606–12.
30. Williams MC, Murchison JT, Edwards LD, Agustí A, Bakke P, Calverley PMA, et al. Coronary artery calcification is increased in patients with COPD and associated with increased morbidity and mortality. Thorax. 2014;69(8):718–23.
31. Dransfield MT, Huang F, Nath H, Singh SP, Bailey WC, Washko GR. CT emphysema predicts thoracic aortic calcification in smokers with and without COPD. COPD. 2010;7(6):404–10.
32. Zagaceta J, Bastarrika G, Zulueta JJ, Colina I, Alcaide AB, Campo A, et al. Prospective comparison of non-invasive risk markers of major cardiovascular events in COPD patients. Respir Res. 2017;18(1):175.
33. Savale L, Chaouat A, Bastuji-Garin S, Marcos E, Boyer L, Maitre B, et al. Shortened telomeres in circulating leukocytes of patients with chronic obstructive pulmonary disease. Am J Respir Crit Care Med. 2009;179(7):566–71.
34. Tsuji T, Aoshiba K, Nagai A. Alveolar cell senescence in patients with pulmonary emphysema. Am J Respir Crit Care Med. 2006;174(8):886–93.
35. Amsellem V, Gary-Bobo G, Marcos E, Maitre B, Chaar V, Validire P, et al. Telomere dysfunction causes sustained inflammation in chronic obstructive pulmonary disease. Am J Respir Crit Care Med. 2011;184(12):1358–66.
36. Kasahara Y, Tuder RM, Cool CD, Lynch DA, Flores SC, Voelkel NF. Endothelial cell death and decreased expression of vascular endothelial growth factor and vascular endothelial growth factor receptor 2 in emphysema. Am J Respir Crit Care Med. 2001;163(3 Pt 1):737–44.
37. Demedts IK, Demoor T, Bracke KR, Joos GF, Brusselle GG. Role of apoptosis in the pathogenesis of COPD and pulmonary emphysema. Respir Res. 2006;7(1):53.
38. Rajendrasozhan S, Yang S-R, Kinnula VL, Rahman I. SIRT1, an antiinflammatory and anti-aging protein, is decreased in lungs of patients with chronic obstructive pulmonary disease. Am J Respir Crit Care Med. 2008;177(8):861–70.

39. Yao H, Chung S, Hwang J, Rajendrasozhan S, Sundar IK, Dean DA, et al. SIRT1 protects against emphysema via FOXO3-mediated reduction of premature senescence in mice. J Clin Invest. 2012;122(6):2032–45.
40. Conti V, Corbi G, Manzo V, Pelaia G, Filippelli A, Vatrella A. Sirtuin 1 and aging theory for chronic obstructive pulmonary disease. Anal Cell Pathol (Amst) [Internet]. 2015 [cited 2018 Feb 27]. Available from: https://www.ncbi.nlm.nih.gov/pmc/articles/PMC4506835/.
41. Nyunoya T, Monick MM, Klingelhutz AL, Glaser H, Cagley JR, Brown CO, et al. Cigarette smoke induces cellular senescence via Werner's syndrome protein down-regulation. Am J Respir Crit Care Med. 2009;179(4):279–87.
42. Benetos A, Okuda K, Lajemi M, Kimura M, Thomas F, Skurnick J, et al. Telomere length as an indicator of biological aging: the gender effect and relation with pulse pressure and pulse wave velocity. Hypertensions. 2001;37(2 Pt 2):381–5.
43. Brouilette SW, Moore JS, McMahon AD, Thompson JR, Ford I, Shepherd J, et al. Telomere length, risk of coronary heart disease, and statin treatment in the West of Scotland Primary Prevention Study: a nested case-control study. Lancet. 2007;369(9556):107–14.
44. Minamino T, Miyauchi H, Yoshida T, Ishida Y, Yoshida H, Komuro I. Endothelial cell senescence in human atherosclerosis: role of telomere in endothelial dysfunction. Circulation. 2002;105(13):1541–4.
45. Gan WQ, Man SFP, Senthilselvan A, Sin DD. Association between chronic obstructive pulmonary disease and systemic inflammation: a systematic review and a meta-analysis. Thorax. 2004;59(7):574–80.
46. Garcia-Rio F, Miravitlles M, Soriano JB, Muñoz L, Duran-Tauleria E, Sánchez G, et al. Systemic inflammation in chronic obstructive pulmonary disease: a population-based study. Respir Res. 2010;11:63.
47. Coulson JM, Rudd JHF, Duckers JM, Rees JIS, Shale DJ, Bolton CE, et al. Excessive aortic inflammation in chronic obstructive pulmonary disease: an 18F-FDG PET pilot study. J Nucl Med. 2010;51(9):1357–60.
48. Miller J, Edwards LD, Agustí A, Bakke P, Calverley PMA, Celli B, et al. Comorbidity, systemic inflammation and outcomes in the ECLIPSE cohort. Respir Med. 2013;107(9):1376–84.
49. Libby P, Tabas I, Fredman G, Fisher EA. Inflammation and its resolution as determinants of acute coronary syndromes. Circ Res. 2014;114(12):1867–79.
50. Hansson GK. Inflammation, atherosclerosis, and coronary artery disease. N Engl J Med. 2005;352(16):1685–95.
51. Torzewski M, Rist C, Mortensen RF, Zwaka TP, Bienek M, Waltenberger J, et al. C-reactive protein in the arterial intima: role of C-reactive protein receptor-dependent monocyte recruitment in atherogenesis. Arterioscler Thromb Vasc Biol. 2000;20(9):2094–9.
52. Ross R. Atherosclerosis – an inflammatory disease. N Engl J Med. 1999;340(2):115–26.
53. Sin DD, Man SFP. Why are patients with chronic obstructive pulmonary disease at increased risk of cardiovascular diseases? The potential role of systemic inflammation in chronic obstructive pulmonary disease. Circulation. 2003;107(11):1514–9.
54. Park HY, Lim SY, Hwang JH, Choi J-H, Koh W-J, Sung J, et al. Lung function, coronary artery calcification, and metabolic syndrome in 4905 Korean males. Respir Med. 2010;104(9):1326–35.
55. Nikolakopoulou S, Hillas G, Perrea D, Tentolouris N, Loukides S, Kostikas K, et al. Serum angiopoietin-2 and CRP levels during COPD exacerbations. COPD. 2014;11(1):46–51.
56. Liu X, Liu Y, Huang X, Lin G, Xie C. Endothelial progenitor cell dysfunction in acute exacerbation of chronic obstructive pulmonary disease. Mol Med Rep. 2017;16(4):5294–302.
57. Kirkham PA, Barnes PJ. Oxidative stress in COPD. Chest. 2013;144(1):266–73.
58. MacNee W. Pulmonary and systemic oxidant/antioxidant imbalance in chronic obstructive pulmonary disease. Proc Am Thorac Soc. 2005;2(1):50–60.
59. Barnes PJ. Inflammatory mechanisms in patients with chronic obstructive pulmonary disease. J Allergy Clin Immunol. 2016;138(1):16–27.

60. Tanrikulu AC, Abakay A, Evliyaoglu O, Palanci Y. Coenzyme Q10, copper, zinc, and lipid peroxidation levels in serum of patients with chronic obstructive pulmonary disease. Biol Trace Elem Res. 2011;143(2):659–67.

61. Can U, Yerlikaya FH, Yosunkaya S. Role of oxidative stress and serum lipid levels in stable chronic obstructive pulmonary disease. J Chin Med Assoc. 2015;78(12):702–8.

62. Singhal SS, Singh SP, Singhal P, Horne D, Singhal J, Awasthi S. Antioxidant role of glutathione S-transferases: 4-hydroxynonenal, a key molecule in stress-mediated signaling. Toxicol Appl Pharmacol. 2015;289(3):361–70.

63. Shukla RK, Kant S, Bhattacharya S, Mittal B. Association of genetic polymorphism of GSTT1, GSTM1 and GSTM3 in COPD patients in a north Indian population. COPD. 2011;8(3):167–72.

64. Senior RM, Tegner H, Kuhn C, Ohlsson K, Starcher BC, Pierce JA. The induction of pulmonary emphysema with human leukocyte elastase. Am Rev Respir Dis. 1977;116(3):469–75.

65. Dinerman JL, Mehta JL, Saldeen TG, Emerson S, Wallin R, Davda R, et al. Increased neutrophil elastase release in unstable angina pectoris and acute myocardial infarction. J Am Coll Cardiol. 1990;15(7):1559–63.

66. Dollery CM, Owen CA, Sukhova GK, Krettek A, Shapiro SD, Libby P. Neutrophil elastase in human atherosclerotic plaques: production by macrophages. Circulation. 2003;107(22):2829–36.

67. Vandenbroucke RE, Dejonckheere E, Libert C. A therapeutic role for matrix metalloproteinase inhibitors in lung diseases? Eur Respir J. 2011;38(5):1200–14.

68. Yasmin, McEniery CM, Wallace S, Dakham Z, Pulsalkar P, Pusalkar P, et al. Matrix metalloproteinase-9 (MMP-9), MMP-2, and serum elastase activity are associated with systolic hypertension and arterial stiffness. Arterioscler Thromb Vasc Biol. 2005;25(2):372.

69. Abilleira S, Bevan S, Markus HS. The role of genetic variants of matrix metalloproteinases in coronary and carotid atherosclerosis. J Med Genet. 2006;43(12):897–901.

70. Golovatch P, Mercer BA, Lemaître V, Wallace A, Foronjy RF, D'Armiento J. Role for cathepsin K in emphysema in smoke-exposed guinea pigs. Exp Lung Res. 2009;35(8):631–45.

71. Li X, Li Y, Jin J, Jin D, Cui L, Li X, et al. Increased serum cathepsin K in patients with coronary artery disease. Yonsei Med J. 2014;55(4):912–9.

72. Platt MO, Ankeny RF, Shi G-P, Weiss D, Vega JD, Taylor WR, et al. Expression of cathepsin K is regulated by shear stress in cultured endothelial cells and is increased in endothelium in human atherosclerosis. Am J Physiol Heart Circ Physiol. 2007;292(3):H1479–86.

73. Hua Y, Robinson TJ, Cao Y, Shi G-P, Ren J, Nair S. Cathepsin K knockout alleviates aging-induced cardiac dysfunction. Aging Cell. 2015;14(3):345–51.

74. Vlahakos DV, Kosmas EN, Dimopoulou I, Ikonomou E, Jullien G, Vassilakos P, et al. Association between activation of the renin-angiotensin system and secondary erythrocytosis in patients with chronic obstructive pulmonary disease. Am J Med. 1999;106(2):158–64.

75. Wang J, Chen L, Chen B, Meliton A, Liu SQ, Shi Y, et al. Chronic activation of the renin-angiotensin system induces lung fibrosis. Sci Rep. 2015;5:15561.

76. Pacurari M, Kafoury R, Tchounwou PB, Ndebele K. The renin-angiotensin-aldosterone system in vascular inflammation and remodeling. Int J Inflamm. 2014;2014:689360.

77. Montecucco F, Pende A, Mach F. The renin-angiotensin system modulates inflammatory processes in atherosclerosis: evidence from basic research and clinical studies. Mediators Inflamm [Internet]. 2009 [cited 2018 Mar 5]. Available from: https://www.ncbi.nlm.nih.gov/pmc/articles/PMC2668935/.

78. da Cunha V, Martin-McNulty B, Vincelette J, Choy DF, Li W-W, Schroeder M, et al. Angiotensin II induces histomorphologic features of unstable plaque in a murine model of accelerated atherosclerosis. J Vasc Surg. 2006;44(2):364–71.

79. Sabit R, Thomas P, Shale DJ, Collins P, Linnane SJ. The effects of hypoxia on markers of coagulation and systemic inflammation in patients with COPD. Chest. 2010;138(1):47–51.

80. Alessandri C, Basili S, Violi F, Ferroni P, Gazzaniga PP, Cordova C. Hypercoagulability state in patients with chronic obstructive pulmonary disease. Chronic Obstructive Bronchitis and Haemostasis Group. Thromb Haemost. 1994;72(3):343–6.
81. Ashitani J-I, Mukae H, Arimura Y, Matsukura S. Elevated plasma procoagulant and fibrinolytic markers in patients with chronic obstructive pulmonary disease. Intern Med. 2002;41(3):181–5.
82. Jatene T, Biering-Sørensen T, Nochioka K, Mangione FM, Hansen KW, Sørensen R, et al. Frequency of cardiac death and stent thrombosis in patients with chronic obstructive pulmonary disease undergoing percutaneous coronary intervention (from the BASKET-PROVE I and II trials). Am J Cardiol. 2017;119(1):14–9.
83. Harrison MT, Short P, Williamson PA, Singanayagam A, Chalmers JD, Schembri S. Thrombocytosis is associated with increased short and long term mortality after exacerbation of chronic obstructive pulmonary disease: a role for antiplatelet therapy? Thorax. 2014;69(7):609–15.
84. Klausen T, Olsen NV, Poulsen TD, Richalet JP, Pedersen BK. Hypoxemia increases serum interleukin-6 in humans. Eur J Appl Physiol. 1997;76(5):480–2.
85. Tyagi T, Ahmad S, Gupta N, Sahu A, Ahmad Y, Nair V, et al. Altered expression of platelet proteins and calpain activity mediate hypoxia-induced prothrombotic phenotype. Blood. 2014;123(8):1250–60.
86. Yamaji-Kegan K, Takimoto E, Zhang A, Weiner NC, Meuchel LW, Berger AE, et al. Hypoxia-induced mitogenic factor (FIZZ1/RELMα) induces endothelial cell apoptosis and subsequent interleukin-4-dependent pulmonary hypertension. Am J Physiol Lung Cell Mol Physiol. 2014;306(12):L1090–103.
87. Fan L, Feng Y, Wan HY, Ni L, Qian YR, Guo Y, et al. Hypoxia induces dysregulation of local renin-angiotensin system in mouse Lewis lung carcinoma cells. Genet Mol Res. 2014;13(4):10562–73.
88. Koechlin C, Maltais F, Saey D, Michaud A, LeBlanc P, Hayot M, et al. Hypoxaemia enhances peripheral muscle oxidative stress in chronic obstructive pulmonary disease. Thorax. 2005;60(10):834–41.
89. Heindl S, Lehnert M, Criée CP, Hasenfuss G, Andreas S. Marked sympathetic activation in patients with chronic respiratory failure. Am J Respir Crit Care Med. 2001;164(4):597–601.
90. Thomson AJ, Drummond GB, Waring WS, Webb DJ, Maxwell SRJ. Effects of short-term isocapnic hyperoxia and hypoxia on cardiovascular function. J Appl Physiol. 2006;101(3):809–16.
91. Morgan BJ, Crabtree DC, Palta M, Skatrud JB. Combined hypoxia and hypercapnia evokes long-lasting sympathetic activation in humans. J Appl Physiol. 1995;79(1):205–13.
92. Hanrahan JP, Grogan DR, Baumgartner RA, Wilson A, Cheng H, Zimetbaum PJ, et al. Arrhythmias in patients with chronic obstructive pulmonary disease (COPD): occurrence frequency and the effect of treatment with the inhaled long-acting beta2-agonists arformoterol and salmeterol. Medicine (Baltimore). 2008;87(6):319–28.
93. Perret-Guillaume C, Joly L, Benetos A. Heart rate as a risk factor for cardiovascular disease. Prog Cardiovasc Dis. 2009;52(1):6–10.
94. Wang X, Jiang Z, Chen B, Zhou L, Kong Z, Zuo S, et al. Cardiac autonomic function in patients with acute exacerbation of chronic obstructive pulmonary disease with and without ventricular tachycardia. BMC Pulm Med. 2016;16(1):124.
95. de Miguel DJ, Morgan JC, García RJ. The association between COPD and heart failure risk: a review. Int J Chron Obstruct Pulmon Dis. 2013;8:305–12.
96. Canepa M, Straburzynska-Migaj E, Drozdz J, Fernandez-Vivancos C, Pinilla JMG, Nyolczas N, et al. Characteristics, treatments and 1-year prognosis of hospitalized and ambulatory heart failure patients with chronic obstructive pulmonary disease in the European Society of Cardiology Heart Failure Long-Term Registry. Eur J Heart Fail. 2018;20(1):100–10.

97. López-Sánchez M, Muñoz-Esquerre M, Huertas D, Gonzalez-Costello J, Ribas J, Manresa F, et al. High prevalence of left ventricle diastolic dysfunction in severe COPD associated with a low exercise capacity: a cross-sectional study. PLoS One. 2013;8(6):e68034.
98. Jörgensen K, Müller MF, Nel J, Upton RN, Houltz E, Ricksten S-E. Reduced intrathoracic blood volume and left and right ventricular dimensions in patients with severe emphysema: an MRI study. Chest. 2007;131(4):1050–7.
99. Watz H, Waschki B, Meyer T, Kretschmar G, Kirsten A, Claussen M, et al. Decreasing cardiac chamber sizes and associated heart dysfunction in COPD: role of hyperinflation. Chest. 2010;138(1):32–8.
100. Alter P, Watz H, Kahnert K, Pfeifer M, Randerath WJ, Andreas S, et al. Airway obstruction and lung hyperinflation in COPD are linked to an impaired left ventricular diastolic filling. Respir Med. 2018;137:14–22.
101. Hohlfeld JM, Vogel-Claussen J, Biller H, Berliner D, Berschneider K, Tillmann H-C, et al. Effect of lung deflation with indacaterol plus glycopyrronium on ventricular filling in patients with hyperinflation and COPD (CLAIM): a double-blind, randomised, crossover, placebo-controlled, single-centre trial. Lancet Respir Med. 2018;6(5):368–78.
102. Stone IS, Barnes NC, James W-Y, Midwinter D, Boubertakh R, Follows R, et al. Lung deflation and cardiovascular structure and function in chronic obstructive pulmonary disease. A randomized controlled trial. Am J Respir Crit Care Med. 2016;193(7):717–26.
103. Come CE, Divo MJ, San José Estépar R, Sciurba FC, Criner GJ, Marchetti N, et al. Lung deflation and oxygen pulse in COPD: results from the NETT randomized trial. Respir Med. 2012;106(1):109–19.
104. Wells JM, Dransfield MT. Pathophysiology and clinical implications of pulmonary arterial enlargement in COPD. Int J Chron Obstruct Pulmon Dis. 2013;8:509–21.
105. Pecci R, De La Fuente Aguado J, Sanjurjo Rivo AB, Sanchez Conde P, Corbacho Abelaira M. Peripheral arterial disease in patients with chronic obstructive pulmonary disease. Int Angiol. 2012;31(5):444–53.
106. Dalleywater W, Powell HA, Hubbard RB, Navaratnam V. Risk factors for cardiovascular disease in people with idiopathic pulmonary fibrosis: a population-based study. Chest. 2015;147(1):150–6.
107. Kim W-Y, Mok Y, Kim GW, Baek S-J, Yun YD, Jee SH, et al. Association between idiopathic pulmonary fibrosis and coronary artery disease: a case-control study and cohort analysis. Sarcoidosis Vasc Diffuse Lung Dis. 2015;31(4):289–96.
108. Nathan SD, Basavaraj A, Reichner C, Shlobin OA, Ahmad S, Kiernan J, et al. Prevalence and impact of coronary artery disease in idiopathic pulmonary fibrosis. Respir Med. 2010;104(7):1035–41.
109. Tattersall MC, Guo M, Korcarz CE, Gepner AD, Kaufman JD, Liu KJ, et al. Asthma predicts cardiovascular disease events: the multi-ethnic study of atherosclerosis. Arterioscler Thromb Vasc Biol. 2015;35(6):1520–5.

Chapter 5
Pathophysiology of Right Heart Disease in Chronic Lung Disease

Indranee Rajapreyar and Deepak Acharya

Key Points/Pearls
- Right heart dysfunction is associated with many types of chronic lung disease.
- Right heart dysfunction in chronic lung disease is often secondary to pulmonary hypertension or hypoxia but may be independent of these factors.
- Pathophysiology of right heart dysfunction in chronic lung disease may be specific to the underlying lung disease.

Introduction

Different chronic lung diseases (CLDs) are associated with varying degrees of right heart dysfunction. The pathophysiology of right heart disease in chronic lung disease is complex, and mechanisms include pulmonary hypertension, hypoxia, neurohormonal alterations, metabolic perturbations, endothelial dysfunction, ischemia, and systemic inflammation. The right ventricle can develop adaptive or maladaptive responses to these processes, and varying degrees of right heart dysfunction can ensue. Clinical management is currently focused on management of underlying

---

I. Rajapreyar
Section of Advanced Heart Failure, Pulmonary Vascular Disease, Heart Transplantation, and Mechanical Circulatory Support, Division of Cardiovascular Diseases, University of Alabama at Birmingham, Birmingham, AL, USA
e-mail: irajapreyar@uabmc.edu

D. Acharya (✉)
Division of Cardiovascular Diseases, Sarver Heart Center, University of Arizona, Tucson, AZ, USA
e-mail: dacharya@shc.arizona.edu

© Springer Nature Switzerland AG 2020
S. P. Bhatt (ed.), *Cardiac Considerations in Chronic Lung Disease*,
Respiratory Medicine, https://doi.org/10.1007/978-3-030-43435-9_5

lung disease and pulmonary hypertension, but as pathophysiologic mechanisms become better understood, new therapeutic targets, including those that focus directly on the right ventricle, may emerge. In this chapter, we provide a comprehensive review of normal physiology as well as the pathophysiology of the right heart and pulmonary circulation in chronic lung disease.

Normal Right Ventricular Anatomy and Physiology

The normal right ventricle (RV) is a crescent-shaped chamber with inlet, trabecular, and outflow components (Fig. 5.1). It has approximately one-sixth the mass of the

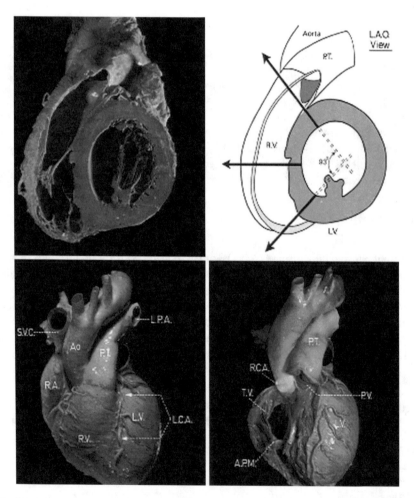

Fig. 5.1 Normal anatomy of the right ventricle. (Reproduced with permission from Mcalpine WA, Heart and Coronary Arteries: An anatomical atlas for clinical diagnosis, radiological investigation, and surgical treatment. Springer 1975)

left ventricle and operates as a high-volume, low-pressure circulation [1]. The normally high capacitance and low afterload of the pulmonary circulation are illustrated by the triangular shape of the right ventricular pressure-volume loop, where isovolumic contraction is not well defined, and ejection continues when RV pressure is falling, with a significant proportion of stroke volume ejected after peak systolic pressure [2] (Fig. 5.2). Right ventricular function is dependent on multiple factors, including filling volumes (preload), pulmonary vascular resistance (afterload), intrinsic RV contractility, interventricular septal contribution, right and left ventricular interaction, and pericardial restraint.

Right Heart Dysfunction in Chronic Lung Disease

Right heart dysfunction associated with CLDs has been recognized since the early 1800s. The World Health Organization (WHO) convened an expert meeting in 1960 in an attempt to provide a more uniform language and consistent classification scheme and defined the term chronic cor pulmonale as "hypertrophy of the right ventricle resulting from diseases affecting the function and/or structure of the lung, except when these pulmonary alterations are the result of diseases that primarily affect the left side of the heart or of congenital heart disease" [3].

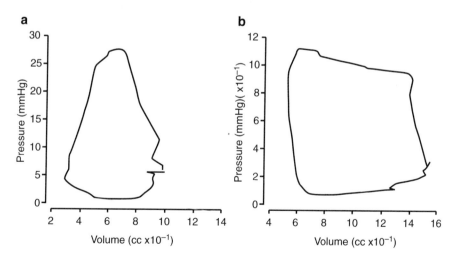

Fig. 5.2 (**a**) Right ventricular pressure-volume loop. (**b**) Left ventricular pressure-volume loop. The right ventricle starts ejecting early in systole and does not have a well-defined isovolemic contraction period. It continues to eject after peak pressure has been achieved, as illustrated by decreasing pressure and volume. In contrast, the left ventricle has well-defined isovolemic contraction and relaxation, and ventricular volume does not decrease after peak systolic pressure. (Reproduced with permission from Ref. [2])

Multiple mechanisms can account for right heart dysfunction in CLD. These include (1) pulmonary hypertension (PH), (2) lung hyperinflation causing reduction of intrathoracic volume, (3) mechanical compression of ventricles, (4) expiratory air-flow limitation resulting in expiratory blood flow limitation in the pulmonary circulation, (5) hypoxia in the setting of higher work and oxygen demands, (6) ischemia, (7) activation of renin-angiotensin-aldosterone system due to hypoxia and/or hypercapnia and resultant volume overload, (8) sympathetic nervous system activation, (9) endothelial dysfunction, and (10) systemic inflammation [4–7]. The relative importance of each of these mechanisms, either in patients with different types of lung disease or in different individuals with the same underlying lung disease, is poorly understood, as is the varying adaptation of the RV to the different forms of physiologic stress.

Pathophysiology of the Pulmonary Vasculature

Pulmonary Vascular Remodeling in PH Due to Chronic Lung Disease

Metabolic remodeling, inflammatory pathway activation, and neurohormonal dysregulation can occur in the pulmonary vasculature in response to the inciting pulmonary insult and, consequently, in the right ventricle due to increased RV pressure afterload. Mechanistic insights to the development and progression of PH are often derived from animal models of PH due to hypoxia, vascular endothelial growth factor inhibitor, and monocrotaline. Pathophysiological mechanisms underlying development of pulmonary hypertension and worsening right ventricular dysfunction in CLD in humans have been extrapolated from animal models of hypoxia.

Pulmonary vascular remodeling was observed in patients with chronic obstructive pulmonary disease (COPD) and PH in varying degrees of severity [8, 9]. A study examining the explanted lungs from patients with COPD who underwent lung transplantation revealed plexiform lesions and medial and intimal fibrosis in small muscular arteries in a subset of COPD patients with severe PH (mPAP >35 mmHg). In the same study, patients with COPD and no PH did not exhibit extensive pulmonary vascular remodeling [8]. Chronic pulmonary vascular remodeling and inability to recruit blood flow during exercise in patients with COPD can result in PH with exercise and progression of PH at rest [10].

Contribution of Inflammatory Pathways to PH in Chronic Lung Disease

Lung injury promotes increased release of the signaling molecule adenosine from inflammatory cells and breakdown of nucleotides like ATP and ADP by CD39 and CD73, respectively, and promotes maladaptive tissue remodeling via adenosine receptor signaling. Adenosine receptor signaling via $A_{2B}R$ stimulates release of cytokines (IL-8, IL-4, IL-13, IL-6, IL-10, TGF-β) from effector cells and growth factors like VEGF that promote angiogenesis and increased fibroblast differentiation promoting fibrosis and progression of disease [11]. Hypoxia, as a result of progressive lung damage, triggers airway inflammation by recruitment of macrophages, with differentiation to M2 phenotype under the influence of Th2 cytokines (IL-4, IL-13), CCL2, and IL-6. Activated macrophages (M2 phenotype) express Found in Inflammatory Zone-1 (Fizzl) and arginase 1, promoting pulmonary artery vascular smooth proliferation and vascular remodeling [12]. Vascular inflammation in PH is predominant in the pulmonary artery adventitia where resident fibroblasts secrete IL −6 and activate STAT 3 signaling in macrophages with increased expression of CD163 + and CD 206+, thereby promoting vascular remodeling. IL-6/STAT3/CEBPβ signaling plays a pivotal role in promoting vascular remodeling by expression of genes that promote fibrosis (arginase-1), altered metabolism and inflammation (HIF1), smooth muscle proliferation and resistance to apoptosis (Pim1, NFAT), and angiogenesis (VEGFa) [13]. HIF1A has been shown to upregulate adenosine receptor 2B in activated macrophages to promote inflammation in idiopathic pulmonary fibrosis (IPF) [14]. There is evidence to suggest that adenosine receptor 2B signaling in COPD and IPF increases hyaluronan synthesis leading to pulmonary vascular remodeling and PH [11, 15, 16]. CD4+ T cells, particularly the TH $_{17}$ subset, have also been implicated in the development in PH due to hypoxia, and IL-6 plays a major role for TH $_{17}$ differentiation [17, 18].

Transforming growth factor beta (TGF-β), a profibrotic cytokine, has been implicated in pathogenesis of fibrotic lung diseases [19]. Bone morphogenetic protein (BMP) and TGFβ signaling (↓BMP/↑TGFβ) impairment plays a role in pulmonary vascular remodeling in animal models of PH [20]. In a detailed study involving explanted lung tissue from patients with IPF and experimental animal model of pulmonary fibrosis, there was a significant decrease inBMPR2A protein with evidence of increased PSMAD 2/PSMAD 3 signaling suggestive of TGFβ activity in human lung tissue with IPF and IPH + PH versus controls. IL-6 was significantly increased in IPF + PH compared to IPF alone, activated STAT3 signaling leading to several expression of miRNAs with the end result of depletion of BMPR2 protein [21].

Mitochondrial Structural and Metabolic Alterations in the Pulmonary Artery

Mitochondrial metabolic remodeling could contribute to pulmonary vascular remodeling and PH disease progression. Oxidative phosphorylation through fatty acid oxidation and glucose oxidation in the mitochondria are sources of energy production. Glucose oxidation in the mitochondria is a minor contributor of energy production [22]. Hypoxia-inducible factor (HIF-1∝), transcription factor, activated in response to hypoxia and inflammation drives the metabolic switch from oxidative phosphorylation to glycolysis, which is a less efficient energy source. Animal models of PAH induced by monocrotaline or chronic hypoxia with Sugen 5416 demonstrated increased FDG-positron emission tomography (PET) uptake in the lungs. Further analysis revealed increased expression of GLUT1 (mediator of increased glucose uptake) in pulmonary artery endothelial cells and pulmonary artery smooth muscle cells (PASMC) but not in airway tissue samples. There is increased expression of HIF-1α in proliferating PAMSC supporting indirect evidence of increased glucose uptake by cells [23]. HIF -1α signaling plays a major role in the glycolytic shift by activating pyruvate dehydrogenase kinase, an enzyme known to inhibit pyruvate dehydrogenase that is involved in glucose oxidation [24]. Glycolytic shift enables cell survival and energy production under hypoxic conditions [25]. Under chronic hypoxic conditions, HIF -1α signaling reduces reactive oxygen species production in mitochondria resulting in inhibition of potassium channels (K_V 1.5), particularly the α subunits altering the membrane potential of mitochondrial membrane with consequent depolarized state. The mitochondrial membrane depolarization allows Ca^{2+} entry through the voltage-gated Ca^{2+} channels causing pulmonary artery vasoconstriction [26]. Elevated intracellular Ca^{2+} levels (cytoplasmic, sarcolemmal, and nuclear) promote pulmonary artery smooth muscle proliferation by activating transcription factors like c-fos, nuclear factor-κ, and c-jun and progression of cell cycle [27, 28]. The increased Ca^{2+} entry also promoted activation of nuclear factor of activated T cells (NFAT), a transcription factor involved in immune response, with increased gene expression of bcl-2 and downregulated potassium channels promoting unopposed cell proliferation [29]. Potassium channel inhibition prevents activation of caspases and mitochondrial cytochrome c release preventing pulmonary artery smooth muscle apoptosis [30]. In addition, increased activity of the glycolytic enzyme, hexokinase-II, results in decreased activity of mitochondrial permeability transition pore (MPTP) preventing cell death [24].

The complex interplay of mitochondrial energetics and electrical remodeling under HIF-1α signaling activated in response to local inflammation and hypoxia creates a self-perpetuating cellular microenvironment promoting cell proliferation and preventing programmed cell death leading to pulmonary vascular remodeling and PH.

Neurohormonal Dysregulation in the Pulmonary Circulation

Adrenergic and cholinergic innervation of pulmonary vasculature mediate vascular tone [31]. In animal models, alveolar hypoxia results in increased pulmonary vascular constriction as a result of sympathetic activation. Human studies demonstrating strong mechanistic links between CLD, sympathetic activation, and progression of pulmonary hypertension are lacking.

Renin-angiotensin aldosterone system (RAAS) activation has been associated with progression of pulmonary artery hypertension. Angiotensin II (Ang II) activates signaling pathways with activation of protein kinases and non-receptor tyrosine kinases with end result of vascular smooth muscle proliferation and fibrosis. Ang II has been implicated in production of reactive oxygen species (ROS) through NAPH oxidase activation resulting in increased vascular inflammation [32]. Pulmonary vascular endothelium is one of the major sites for angiotensin-converting enzyme activity (ACE) [33].

In rats exposed to hypoxia, there was increased ACE mRNA and ACE immunostaining in the small neo-muscularized pulmonary arteries [34]. Administration of captopril and losartan to hypoxic rats improved mean pulmonary artery pressures, decreased right ventricular hypertrophy, and decreased medial thickening and muscularization of small pulmonary arteries providing indirect evidence of the role of Ang II production and activation via angiotensin 1 (AT1) receptor in progression of pulmonary hypertension [34]. In rats exposed to chronic cigarette smoke, pulmonary hypertension developed with increased ACE and Ang II expression in lung tissue [35].

In normal human subjects, ACE immunostaining was highest in the alveolar capillary endothelium, whereas in subjects with PAH, increased ACE immunostaining was seen in large pre-acinar and small acinar arteries. In addition, there was increased ACE immunostaining in arteries with fibrotic and plexiform lesions [36]. In a study of idiopathic PAH patients, there was increased renin activity, angiotensin 1, and Ang II, and increasing trends were associated with risk of death or lung transplantation. Ang II increases pulmonary artery smooth muscle proliferation via AT1 receptor signaling [37].

Ang II via activation of AT1 receptor and increased production of growth factors (TGF-β, PDGF) promotes human lung fibroblast proliferation in patients with idiopathic pulmonary fibrosis [38]. Renal denervation in animal models of PH decreased AT1 receptor density and mineralocorticoid with decreased proliferation of pulmonary arterial smooth muscle suggesting combined role of sympathetic nervous system (SNS), RAAS, and aldosterone in PH disease progression [39].

The endothelin system has been implicated in pathogenesis of WHO group 1 pulmonary arterial hypertension (idiopathic), and one of the major therapeutic targets is endothelin receptor antagonism. Increased expression of endothelin-1 was found in alveolar epithelial cells in lung specimens obtained from patients with pulmonary fibrosis and in muscular pulmonary arteries from patients with concomitant pulmonary fibrosis and pulmonary hypertension [18]. Arterial endothelin-1 levels at rest were significantly elevated in patients with interstitial lung disease (ILD) and emphysema with pulmonary hypertension compared to patients with lung disease without pulmonary hypertension. With exercise, arterial levels of endothelin-1 increased in patients with ILD and correlated significantly with alveolar-arterial oxygen difference [40]. Endothelin-1 increases extra-adrenal synthesis of aldosterone in human pulmonary vascular endothelial cells and animal rodent models of PH by increased expression of aldosterone synthase. Aldosterone increases oxidant stress by increasing NADPH oxidase type 4 (NOX4), and generated reactive oxygen species (ROS) impair endothelin-B (ET$_B$) receptor eNOS (nitric oxide synthase) signaling with decreased nitric oxide synthesis and pulmonary vascular dysfunction. Aldosterone antagonists restored endothelin-1-ET$_B$ receptor signaling to increase nitric oxide availability and potentially prevent adverse pulmonary vascular remodeling [41]. We can speculate from these studies that activation of endothelin system contributes to pathogenesis of pulmonary hypertension in patients with CLD with concomitant pulmonary hypertension.

Pulmonary Hypertension and the Right Ventricle

The classical view of cor pulmonale is that parenchymal lung disease causes hypoxic vasoconstriction and remodeling of the pulmonary vascular bed, which elevates pulmonary vascular resistance, which then leads to PH. The PH increases right ventricular work and causes RV dilation and/or hypertrophy and subsequently RV failure. In other words, PH is the central component in cor pulmonale [42, 43].

In patients with COPD and IPF, the prevalence of PH correlates with the severity of underlying lung disease. The majority of patients who develop PH, however, have PA pressures in the mild range, i.e., mean PAP (mPAP) $\leq$ 35 mmHg. A small minority have severe PH [44]. Some investigators have postulated that these may represent distinct phenotypes, i.e., predominant respiratory limitation with mild PH vs. predominant pulmonary vascular perturbation out of proportion to the degree of lung disease, with important management implications [45, 46]. The development of PH, even mild, is associated with more exercise limitations and worse prognosis [47–51].

Recent evidence, however, challenges some assumptions of the classical view of cor pulmonale. In an important study, Hilde and colleagues evaluated 94 patients with Gold II–IV COPD and 34 controls. Patients were categorized as having PH if mPAP was $\geq$25 mmHg on resting right heart catheterization. Those without PH were further divided into mPAP $\leq$20 and mPAP 21–24 groups. Echocardiographic RV parameters were impaired in both patients with PH and those without PH compared to controls. RV strain, RV myocardial performance index, and RV isovolumic relaxation were impaired compared to controls in patients with mPAP $\leq$20 mmHg, and RV size and wall thickness had already increased in COPD patients with mPAP $\leq$20 mmHg [7]. Similar findings were found in a series of 52 patients with IPF, where impaired RV systolic and diastolic function was observed in patients without PH by echocardiography [52].

This dissociation between RV remodeling and PH suggests that other mechanisms are involved in RV dysfunction and that RV dysfunction is a process that begins long before resting PH. It is also important to note that 50% of the pulmonary vascular bed has to be damaged before resting PA pressures increases, and resting PA pressures may not reflect hemodynamics during exercise or intermittent nocturnal hypoxemia that could lead to altered pulmonary vascular compliance well before manifest pulmonary hypertension [53].

Pathophysiology of the Right Ventricle

Right Ventricular Response

Right ventricular function is a major determinant of prognosis in CLD and pulmonary hypertension [22]. The molecular, metabolic, and adrenergic system alterations in the right ventricle (RV) determine the adaptive versus maladaptive changes in the right ventricle in response to hypoxia or PH. Adaptive changes are characterized by minimal RV dilation, increased concentric hypertrophy, and minimal fibrosis with preserved RV cardiac output. Maladaptive changes in RV result in increased fibrosis, RV dilation, decreased RV systolic function with impaired functional impairment, and decreased survival. As discussed earlier, studies in patients with COPD have revealed that there is dissociation between RV remodeling process and PH suggesting other mechanisms may contribute to RV systolic dysfunction [7]. In a study involving two different animal models of PH, there was a variable degree of RV dilation, fibrosis, and capillary density despite similar increase in RV afterload. Animal model with PH induced by combination of hypoxia and VEGF receptor blocker (SU5416) resulted in more RV fibrosis, decreased capillary density, and decreased VEGF protein expression when compared to PH induced by pulmonary artery banding (PAB) alone. Susceptibility to oxidative stress due to decreased antioxidant transcription factor E2-related factor 2 (Nrf2) and HO-1 gene may contribute to differences in the degree of RV impairment [54]. Right ventricular ischemia has been implicated in the development of RV dysfunction in patients with primary pulmonary arterial hypertension [55]. Right ventricular ischemia could result from decreased right coronary artery perfusion pressure from elevated RV end-diastolic pressure, decreased capillary density from impaired angiogenesis, and hypoxemia [22]. RV ischemia can further trigger a cascade of events leading to neurohormonal activation and metabolic and mitochondrial alterations that promote maladaptive remodeling.

Neurohormonal Activation

Sympathetic nervous activation in chronic left ventricular systolic heart failure leads to maladaptive left ventricular remodeling with decreased long-term survival [56]. Patients with pulmonary arterial hypertension (WHO group 1) with increased muscle sympathetic nerve activity (MSNA) had disease progression with clinical deterioration [57]. Patients with chronic respiratory failure due to COPD and pulmonary fibrosis demonstrated increased MSNA likely due to peripheral arterial chemoreceptor activation providing evidence of increased sympathetic activation in CLD [58]. Patients with COPD have elevated resting heart rate, decreased heart rate variability, and decreased baroreceptor sensitivity indicative of heightened sympathetic activation [59]. In a small study involving COPD patients, increased MSNA activity was significantly higher in patients who died or were hospitalized for COPD exacerbation [60]. The untoward consequences of sympathetic activation seen in PAH (WHO group 1) and COPD may be pertinent to patients with CLD with increased sympathetic activity. There is lack of data regarding long-term consequences of sympathetic nervous system activation in worsening respiratory function, pulmonary hypertension, and RV failure in patients with CLD. The mechanisms of sympathetic activation in COPD are postulated due to peripheral arterial chemoreceptor stimulation from hypoxia, stimulation of central chemoreceptors due to hypercapnia, breathing patterns, chronic hyperinflation resulting in alteration of local pulmonary stretch receptors, diaphragmatic remodeling, use of beta sympathomimetics, and inflammatory state [59, 61, 62]. Plasma norepinephrine levels were elevated twofold in end-stage emphysematous patients and elevated threefold in patients with acute cor pulmonale due to COPD [63, 64]. Data regarding prognostic significance of elevated norepinephrine levels in CLD is lacking.

Remodeling of adrenergic receptor signaling in right ventricle resulted in decreased inotropic reserve in PH in animal models of RVH caused by combination of VEGFR inhibitor and hypoxia or monocrotaline. There was increase in G protein-coupled receptor kinase-2 (GRK2) activity with end result of β1-AR downregulation and decreased contractile reserve in response to inotropes [65].

Role of Renin-Angiotensin System

Activation of renin-angiotensin system in chronic left ventricular systolic heart failure leads to maladaptive remodeling and progression of disease [66]. In animal models with chronic exposure to hypoxia, there is 3.4-fold increase in right ventricular ACE expression and correlated with presence of right ventricular hypertrophy [67]. Activation of renin-angiotensin system and sympathetic nervous system from increased right atrial pressures with exercise and hypoxia in patients with COPD creates a vicious cycle of sodium and fluid retention and worsening RV systolic function [46].

Metabolic Alterations in the Right Ventricle

The right ventricle is a thin-walled structure with one-fifth the energy of the left ventricle due to low pulmonary vascular resistance [68]. The energy source for a normal adult heart is predominantly fatty acids (60–90%) with glucose accounting for 10–40% [22]. With chronic pressure overload to the right ventricle and hypoxia due to CLD, metabolism in the right ventricle shifts from predominantly fatty acid oxidation to glycolysis. Evidence of increased glycolysis has been studied extensively in animal rodent models and human subjects. In patients with iPAH, [18 F]fluorodeoxyglucose (FDG) PET imaging demonstrated increased accumulation in the RV free wall and correlated with increased RV wall stress, and there was a decrease in uptake in treatment responders to pulmonary vasodilators [69]. Patients with PAH with increased FDG uptake in the RV free wall experienced clinical worsening, poor exercise tolerance, and higher all-cause mortality [70]. Impaired RV myocardial fatty acid uptake in patients with RV hypertrophy due to PH (idiopathic and chronic thromboembolic) using iodine-123-labeled 15-(p-iodophenyl)-3-(R,S)-methyl pentadecanoic acid was associated with poor RV contractility and decreased survival [71]. Metabolic shift to glycolysis was mediated by activation of pyruvate dehydrogenase kinase (PDK) which inhibits pyruvate dehydrogenase phosphorylation in rodent models of MCT-induced RVH. There is inefficient energy production with consequent decreased RV systolic function. The expression of PGC-1α protein and mRNA levels, a key regulator of peroxisome proliferator-activated receptor gamma coactivator 1-alpha that is responsible for fatty acid oxidation, is decreased in animal rodent models of PH induced by combination of SU5416 and hypoxia with significant RV dysfunction as opposed to rodents that have right ventricular hypertrophy due to pulmonary artery banding. Human RV tissue samples from patients with PAH undergoing transplantation exhibited a similar decrease of PGC-1αmRNA in failing RVs compared to normal hearts. The findings of increased gene expression (GLUT-1 and hexokinase) responsible for glycolysis and decreased expression of genes responsible for encoding proteins for fatty acid transport into cells and mitochondria, mitochondrial fatty acid oxidation, and glucose oxidation in the failing RV are suggestive of maladaptive metabolic remodeling [72]. Evidence from animal models of PH have shown that increased glutaminolysis by cMyc activation (similar to cancer cells) promotes cell growth causing RVH and supports the increasing metabolic needs of the right ventricle [73]. The findings of decreased high-energy phosphates in the RV myocardium, decreased mitochondrial oxygen consumption, and dysfunction enzyme activity of mitochondrial electron transport chain could reflect a transition from a compensated to a decompensated state of RV dysfunction [74]. Mitochondrial DNA damage by reactive oxygen species, changes to the mitochondrial structure, decreased mitochondrial content, and abnormal cellular respiration are seen in RV dysfunction due to PH. Right ventricular hypertrophy due to pulmonary artery banding which is a more adaptive remodeling of RV has less pronounced mitochondrial dysfunction [72]. Right ventricular myocardial gene remodeling with decreased angiogenic factors VEGF, Ang 1, and apelin contributes to decreased capillary density and consequent myocardial ischemia in failing right ventricle [75]. In addition, impaired hypoxia-inducible factor (HIF1 α) signaling due to increased mitochondrial reactive oxygen species production impairs angiogenesis leading to decompensated RV failure. Finally, into metabolic remodeling, there is evidence of electrical remodeling with prolonged QTc interval due to decreased expression of potassium channels [73].

Hypoxia and Right Ventricular Dysfunction

Acute hypoxia can cause pulmonary vasoconstriction, whereas chronic hypoxia is associated with remodeling. The mechanisms of remodeling are complex and include myofibroblast differentiation, release of growth factors, vasoconstrictors, adhesion molecules, matrix proteins, altered calcium handling, and inflammatory mediators. A detailed review is provided by Stenmark et al. [76]. Hypoxia is a marker of the severity of lung disease, is associated with worse outcomes, and may lead to pulmonary hypertension and secondary RV failure.

However, the role of hypoxia in primary RV dysfunction is unclear, and hypoxia may not be a necessary prerequisite for RV dysfunction. In one study, right ventricular hypertrophy was observed in 25 patients, of whom the majority [19] had resting normoxia (PaO2 > 80 mmHg) and the rest had mild hypoxia (PaO2 60–80). Therefore, RV structural abnormalities occur well before resting hypoxemia. It should be noted that dynamic changes in oxygenation during exercise or sleep were not evaluated in this study [77].

Disease-Specific Pathophysiologic Responses

A large proportion of early human clinical research on RHD in CLD focused on cor pulmonale from COPD, which accounts for 80–90% of cor pulmonale [42]. More recently, investigation on other causes, including IPF, interstitial lung diseases related to connective tissue diseases, cardiac sarcoidosis, and cystic fibrosis, has increased. The RV pathology as well as response to hypoxemia, pressure, and volume overload may vary based on the underlying condition. For some processes, there may also be direct involvement of the right ventricle in addition to the parenchymal lung disease. For example, pathologic analysis of the right ventricles of patients who died of idiopathic PH vs. systemic sclerosis-related PH (SScPAH) revealed that those with systemic sclerosis had significantly more inflammatory cells than IPAH but a similar degree of fibrosis [78]. SScPAH patients also have higher pro-BNP levels than IPAH patients despite less severe hemodynamic abnormalities, and pro-BNP is a stronger predictor of survival in SScPAH than IPAH, suggesting differences in neurohormonal responses between the two conditions [79]. Patients with systemic sclerosis also have increase in RA area, increase in RV wall thickness, and impaired diastolic function compared to controls despite similar resting pulmonary pressures and RV systolic function [80]. Other conditions, such as sarcoidosis, also have demonstrated pathophysiologic heterogeneity [44]. It is beyond the scope of this manuscript to discuss the details of all such pathophysiologic differences, but these types of disease-specific responses may lead to distinct phenotypes that are currently poorly understood but may have implications regarding need for close surveillance, aggressiveness of therapy, and in some cases treatment and response to pulmonary vasodilators.

Diagnosis of Right Heart Dysfunction in Chronic Lung Disease

The diagnosis of right heart dysfunction in CLD is not always straightforward and reflects the pathophysiologic complexity and heterogeneity of the condition. Symptoms of dyspnea, exertional intolerance, and fatigue can be nonspecific and potentially related to the underlying CLD rather than RHD. The development of peripheral edema can be due to activation of the renin-angiotensin-aldosterone system from hypoxia and/or hypercapnia and subsequent altered sodium and fluid hemodynamics and does not necessarily indicate right heart dysfunction. Physical exam findings of jugular venous distension, tricuspid regurgitation, right ventricular heave, epigastric pulsation, and pulsatile liver are more specific, but by the time these findings occur the RV dysfunction is advanced.

Echocardiography is the most important screening test for early as well as advanced RV dysfunction or PH. Standard measurements include ventricular and atrial size, RV wall thickness, systolic and diastolic measurements, and RA pressure estimation using IVC diameter and collapsibility. Pulmonary artery systolic pressure is estimated using tricuspid regurgitation velocity and RA pressure. Reference values from the American Society of Echocardiography are listed in Tables 5.1 and 5.2 [81]. Early pathophysiologic changes may not be detected by standard

Table 5.1 Summary of reference limits for recommended measures of right heart structure and function

Variable	Unit	Abnormal
Chamber dimensions		
RV basal diameter	cm	>4.2
RV subcostal wall thickness	cm	>0.5
RVOT PSAX distal diameter	cm	>2.7
RVOT PLAX proximal diameter	cm	>3.3
RA major dimension	cm	>5.3
RA minor dimension	cm	>4.4
RA end-systolic area	cm²	>18
Systolic function		
TAPSE	cm	<1.6
Pulsed Doppler peak velocity at the annulus	cm/s	<10
Pulsed Doppler MPI	–	>0.40
Tissue Doppler MPI	–	>0.55
FAC (%)	%	<35
Diastolic function		
E/A ratio	–	<0.8 or > 2.1
E/E' ratio	–	>6
Deceleration time (ms)	ms	<120

Reproduced with permission from Ref [81]
FAC fractional area change, *MPI* myocardial performance index, *PLAX* parasternal long axis, *PSAX* parasternal short axis, *RA* right atrium, *RV* right ventricle, *RVD* right ventricular diameter, *RVOT* right ventricular outflow tract, *TAPSE*, tricuspid annular plane systolic excursion

Table 5.2 Estimation of RA pressure on the basis of IVC diameter and collapsibility

Variable	Normal (0–5 [3] mm Hg)	Intermediate (5–10 [8] mm Hg)	High (15 mm Hg)	
IVC diameter	≤2.1 cm	≤2.1 cm	>2.1 cm	>2.1 cm
Collapse with sniff	>50%	<50%	>50%	<50%
Secondary indices of elevated RA pressure				Restrictive filling
				Tricuspid E/E′ > 6
				Diastolic flow predominance in hepatic veins (systolic filling fraction <55%)

Reproduced with permission from Ref. [81]

Ranges are provided for low and intermediate categories, but for simplicity, midrange values of 3 mm Hg for normal and 8 mm Hg for intermediate are suggested. Intermediate (8 mm Hg) RA pressures may be downgraded to normal (3 mm Hg) if no secondary indices of elevated RA pressure are present, upgraded to high if minimal collapse with sniff (<35%) and secondary indices of elevated RA pressure are present, or left at 8 mm Hg if uncertain

IVC inferior vena cava, *RA* right atrial

Fig. 5.3 Stages of pulmonary hypertension. As pulmonary hypertension progresses, pulmonary vascular resistance continues to rise. When the right ventricle fails, the systolic pulmonary pressure decreases, as does the cardiac output. (Reproduced with permission from Ref. [82])

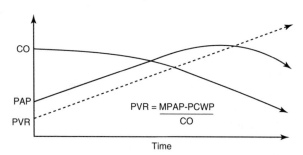

measures, and tissue deformation/strain rate imaging may detect more subtle ventricular dysfunction and may be less load-dependent.

It is important to recognize that echocardiography may not accurately diagnose PH if there are poor windows, if the probe angulation is not parallel to the tricuspid jet, or if there is no tricuspid regurgitation jet. Also, we advise caution in using echo-derived PA systolic pressure alone to longitudinally evaluate pulmonary pressures, because a decrease in PA systolic pressure could reflect either improvement in PH or worsening PH with RV failure and inability of the RV to generate high pressure [82](Fig. 5.3).

Cardiac magnetic resonance imaging provides accurate, comprehensive assessment of the heart but is not widely available, is time-consuming, and is not cost-effective as an initial screening test for all patients with CLD. However, it can be valuable to provide detailed ventricular size and volume measurements in order to track subtle changes and assess responses to therapy or for research purposes. It can also be a useful noninvasive exam when echocardiographic images are suboptimal or there is still clinical uncertainty after echocardiogram.

Hemodynamic assessment with a right heart catheterization (RHC) is the most direct physiologic assessment of the right heart, left heart, and the pulmonary circulation. The degree of RV failure, the severity of pulmonary hypertension, the pulmonary vascular resistance, the relationship between the pulmonary vasculature and right heart dysfunction, and the left ventricular contribution to pulmonary pressures by the pulmonary capillary wedge pressure can all be measured. Exercise RHC may provide important information regarding changes in pulmonary pressure with exertion and/or hypoxia and can sometimes unmask mild left ventricular diastolic dysfunction. Careful measurement of pressures at end expiration (but avoiding Valsalva maneuver) is crucial, since there are often very wide respiratory variations in intrathoracic pressures in patients with COPD, OSA, and other lung diseases, and automated measurements or inadequate attention can make the measurements uninterpretable.

Conclusion

Right heart dysfunction in chronic lung disease is a complex, multifaceted process, both related to and independent of PH. Large-scale human studies are limited, and pathway redundancies and relationships are not well understood. Further investigation into these processes may provide new models and innovative therapeutic targets for right heart dysfunction in chronic lung diseases.

References

1. Dell'Italia LJ. Anatomy and physiology of the right ventricle. Cardiol Clin. 2012;30(2):167–87.
2. Redington AN, Gray HH, Hodson ME, Rigby ML, Oldershaw PJ. Characterisation of the normal right ventricular pressure-volume relation by biplane angiography and simultaneous micromanometer pressure measurements. Br Heart J. 1988;59(1):23–30.
3. Organization WH. Chronic Cor Pulmonale: report of an expert committee. World Health Organization Technical Report Series 1961;No. 213.
4. MacNee W. Pathophysiology of cor pulmonale in chronic obstructive pulmonary disease. Part one. Am J Respir Crit Care Med. 1994;150(3):833–52.
5. MacNee W. Pathophysiology of cor pulmonale in chronic obstructive pulmonary disease. Part two. Am J Respir Crit Care Med. 1994;150(4):1158–68.
6. Zangiabadi A, De Pasquale CG, Sajkov D. Pulmonary hypertension and right heart dysfunction in chronic lung disease. Biomed Res Int. 2014;2014:739674.
7. Hilde JM, Skjorten I, Grotta OJ, Hansteen V, Melsom MN, Hisdal J, et al. Right ventricular dysfunction and remodeling in chronic obstructive pulmonary disease without pulmonary hypertension. J Am Coll Cardiol. 2013;62(12):1103–11.
8. Carlsen J, Hasseriis Andersen K, Boesgaard S, Iversen M, Steinbruchel D, Bogelund AC. Pulmonary arterial lesions in explanted lungs after transplantation correlate with severity of pulmonary hypertension in chronic obstructive pulmonary disease. J Heart Lung Transplant. 2013;32(3):347–54.

9. Andersen KH, Andersen CB, Gustafsson F, Carlsen J. Pulmonary venous remodeling in COPD-pulmonary hypertension and idiopathic pulmonary arterial hypertension. Pulm Circ. 2017;7(2):514–21.
10. Matthay RA, Arroliga AC, Wiedemann HP, Schulman DS, Mahler DA. Right ventricular function at rest and during exercise in chronic obstructive pulmonary disease. Chest. 1992;101(5 Suppl):255S–62S.
11. Karmouty-Quintana H, Xia Y, Blackburn MR. Adenosine signaling during acute and chronic disease states. J Mol Med. 2013;91(2):173–81.
12. Vergadi E, Chang MS, Lee C, Liang OD, Liu X, Fernandez-Gonzalez A, et al. Early macrophage recruitment and alternative activation are critical for the later development of hypoxia-induced pulmonary hypertension. Circulation. 2011;123(18):1986–95.
13. El Kasmi KC, Pugliese SC, Riddle SR, Poth JM, Anderson AL, Frid MG, et al. Adventitial fibroblasts induce a distinct proinflammatory/profibrotic macrophage phenotype in pulmonary hypertension. J Immunol. 2014;193(2):597–609.
14. Philip K, Mills TW, Davies J, Chen NY, Karmouty-Quintana H, Luo F, et al. HIF1A upregulates the ADORA2B receptor on alternatively activated macrophages and contributes to pulmonary fibrosis. FASEB J. 2017;31(11):4745–58.
15. Karmouty-Quintana H, Zhong H, Acero L, Weng T, Melicoff E, West JD, et al. The A2B adenosine receptor modulates pulmonary hypertension associated with interstitial lung disease. FASEB J. 2012;26(6):2546–57.
16. Karmouty-Quintana H, Weng T, Garcia-Morales LJ, Chen NY, Pedroza M, Zhong H, et al. Adenosine A2B receptor and hyaluronan modulate pulmonary hypertension associated with chronic obstructive pulmonary disease. Am J Respir Cell Mol Biol. 2013;49(6):1038–47.
17. Maston LD, Jones DT, Giermakowska W, Howard TA, Cannon JL, Wang W, et al. Central role of T helper 17 cells in chronic hypoxia-induced pulmonary hypertension. Am J Physiol Lung Cell Mol Physiol. 2017;312(5):L609–L24.
18. Giaid A, Yanagisawa M, Langleben D, Michel RP, Levy R, Shennib H, et al. Expression of endothelin-1 in the lungs of patients with pulmonary hypertension. N Engl J Med. 1993;328(24):1732–9.
19. Tatler AL, Jenkins G. TGF-beta activation and lung fibrosis. Proc Am Thorac Soc. 2012;9(3):130–6.
20. Long L, Crosby A, Yang X, Southwood M, Upton PD, Kim DK, et al. Altered bone morphogenetic protein and transforming growth factor-beta signaling in rat models of pulmonary hypertension: potential for activin receptor-like kinase-5 inhibition in prevention and progression of disease. Circulation. 2009;119(4):566–76.
21. Chen NY, Chen NY, D Collum S, Luo F, Weng T, Le TT, M Hernandez A, et al. Macrophage bone morphogenic protein receptor 2 depletion in idiopathic pulmonary fibrosis and group III pulmonary hypertension. Am J Physiol Lung Cell Mol Physiol. 2016;311(2):L238–54.
22. Ryan JJ, Archer SL. The right ventricle in pulmonary arterial hypertension: disorders of metabolism, angiogenesis and adrenergic signaling in right ventricular failure. Circ Res. 2014;115(1):176–88.
23. Marsboom G, Wietholt C, Haney CR, Toth PT, Ryan JJ, Morrow E, et al. Lung (1)(8)F-fluorodeoxyglucose positron emission tomography for diagnosis and monitoring of pulmonary arterial hypertension. Am J Respir Crit Care Med. 2012;185(6):670–9.
24. Cottrill KA, Chan SY. Metabolic dysfunction in pulmonary hypertension: the expanding relevance of the Warburg effect. Eur J Clin Investig. 2013;43(8):855–65.
25. Xu W, Koeck T, Lara AR, Neumann D, DiFilippo FP, Koo M, et al. Alterations of cellular bioenergetics in pulmonary artery endothelial cells. Proc Natl Acad Sci U S A. 2007;104(4):1342–7.
26. Platoshyn O, Yu Y, Golovina VA, McDaniel SS, Krick S, Li L, et al. Chronic hypoxia decreases K(V) channel expression and function in pulmonary artery myocytes. Am J Physiol Lung Cell Mol Physiol. 2001;280(4):L801–12.

27. Platoshyn O, Golovina VA, Bailey CL, Limsuwan A, Krick S, Juhaszova M, et al. Sustained membrane depolarization and pulmonary artery smooth muscle cell proliferation. Am J Physiol Cell Physiol. 2000;279(5):C1540–9.
28. Burg ED, Remillard CV, Yuan JX. Potassium channels in the regulation of pulmonary artery smooth muscle cell proliferation and apoptosis: pharmacotherapeutic implications. Br J Pharmacol. 2008;153(Suppl 1):S99–S111.
29. Bonnet S, Rochefort G, Sutendra G, Archer SL, Haromy A, Webster L, et al. The nuclear factor of activated T cells in pulmonary arterial hypertension can be therapeutically targeted. Proc Natl Acad Sci U S A. 2007;104(27):11418–23.
30. Krick S, Platoshyn O, McDaniel SS, Rubin LJ, Yuan JX. Augmented K(+) currents and mitochondrial membrane depolarization in pulmonary artery myocyte apoptosis. Am J Physiol Lung Cell Mol Physiol. 2001;281(4):L887–94.
31. Vaillancourt M, Chia P, Sarji S, Nguyen J, Hoftman N, Ruffenach G, et al. Autonomic nervous system involvement in pulmonary arterial hypertension. Respir Res. 2017;18(1):201.
32. Mehta PK, Griendling KK. Angiotensin II cell signaling: physiological and pathological effects in the cardiovascular system. Am J Physiol Cell Physiol. 2007;292(1):C82–97.
33. Studdy PR, Lapworth R, Bird R. Angiotensin-converting enzyme and its clinical significance– a review. J Clin Pathol. 1983;36(8):938–47.
34. Morrell NW, Atochina EN, Morris KG, Danilov SM, Stenmark KR. Angiotensin converting enzyme expression is increased in small pulmonary arteries of rats with hypoxia-induced pulmonary hypertension. J Clin Invest. 1995;96(4):1823–33.
35. Yuan YM, Luo L, Guo Z, Yang M, Ye RS, Luo C. Activation of renin-angiotensin-aldosterone system (RAAS) in the lung of smoking-induced pulmonary arterial hypertension (PAH) rats. J Renin Angiotensin Aldosterone Syst. 2015;16(2):249–53.
36. Orte C, Polak JM, Haworth SG, Yacoub MH, Morrell NW. Expression of pulmonary vascular angiotensin-converting enzyme in primary and secondary plexiform pulmonary hypertension. J Pathol. 2000;192(3):379–84.
37. de Man FS, Tu L, Handoko ML, Rain S, Ruiter G, Francois C, et al. Dysregulated renin-angiotensin-aldosterone system contributes to pulmonary arterial hypertension. Am J Respir Crit Care Med. 2012;186(8):780–9.
38. Marshall RP, McAnulty RJ, Laurent GJ. Angiotensin II is mitogenic for human lung fibroblasts via activation of the type 1 receptor. Am J Respir Crit Care Med. 2000;161(6):1999–2004.
39. da Silva Goncalves Bos D, Happe C, Schalij I, Pijacka W, Paton JFR, Guignabert C, et al. Renal denervation reduces pulmonary vascular remodeling and right ventricular diastolic stiffness in experimental pulmonary hypertension. JACC Basic Transl Sci. 2017;2(1):22–35.
40. Yamakami T, Taguchi O, Gabazza EC, Yoshida M, Kobayashi T, Kobayashi H, et al. Arterial endothelin-1 level in pulmonary emphysema and interstitial lung disease. Relation with pulmonary hypertension during exercise. Eur Respir J. 1997;10(9):2055–60.
41. Maron BA, Zhang YY, White K, Chan SY, Handy DE, Mahoney CE, et al. Aldosterone inactivates the endothelin-B receptor via a cysteinyl thiol redox switch to decrease pulmonary endothelial nitric oxide levels and modulate pulmonary arterial hypertension. Circulation. 2012;126(8):963–74.
42. Weitzenblum E. Chronic cor pulmonale. Heart. 2003;89(2):225–30.
43. Fishman AP. State of the art: chronic cor pulmonale. Am Rev Respir Dis. 1976;114(4):775–94.
44. Seeger WAY, Barberà JA, Champion H, Coghlan JG, Cottin V, De Marco T, Galiè N, Ghio S, Gibbs S, Martinez FJ, Semigran MJ, Simonneau G, Wells AU, Vachiéry JL. Pulmonary hypertension in chronic lung diseases. J Am Coll Cardiol. 2013;62(25 (Suppl)):D109–16.
45. Forfia PR, Vaidya A, Wiegers SE. Pulmonary heart disease: the heart-lung interaction and its impact on patient phenotypes. Pulm Circ. 2013;3(1):5–19.
46. Naeije R. Pulmonary hypertension and right heart failure in chronic obstructive pulmonary disease. Proc Am Thorac Soc. 2005;2(1):20–2.

47. Oswald-Mammosser M, Weitzenblum E, Quoix E, Moser G, Chaouat A, Charpentier C, et al. Prognostic factors in COPD patients receiving long-term oxygen therapy. Importance of pulmonary artery pressure. Chest. 1995;107(5):1193–8.
48. Lettieri CJ, Nathan SD, Barnett SD, Ahmad S, Shorr AF. Prevalence and outcomes of pulmonary arterial hypertension in advanced idiopathic pulmonary fibrosis. Chest. 2006;129(3):746–52.
49. Boutou AK, Pitsiou GG, Trigonis I, Papakosta D, Kontou PK, Chavouzis N, et al. Exercise capacity in idiopathic pulmonary fibrosis: the effect of pulmonary hypertension. Respirology. 2011;16(3):451–8.
50. Minai OA, Santacruz JF, Alster JM, Budev MM, McCarthy K. Impact of pulmonary hemodynamics on 6-min walk test in idiopathic pulmonary fibrosis. Respir Med. 2012;106(11):1613–21.
51. Weitzenblum EHC, Ducolone A, Mirhom R, Rasaholinjanahary R, Ehrhart M. Prognostic value of pulmonary artery pressure in chronic obstructive pulmonary disease. Thorax. 1981;36:752–8.
52. D'Andrea A, Stanziola A, Di Palma E, Martino M, D'Alto M, Dellegrottaglie S, et al. Right ventricular structure and function in idiopathic pulmonary fibrosis with or without pulmonary hypertension. Echocardiography. 2016;33(1):57–65.
53. Rubin LJ. Cor pulmonale revisited. J Am Coll Cardiol. 2013;62(12):1112–3.
54. Bogaard HJ, Natarajan R, Henderson SC, Long CS, Kraskauskas D, Smithson L, et al. Chronic pulmonary artery pressure elevation is insufficient to explain right heart failure. Circulation. 2009;120(20):1951–60.
55. Gomez A, Bialostozky D, Zajarias A, Santos E, Palomar A, Martinez ML, et al. Right ventricular ischemia in patients with primary pulmonary hypertension. J Am Coll Cardiol. 2001;38(4):1137–42.
56. Triposkiadis F, Karayannis G, Giamouzis G, Skoularigis J, Louridas G, Butler J. The sympathetic nervous system in heart failure physiology, pathophysiology, and clinical implications. J Am Coll Cardiol. 2009;54(19):1747–62.
57. Ciarka A, Doan V, Velez-Roa S, Naeije R, van de Borne P. Prognostic significance of sympathetic nervous system activation in pulmonary arterial hypertension. Am J Respir Crit Care Med. 2010;181(11):1269–75.
58. Heindl S, Lehnert M, Criee CP, Hasenfuss G, Andreas S. Marked sympathetic activation in patients with chronic respiratory failure. Am J Respir Crit Care Med. 2001;164(4):597–601.
59. van Gestel AJ, Steier J. Autonomic dysfunction in patients with chronic obstructive pulmonary disease (COPD). J Thorac Dis. 2010;2(4):215–22.
60. Andreas S, Haarmann H, Klarner S, Hasenfuss G, Raupach T. Increased sympathetic nerve activity in COPD is associated with morbidity and mortality. Lung. 2014;192(2):235–41.
61. Dempsey JA, Sheel AW, St Croix CM, Morgan BJ. Respiratory influences on sympathetic vasomotor outflow in humans. Respir Physiol Neurobiol. 2002;130(1):3–20.
62. Levine S, Nguyen T, Kaiser LR, Rubinstein NA, Maislin G, Gregory C, et al. Human diaphragm remodeling associated with chronic obstructive pulmonary disease: clinical implications. Am J Respir Crit Care Med. 2003;168(6):706–13.
63. Hofford JM, Milakofsky L, Vogel WH, Sacher RS, Savage GJ, Pell S. The nutritional status in advanced emphysema associated with chronic bronchitis. A study of amino acid and catecholamine levels. Am Rev Respir Dis. 1990;141(4 Pt 1):902–8.
64. Anand IS, Chandrashekhar Y, Ferrari R, Sarma R, Guleria R, Jindal SK, et al. Pathogenesis of congestive state in chronic obstructive pulmonary disease. Studies of body water and sodium, renal function, hemodynamics, and plasma hormones during edema and after recovery. Circulation. 1992;86(1):12–21.
65. Piao L, Fang YH, Parikh KS, Ryan JJ, D'Souza KM, Theccanat T, et al. GRK2-mediated inhibition of adrenergic and dopaminergic signaling in right ventricular hypertrophy: therapeutic implications in pulmonary hypertension. Circulation. 2012;126(24):2859–69.
66. Cohn JN, Ferrari R, Sharpe N. Cardiac remodeling–concepts and clinical implications: a consensus paper from an international forum on cardiac remodeling. Behalf of an International Forum on Cardiac Remodeling. J Am Coll Cardiol. 2000;35(3):569–82.

67. Morrell NW, Danilov SM, Satyan KB, Morris KG, Stenmark KR. Right ventricular angiotensin converting enzyme activity and expression is increased during hypoxic pulmonary hypertension. Cardiovasc Res. 1997;34(2):393–403.
68. Friedberg MK, Redington AN. Right versus left ventricular failure: differences, similarities, and interactions. Circulation. 2014;129(9):1033–44.
69. Oikawa M, Kagaya Y, Otani H, Sakuma M, Demachi J, Suzuki J, et al. Increased [18F]fluorodeoxyglucose accumulation in right ventricular free wall in patients with pulmonary hypertension and the effect of epoprostenol. J Am Coll Cardiol. 2005;45(11):1849–55.
70. Tatebe S, Fukumoto Y, Oikawa-Wakayama M, Sugimura K, Satoh K, Miura Y, et al. Enhanced [18F]fluorodeoxyglucose accumulation in the right ventricular free wall predicts long-term prognosis of patients with pulmonary hypertension: a preliminary observational study. Eur Heart J Cardiovasc Imaging. 2014;15(6):666–72.
71. Nagaya N, Goto Y, Satoh T, Uematsu M, Hamada S, Kuribayashi S, et al. Impaired regional fatty acid uptake and systolic dysfunction in hypertrophied right ventricle. J Nucl Med. 1998;39(10):1676–80.
72. Gomez-Arroyo J, Mizuno S, Szczepanek K, Van Tassell B, Natarajan R, dos Remedios CG, et al. Metabolic gene remodeling and mitochondrial dysfunction in failing right ventricular hypertrophy secondary to pulmonary arterial hypertension. Circ Heart Fail. 2013;6(1):136–44.
73. Piao L, Fang YH, Cadete VJ, Wietholt C, Urboniene D, Toth PT, et al. The inhibition of pyruvate dehydrogenase kinase improves impaired cardiac function and electrical remodeling in two models of right ventricular hypertrophy: resuscitating the hibernating right ventricle. J Mol Med. 2010;88(1):47–60.
74. Daicho T, Yagi T, Abe Y, Ohara M, Marunouchi T, Takeo S, et al. Possible involvement of mitochondrial energy-producing ability in the development of right ventricular failure in monocrotaline-induced pulmonary hypertensive rats. J Pharmacol Sci. 2009;111(1):33–43.
75. Drake JI, Bogaard HJ, Mizuno S, Clifton B, Xie B, Gao Y, et al. Molecular signature of a right heart failure program in chronic severe pulmonary hypertension. Am J Respir Cell Mol Biol. 2011;45(6):1239–47.
76. Stenmark KR, Fagan KA, Frid MG. Hypoxia-induced pulmonary vascular remodeling: cellular and molecular mechanisms. Circ Res. 2006;99(7):675–91.
77. Vonk-Noordegraaf A, Marcus JT, Holverda S, Roseboom B, Postmus PE. Early changes of cardiac structure and function in COPD patients with mild hypoxemia. Chest. 2005;127(6):1898–903.
78. Overbeek MJ, Mouchaers KT, Niessen HM, Hadi AM, Kupreishvili K, Boonstra A, et al. Characteristics of interstitial fibrosis and inflammatory cell infiltration in right ventricles of systemic sclerosis-associated pulmonary arterial hypertension. Int J Rheumatol. 2010;2010. pii: 604615. https://doi.org/10.1155/2010/604615. Epub 2010 Sep 30.
79. Mathai SC, Bueso M, Hummers LK, Boyce D, Lechtzin N, Le Pavec J, et al. Disproportionate elevation of N-terminal pro-brain natriuretic peptide in scleroderma-related pulmonary hypertension. Eur Respir J. 2010;35(1):95–104.
80. Lindqvist P, Caidahl K, Neuman-Andersen G, Ozolins C, Rantapaa-Dahlqvist S, Waldenstrom A, et al. Disturbed right ventricular diastolic function in patients with systemic sclerosis: a Doppler tissue imaging study. Chest. 2005;128(2):755–63.
81. Rudski LG, Lai WW, Afilalo J, Hua L, Handschumacher MD, Chandrasekaran K, et al. Guidelines for the echocardiographic assessment of the right heart in adults: a report from the American Society of Echocardiography endorsed by the European Association of Echocardiography, a registered branch of the European Society of Cardiology, and the Canadian Society of Echocardiography. J Am Soc Echocardiogr. 2010;23(7):685–713. quiz 86–8
82. Haddad F, Hunt SA, Rosenthal DN, Murphy DJ. Right ventricular function in cardiovascular disease, part I: anatomy, physiology, aging, and functional assessment of the right ventricle. Circulation. 2008;117(11):1436–48.

Chapter 6
Pulmonary Hypertension Associated with Chronic Lung Diseases: Treatment Considerations

Jason Weatherald, David Montani, and Olivier Sitbon

Key Pearls
- Pulmonary hypertension (PH) is associated with worse survival in patients with chronic lung diseases, but treatment consists of optimizing the underlying lung disease, long-term oxygen, and consideration of lung transplantation.
- Pulmonary arterial hypertension (PAH) therapies have been studied in a small number of randomized controlled trials including patients with COPD, interstitial lung disease, and sarcoidosis-associated PH with no consistent therapeutic benefits on symptoms, exercise capacity, or clinical outcomes. In one trial of patients with idiopathic pulmonary fibrosis, ambrisentan was harmful.
- Patients with mild lung disease and severe PH without another explanation should be evaluated in centers with expertise in the diagnosis and treatment of PAH.

J. Weatherald (✉)
University of Calgary, Department of Medicine, Division of Respiratory Medicine, Calgary, AB, Canada

Libin Cardiovascular Institute of Alberta, Calgary, AB, Canada
e-mail: jcweathe@ucalgary.ca

D. Montani · O. Sitbon
Université Paris-Sud, Faculté de Médecine, Université Paris-Saclay, Le Kremlin-Bicêtre, France

Service de Pneumologie, Hôpital Bicêtre, AP-HP, Le Kremlin-Bicêtre, France

INSERM UMR_S 999, Hôpital Marie Lannelongue, Le Plessis Robinson, France
e-mail: david.montani@aphp.fr; olivier.sitbon@aphp.fr

© Springer Nature Switzerland AG 2020
S. P. Bhatt (ed.), *Cardiac Considerations in Chronic Lung Disease*,
Respiratory Medicine, https://doi.org/10.1007/978-3-030-43435-9_6

Introduction

Pulmonary hypertension (PH) is an important complication of chronic parenchymal lung diseases. The current definition of PH requires an abnormal resting mean pulmonary arterial pressure > 20 mmHg during right heart catheterization (RHC) [1, 2]. The most common chronic lung conditions that cause PH are chronic obstructive pulmonary disease (COPD) and idiopathic pulmonary fibrosis (IPF), but PH can occur in the context of other parenchymal lung diseases including combined pulmonary fibrosis and emphysema (CPFE), sarcoidosis, lymphangioleiomyomatosis (LAM), and pulmonary Langerhans cell histiocytosis (PLCH). PH that occurs due to chronic lung diseases or chronic hypoxia (high altitude or severe sleep-disordered breathing) comprises Group 3 PH, whereas conditions such as sarcoidosis, LAM, and PLCH have multiple or multifactorial mechanisms and are classified into Group 5 PH [3].

When present, PH contributes to more severe symptoms and exercise intolerance and can lead to right heart failure, which portends a worse prognosis in patients with chronic lung disease. Most patients have mild elevations in mPAP, but a smaller proportion develop severe PH, which is defined by a resting mPAP $\geq$35 mmHg or mPAP $\geq$25 mmHg with a low cardiac index (CI) < 2.0–2.5 L.min.m^{-2} [2–4]. Usually, the severity of PH is proportional to the severity of lung disease; however, in some cases, severe PH is present with only mild parenchymal lung disease or mild to moderately impaired pulmonary function testing, making it difficult to determine whether there are two conditions present (i.e., Group 1 pulmonary arterial hypertension with comorbid mild lung disease).

In patients with Group 1 PAH, targeted medical therapies improve endothelial cell dysfunction, have vasodilatory and anti-proliferative effects on the pulmonary vasculature, reduce the right ventricular afterload, and improve symptoms, exercise capacity, and clinical outcomes in randomized trials. Given the similar pre-capillary hemodynamic profile (elevated mPAP $\geq$20 mmHg, pulmonary arterial wedge pressure $\leq$ 15 mmHg, and pulmonary vascular resistance >3 Wood units) and common histopathological changes in patients with PAH and some patients with PH due to chronic lung disease, there has been interest in studying the effects of PAH therapies in these patients. In general, treatment of PH in chronic lung disease should be directed at the underlying condition and contributing etiologies such as left heart disease, thromboembolic disease, and sleep-disordered breathing (Fig. 6.1). Because of the negative impact of PH on survival in most chronic lung diseases, those who develop PH should be considered for lung transplantation if they are appropriate candidates [5]. In this chapter, we will focus on literature regarding therapies that target the pulmonary vasculature in chronic lung diseases. However, it is important to state from the outset that no PAH therapies are proven to be effective in chronic lung diseases and there is clear evidence that worsening gas exchange can occur due to the effects of these therapies on hypoxic vasoconstriction and worsening ventilation-perfusion matching. Therefore, the use of PAH therapies in patients with chronic lung disease-associated PH should be restricted to trial protocols, registries, and centers with considerable expertise.

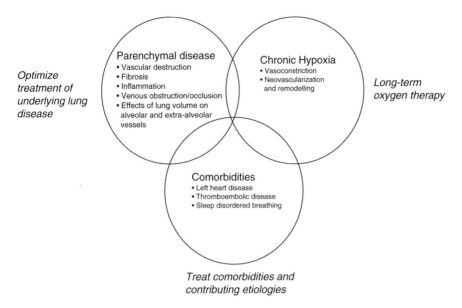

Fig. 6.1 Management of pulmonary hypertension in chronic lung diseases

PH Associated with Chronic Obstructive Pulmonary Disease

Treatment of PH in COPD begins with optimization of medical therapy for COPD according to guidelines [6]. Several factors can lead to the development of an increased mPAP and pulmonary vascular resistance (PVR) in COPD, including airflow limitation, alveolar hypoxia and vasoconstriction, destruction of the pulmonary vascular bed due to emphysema, polycythemia, and inflammation (Fig. 6.1) [7]. Long-term oxygen treatment improves survival in hypoxemic COPD patients but was unrelated to the degree of PH in the Nocturnal Oxygen Therapy Trial [8]. Continuously administered oxygen for at least 18 hours per day does not fully correct PH to normal but improves the pulmonary vascular resistance and cardiac function [9] and may prevent progressive mPAP elevation [10].

Other than long-term oxygen therapy, there has been significant interest in PAH therapies for treating PH in COPD, particularly those with severe PH, which has usually been defined by the presence of mPAP >35–40 mmHg or a low CI < 2.0–2.5 L. min.m^{-2} [4, 7]. Severe PH is present in less than 5% of COPD patients, and many have other explanations for a severely elevated mPAP such as concurrent left ventricular dysfunction, pulmonary embolism, pulmonary fibrosis, or sleep-disordered breathing [11]. However, a small proportion (approximately 1%) of COPD patients have severe PH without an alternative explanation or have severe PH in the presence of only mild lung disease. COPD patients with severe PH, relatively preserved pulmonary function, and little-to-no emphysema often exhibit cardiovascular limitation to exercise rather than ventilatory mechanical limitation to exercise, which may be a "pulmonary vascular phenotype" of COPD [12]. Pulmonary vasodilator therapies could potentially be beneficial in this group of patients; however, the evidence to support this is limited [2, 12, 13].

An uncontrolled study by Girard et al. included 26 patients with moderate-to-severe COPD (mean FEV_1 57 ± 20% predicted) and severe PH (mean mPAP 48 ± 9 mmHg) who were treated with PAH-targeted medications and found that PVR and mPAP decreased, CI increased, but there were no significant improvements in exercise capacity or NT-pro-BNP [14]. Calcaianu et al. reported similar findings in 28 patients with mild-to-moderate airflow limitation and severe precapillary PH [15]. Targeted PAH therapy improved PVR and CI but had no effect on exercise capacity or functional class. A study from the ASPIRE registry found no difference in survival for patients with COPD (mean FEV_1 65 ± 23% predicted) and severe PH (mPAP ≥40 mmHg) who were treated with PAH treatments and those who were not treated [16]. However, 8 of the 43 patients who were treated with PAH therapies in this study demonstrated a clinical improvement, defined as decrease in PVR of >20% or an improvement in WHO functional class, and these individuals had better survival than those not demonstrating clinical improvement. Relatively few prospective clinical studies of specific PAH therapies have been performed in COPD patients despite the relative burden and prognostic importance of PH in this population. Unfortunately, most of the available trials in COPD-associated PH have been small and have shown no convincing benefit of PAH therapies.

Calcium Channel Blockers

Calcium channel blockers, such as nifedipine, cause pulmonary arterial vasodilation and improve hemodynamics acutely in patients with COPD but have no demonstrated long-term benefits [17, 18]. Furthermore, nifedipine may worsen arterial oxygenation at rest and during exercise by inhibiting normal hypoxic vasoconstriction in lungs of COPD patients, leading to worsened ventilation-perfusion matching and worsening gas exchange [19].

Inhaled Vasodilators

Similar to calcium channel blockers, inhaled nitric oxide (NO) causes pulmonary vasodilation, which may be advantageous in COPD-associated PH by theoretically causing vasodilation only in ventilated lung units. However, studies have shown that inhaled NO decreases PaO_2 in COPD by impairing hypoxic regulation of ventilation-perfusion matching [20]. However, when added to oxygen, inhaled nitric oxide reduces PVR and mPAP and improves cardiac function in COPD patients with pulmonary hypertension compared to oxygen alone, without causing arterial desaturation [21]. Despite these promising findings, no long-term studies of inhaled NO in COPD-associated PH have been performed. Iloprost is an inhaled prostacyclin analogue with potent acute vasodilatory effects, which should act preferentially in well-ventilated lung regions. In ten moderate-to-severe COPD patients (FEV_1 $47.4 \pm 8.2\%$ predicted), 5.0 µg of inhaled iloprost improved ventilatory efficiency (V_E/VCO_2) during exercise and 6-minute walk distance (6MWD) with a reduction in the alveolar-arterial O_2 gradient ($PA\text{-}aO_2$) and no arterial desaturation [22]. However, in contrast, a randomized double-blind crossover study including 16 patients with COPD-associated PH found inhaled iloprost had no effect on 6MWD, caused a reduction in peak VO_2, and a 2.2% reduction in resting SpO_2 with a 10 µg dose of iloprost [23]. Although no long-term studies of inhaled prostacyclins have been performed to date, the existing evidence suggests no benefit in COPD-associated PH.

Phosphodiesterase-5 Inhibitors in COPD-Associated PH

The acute effects of sildenafil, a phosphodiesterase-5 inhibitor (PDE5i), were studied in 20 patients with severe or very severe COPD, 17 of whom had an mPAP >20 mmHg at rest (mean mPAP 27 ± 10 mmHg) and all of whom had PH during exercise [24]. Sildenafil given at 20 mg or 40 mg reduced mPAP and PVR acutely and improved hemodynamics during exercise but caused mild worsening of gas exchange at rest, which was related to increased pulmonary blood flow to poorly ventilated lung units as measured with the multiple inert gas technique. Several longer-term randomized controlled trials (RCTs) have evaluated PDE5i therapy in COPD-associated PH with disappointing results (Table 6.1) [25–29]. Only one study by Rao et al. [25], which only used echocardiography-derived estimates of PH, found a significant improvement in exercise capacity, while all other studies have found no improvement in exercise tolerance using peak VO_2 or 6MWD. The largest study by Goudie et al. compared a low dose of tadalafil (10 mg) to placebo in 120 patients with COPD and evidence of PH on echocardiogram and found no effect on 6MWD, quality of life, or B-natriuretic peptide levels [28]. It is unclear whether the usual dose of 40 mg used in treating PAH would have more significant clinical effects. Only one randomized study by Vitulo et al. reported long-term hemodynamic effects of PDE5i compared to placebo in COPD patients with severe PH, which were modest but significant (PVR – 1.38 Wood units and CI +0.4 L.min. m^{-2}) [29]. Interestingly, while 6MWD did not significantly improve in this study at 16 weeks, dyspnea scores improved, there was no worsening in PaO_2, and quality of life scores on the Short Form-36 improved by a clinically significant 9.85 units [29]. Therefore, sildenafil could be considered in patients with COPD and severe PH who have refractory breathlessness despite optimal medical therapy.

Table 6.1 Randomized trials of PDE5i in COPD-associated PH

Author	Ref	N	Drug	Severity of PH	Follow-up	Endpoints
Rao (2011)	[25]	33	Sildenafil 20 mg TID vs. placebo	sPAP >40 mmHg on echo	12 weeks	6MWD: +190 m vs. placebo sPAP decreased
Lederer (2012)	[26]	10	Sildenafil 25 mg TID vs. placebo	No PH	4 weeks	6MWD: no effect VO$_2$: no effect QoL: worsened
Blanco (2013)	[27]	60	Sildenafil 20 mg TID vs. placebo added to pulmonary rehabilitation	mPAP 31 ± 5 mmHg	12 weeks	Cycle endurance time: no effect VO$_2$: no effect 6MWD: no effect
Goudie (2014)	[28]	120	Tadalafil 10 mg daily vs. placebo	sPAP 42 ± 10 mmHg (echo estimated)	12 weeks	sPAP: decreased −12.3 mmHg 6MWD: no effect QoL: no effect BNP: no effect
Vitulo (2017)	[29]	28	Sildenafil 20 mg TID vs. placebo	mPAP 25 mmHg in 68%, mPAP 39 ± 8 mmHg, PVR 7 ± 2.6 WU	16 weeks	PVR: −1.38 WU CI: +0.42 L.min.m^{-2} BODE: improved 6MWD: no effect SF-36: +9.85 units

PH pulmonary hypertension, *TID* thrice daily, *6MWD* 6- minute walk distance, *sPAP* systolic pulmonary arterial pressure, *VO$_2$* maximum oxygen consumption measured during incremental exercise, *QoL* quality of life, *mPAP* mean pulmonary arterial pressure, *BNP* brain natriuretic peptide, *PVR* pulmonary vascular resistance, *WU* Wood unit, *BODE* body-mass-index, airflow obstruction, dyspnea, exercise capacity

Endothelin Receptor Antagonists in COPD-Associated PH

Two randomized trials have evaluated bosentan, an endothelin receptor antagonist (ERA), in patients with COPD. Stolz et al. randomized 20 patients with severe or very severe COPD to bosentan 125 mg twice daily and 10 to placebo with a primary endpoint of change in 6MWD at 12 weeks [30]. While most patients had echocardiographic evidence of PH, right heart catheterizations were not performed in this study. Six patients in the bosentan arm dropped out due to adverse effects compared to only one in the placebo group. There were no differences in 6MWD, echocardiographic parameters, or Borg dyspnea index, while PaO$_2$ decreased significantly and quality of life deteriorated in the bosentan group. In another randomized non-blinded trial of 32 patients, Valerio et al. found reductions in mPAP and PVR and an improvement in 6MWD for bosentan-treated patients with no significant changes in either variable in the standard care group at 18 months [31]. There have been no reported trials with the other ERAs (macitentan, ambrisentan, sitaxsentan) in COPD-associated PH. Based on the available data, ERAs are not recommended in patients with COPD and PH.

Other PAH Therapies in COPD-Associated PH

Epoprostenol is an intravenously administered prostacyclin that revolutionized the treatment of PAH, improving symptoms, hemodynamics, and survival [32]. There are no long-term randomized trials of parenteral epoprostenol in COPD-associated PH; however, one small, short-term randomized study used epoprostenol in COPD patients with PH and acute respiratory requiring mechanical ventilation [33]. Small uncontrolled studies suggested hemodynamic benefits, but worsening oxygenation frequently occurs with epoprostenol in stable COPD patients or those with PH and acute respiratory failure [33, 34]. Riociguat is a soluble guanylate cyclase stimulator approved for use in PAH and chronic thromboembolic pulmonary hypertension (Group IV). An open-label pilot study of 23 patients with COPD-associated PH found acute decreases in mPAP and PVR and improvements in CI with riociguat, but PaO_2 decreased on average by 10–15 mmHg [35]. Although PAH therapies consistently worsen oxygenation in COPD, total oxygen delivery may conceivably increase if cardiac output improves to a greater extent; furthermore, administration of supplemental oxygen may mitigate the hypoxemia. Thus, future studies should consider the effects of these medications with or without supplemental oxygen on important endpoints such as quality of life, exercise tolerance, and clinical events.

PH Associated with Interstitial Lung Diseases

PH can occur in association with most fibrotic interstitial lung diseases (ILD), of which IPF is the most frequent. Importantly, PH can result due to several potential mechanisms in ILD patients including as a direct result of parenchymal fibrosis and vascular destruction, venous and venular involvement, and other comorbidities including thromboembolism, sleep-disordered breathing, and left heart disease with post-capillary PH [36–39]. Therefore, it is important to search for and treat other contributing causes before even considering further treatment with PAH therapies.

In a registry-based study, patients with PH associated with chronic fibrosing idiopathic interstitial pneumonias had worse survival than patients with PAH, and while some short-term improvements in 6MWD were seen in patients treated with PAH therapies, it is unclear whether treatment of PH improves outcomes [40]. Systemic sclerosis can cause PH through multiple mechanisms, including left ventricular dysfunction (post-capillary, Group 2), pre-capillary PH secondary to ILD (Group 3), pulmonary veno-occlusive disease, and Group 1 PAH [41]. Patients with systemic sclerosis and ILD-associated PH have worse outcomes than those who have PAH and no ILD [42, 43]. While PAH therapies are effective in systemic sclerosis patients with Group 1 PAH, observational studies have shown no clear benefit of PAH therapies in systemic sclerosis ILD-associated PH in terms of functional capacity, 6MWD, or hemodynamics, but arterial oxygenation significantly worsened [44].

Several open-label, uncontrolled, and retrospective studies had suggested potentially favorable effects of sildenafil, endothelin receptor antagonists, and prostacyclins in patients with ILD. Several RCTs have subsequently evaluated PAH therapies in IPF, and one RCT has evaluated bosentan in the treatment of ILD secondary to systemic sclerosis. However, the inclusion of patients with PH in these studies was variable, and no studies have demonstrated clinical efficacy (Table 6.2). Pre-clinical

Table 6.2 Randomized controlled trials of PAH therapies in ILD with or without associated PH

Author	Ref	N	Lung disease	Drug	PH patients included?	Duration	Endpoints
Krowka (2007)	[54]	51	IPF	Iloprost vs. placebo	Yes	12 weeks	Safety: similar rate of adverse events 6MWD: no difference NYHA: no difference in proportion who improved
King (2008)	[45]	158	IPF	Bosentan 125 mg BID (starting dose 62.5 mg BID × 4 weeks) vs. placebo	Yes – mild PH on echo (RVSP <50 mmHg) included	12 months	6MWD: no difference Disease progression: trend in favor of bosentan Lung function: no difference Dyspnea and QoL: trends in favor of bosentan
Zisman (2010)	[49]	180	IPF	Sildenafil 20 mg TID vs. placebo	Yes	12 weeks	6MWD improvement of >20%: no significant difference Secondary endpoints: Improved dyspnea scores, DLCO, and PaO$_2$
Jackson (2010)	[55]	29	IPF	Sildenafil 20 mg TID vs. placebo	Yes – mild PH on echo (RVSP <50 mmHg) included	6 months	6MWD: no difference Dyspnea scores: no difference Lung function no difference RVSP: no difference Adverse effects higher in sildenafil group

Table 6.2 (continued)

Author	Ref	N	Lung disease	Drug	PH patients included?	Duration	Endpoints
Seibold (2010)	[56]	163	Systemic sclerosis ILD	Bosentan 125 mg BID (starting dose 62.5 mg BID × 4 weeks) vs. placebo	Excluded	12 months	6MWD: no difference Time to death or worsening PFTs: no difference Change in FVC or DLCO: no difference
King (2011)	[46]	616	IPF	Bosentan 125 mg BID (starting dose 62.5 mg BID × 4 weeks) vs. placebo	Yes	20 months	Time to IPF worsening or death: no difference QoL: no difference Dyspnea: no difference Change in FVC: no difference
Raghu (2013a)	[47]	494	IPF	Ambrisentan 10 mg daily vs. placebo	Yes excluded patients on other long-term PH therapies	34 weeks	Time to IPF progression: terminated early due to higher disease progression in ambrisentan group Hospitalizations: increased in ambrisentan group 6MWD: no difference Lung function decline: no difference
Raghu (2013b)	[48]	178	IPF	Macitentan 10 mg vs. placebo	Yes	12 months	Change in FVC: no difference Time to IPF worsening or death: no difference Dyspnea: no difference Adverse events: no difference

(continued)

Table 6.2 (continued)

Author	Ref	N	Lung disease	Drug	PH patients included?	Duration	Endpoints
Corte (2014)	[51]	60	Fibrotic IIP (IPF *n* = 46, fibrotic NSIP *n* = 14)	Bosentan 125 mg BID (starting dose 62.5 mg BID × 4 weeks) vs. placebo	Yes – Only included PH confirmed on RHC	16 weeks	Decrease in PVRi >20%: no difference 6MWD: no difference Symptoms and QoL: no difference RV function on echo: no difference BNP: no difference O_2 requirements: trend toward increased O_2 needs in bosentan group Disease progression: no difference

IPF idiopathic pulmonary fibrosis, *6MWD* 6-minute walk distance, *NYHA* New York Heart Association, *PH* pulmonary hypertension, *TID* thrice daily, *BID* twice daily, *RVSP* right ventricular systolic pressure, *QoL* quality of life, *DLCO* diffusing capacity of carbon monoxide, *PaO₂* partial pressure of oxygen in arterial blood, *PFT* pulmonary function test, *FVC* forced vital capacity, *NSIP* non-specific interstitial pneumonitis, *BNP* brain natriuretic peptide, *RHC* right heart catheterization, *PVR* pulmonary vascular resistance

studies showed that endothelin-1 is involved in the pathogenesis of IPF and that endothelin-1 blockade may have anti-fibrotic effects, but all major trials of endothelin receptor antagonists in IPF have been negative: bosentan (BUILD-1 and BUILD-3) [45, 46], ambrisentan (ARTEMIS-IPF) [47], and macitentan (MUSIC) [48]. Beyond the absent signal for efficacy, there are also potential safety concerns with endothelin receptor antagonists in IPF. The ARTEMIS-IPF trial was actually stopped prematurely, as there was a signal for harm in the ambrisentan group, with 1.74-fold increase in the risk of disease progression and 2.6-fold increase in the risk of hospitalization [47]. The STEP-IPF trial evaluated sildenafil in IPF, which did have some positive secondary outcomes including improvements in symptoms and gas exchange, but the primary outcome (improvement in 6MWD) was negative [49]. In a subgroup analysis of patients from the Sildenafil Trial of Exercise Performance in Idiopathic Pulmonary Fibrosis (STEP-IPF) study who had echocardiography performed, those with baseline right ventricular dysfunction had improved exercise capacity (+99 m) and better quality of life with sildenafil compared to placebo, suggesting these IPF patients might still benefit from sildenafil [50].

Unfortunately, there have been very few RCTs specifically evaluating the efficacy of PAH therapies in patients with ILD-associated PH. The only RCT to study the effect of PAH therapies specifically in patients with ILD and PH was by Corte et al. who compared bosentan to placebo in 60 patients with IPF (n = 46) or fibrotic non-specific interstitial pneumonia (n = 14) [51]. Patients in this study had severe ILD as evidenced by a forced vital capacity of 54.2 ± 21.2% predicted and severe reduction in diffusion capacity for carbon monoxide <30% predicted and moderate-to-severe PH (mean mPAP 36.0 ± 8.9 mmHg and PVRi 13.0 ± 6.7 Wood units/m^2). There was no benefit with bosentan over placebo with regard to hemodynamics, exercise capacity, symptoms, lung function, or right ventricular function on echocardiography.

Based on the available evidence, PAH therapies are not recommended in IPF irrespective of whether PH is present and treatment should consist of treating the underlying condition according to current guidelines, which consists of oxygen and anti-fibrotic agents, such as pirfenidone or nintedanib, in appropriate patients [52]. It remains unclear whether patients with mild-to-moderate IPF and severe, dispro-portionate PH may benefit from PAH therapies. This population is uncommon and has not been specifically studied in an RCT. It may be that these patients have two diseases, PAH and IPF, and they may be candidates for PAH therapy. However, a post hoc analysis of patients from the ARTEMIS-IPF study who had <5% honey-combing on high-resolution CT scan, mild-to-moderate restriction, and severe PH on baseline right heart catheterization (mPAP ≥35 mmHg) found no differences in progression-free survival between ambrisentan and placebo [53]. Patients with sys-temic sclerosis and mild ILD associated with pre-capillary PH have similar out-comes to systemic sclerosis PAH without ILD, whereas those with extensive ILD have a much worse prognosis [43]. Therefore, patients with systemic sclerosis and severe PH and only mild extent of ILD might be considered for treatment with tar-geted therapies according to guidelines for PAH [3].

Other PAH Therapies in ILD-Associated PH

A randomized open-label trial by Ghofrani et al. compared the acute effects of silde-nafil and epoprostenol infusion in 16 patients with fibrotic lung disease and PH [57]. While epoprostenol improved CI by 42% and reduced mPAP and PVR, there was a significant effect on ventilation-perfusion inequality and pulmonary shunt flow, with resultant hypoxemia. Similarly, sildenafil acutely reduced mPAP and PVR with an increase in CI by 9.1% but with, in contrast to epoprostenol, a considerable improvement in PaO$_2$ [57]. There have been no further studies using epoprostenol in fibrotic lung disease; however, a small, non-randomized, open-label study described long-term hemodynamic benefits, echocardiographic improvements in right ven-tricular function, some improvement in quality of life scores, and an increase in 6MWD with parenteral administration of treprostinil [58]. There was a trend to worsening oxygenation in this study, but room air oxygen saturation and oxygen delivery were not significantly different after 12 weeks of treatment. The effects of riociguat have also been assessed in a small pilot study including 22 patients with ILD-associated PH [59]. Riociguat was generally well tolerated (three patients dis-continued therapy due to side effects), and there was a modest improvement in

6MWD by 25 m. Hemodynamics improved with an increase in CI by 0.7 L.min. m^{-2}, and there was not a major concerning effect on gas exchange at 12 weeks. However, the RISE-IIP study found no improvements, more adverse effects, and more deaths in the group treated with riociguat versus placebo (eight deaths with riociguat versus three) [60]. Thus, PAH therapies should generally not be used in patients with ILD unless future placebo-controlled trials demonstrate convincing benefit.

PH Due to Other Parenchymal Lung Diseases (Group 5 PH)

Group 5 PH includes several chronic parenchymal lung diseases that cause PH through multiple and/or poorly understood mechanisms [61].

Sarcoidosis-Associated PH

Pulmonary vascular disease is frequently observed in sarcoidosis, particularly in the advanced stages of the disease. The mechanisms of PH in sarcoidosis are multiple and often combined. In cases of post-capillary PH on right heart catheterization (mPAP ≥20 mmHg and pulmonary artery wedge pressure > 15 mmHg), left heart involvement and fibrosing mediastinitis with venous compression are potential explanations. In the setting of pre-capillary PH (mPAP >20 mmHg, PVR ≥3 Wood Units and PAWP ≤15 mmHg), three main mechanisms have been identified which warrant different treatment strategies [62]. Severe pre-capillary PH may be secondary to granulomatous pulmonary vasculopathy, vascular bed destruction, and/or vascular remodeling due to chronic hypoxia. Significant pulmonary venous involvement may occur, mimicking pulmonary veno-occlusive disease, which carries a risk of pulmonary edema when PAH therapies are given. The presence of PH is associated with impaired functional capacity and worse survival in patients with sarcoidosis [63, 64]. However, data supporting specific treatment strategies are few due to its rarity and the heterogeneous mechanisms of PH in sarcoidosis. There has been only one randomized controlled trial in sarcoidosis-associated PH, which reported improvements in mPAP and PVR at 16 weeks in bosentan-treated patients compared to placebo; however, there was no improvement in 6MWD [65]. Observational studies have reported similar effects of oral PAH-targeted medications or parenteral prostacyclin therapy on hemodynamics without improvements in exercise capacity [64, 66, 67]. A study of 126 patients with sarcoidosis-associated PH from the French PH Registry found that PAH therapies improved PVR significantly from 9.7 ± 4.4 to 6.9 ± 3.0 Wood units and NYHA functional class improved, but there was no improvement in 6MWD [64]. Immunosuppressive therapies may be useful in specific cases of sarcoidosis-associated PH caused by compression of pulmonary arteries from mediastinal lymphadenopathy and mediastinitis or in those with pulmonary vascular granulomatous inflammation [62, 64, 68]. Pulmonary angioplasty with stenting is also an option when PH is attributable to vascular stenoses [69].

Pulmonary Langerhans Cell Histiocytosis-Associated PH

A rare smoking-related parenchymal lung disease, pulmonary Langerhans cell histiocytosis (PLCH), is characterized by airflow obstruction, granulomatous inflammation, parenchymal nodules, and cysts. A diffuse vasculopathy and venous fibrotic obliteration with capillary dilatation evocative of pulmonary veno-occlusive disease can be present in regions unaffected by parenchymal lesions [70]. The primary management of PH in PLCH is to treat the underlying lung disease, which involves smoking cessation and potentially cladribine [71, 72]. Although there have been no prospective randomized studies of PAH-specific therapies in PLCH, long-term improvements in hemodynamics and symptoms have been reported with oral therapies. A retrospective observational study by Le Pavec et al. described 14 patients with PLCH-associated PH who received PAH therapies [73]. Functional capacity improved in 67% of patients, 6MWD increased ≥10% in 45% of patients, and there was a 33% decrease in PVR, which was sustained over the long-term. Although PH is common in advanced PLCH, because of the potential venous involvement, PAH therapies must be used cautiously due to the risk of inducing pulmonary edema.

Lymphangioleiomyomatosis-Associated PH

Lymphangioleiomyomatosis (LAM) is a rare condition almost exclusively affecting females that is characterized by diffuse cystic lung disease, chylous effusions and ascites, renal angiomyolipomas, and lymphangioleiomyomas [74]. Arteriolar, bronchial, and venous infiltration with LAM cells can lead to PH through multiple mechanisms, justifying its inclusion Group 5 of the PH classification [75]. PH occurs in approximately 8% of patients with LAM although the proportion is higher (45%) in LAM patients referred for lung transplantation [76]. In 44 women with LAM undergoing lung transplantation, most patients had mild-to-moderate PH (average mPAP 33 ± 8.3 mmHg), but mPAP was as high as 47 mmHg [76].

There have been no prospective studies or RCTs of PAH therapy in LAM-associated PH. Cottin et al. described the management and outcomes of 20 patients with LAM-associated PH, most of whom had severe airflow obstruction (FEV_1 < 50% predicted) and mild-moderate PH (mPAP 32 ± 6 mmHg and PVR 4.7 ± 2.3 Wood units) [75]. Two patients in this study, however, had severe PH (mPAP >35 mmHg) with a normal FEV_1. Six patients (30%) received PAH therapies (bosentan or sildenafil) with hemodynamic improvements and no detrimental effect on gas exchange or episodes of pulmonary edema, but no improvements in dyspnea or 6MWD. Current guidelines recommend the use of sirolimus or everolimus in LAM patients with abnormal or worsening lung function; however, the effects of these therapies on hemodynamics or exercise capacity in LAM-associated PH are unknown [74].

Conclusions

Pulmonary hypertension is a complication of chronic lung disease, which adversely impacts survival and causes further disability. Management of PH in patients with chronic lung disease should be directed toward optimization of the underlying lung condition, the administration of supplemental oxygen in hypoxemic patients, and consideration of lung transplantation where appropriate. Despite promising results from observational studies, randomized controlled trials do not support the use of PAH therapies in PH due to chronic lung diseases, and they indeed may be harmful in some groups. Therefore, current guidelines recommend against the use of PAH therapies in PH due to lung disease. Although PH occurs frequently in the context of severe lung disease, it may also manifest with severe hemodynamic impairment with only mild-moderate lung disease. Other contributing causes such as left heart disease, thromboembolic disease, and sleep-disordered breathing should be systematically sought, and such patients should be evaluated in expert referral centers and/ or considered for clinical trials.

References

1. Simonneau G, Montani D, Celermajer DS, Denton CP, Gatzoulis MA, Krowka M, et al. Haemodynamic definitions and updated clinical classification of pulmonary hypertension. Eur Respir J. 2019;53(1):1801913.
2. Nathan SD, Barbera JA, Gaine SP, Harari S, Martinez FJ, Olschewski H, et al. Pulmonary hypertension in chronic lung disease and hypoxia. Eur Respir J. 2019;53(1):1801914.
3. Galiè N, Humbert M, Vachiery J-L, Gibbs S, Lang I, Torbicki A, et al. 2015 ESC/ERS guidelines for the diagnosis and treatment of pulmonary hypertension: the Joint Task Force for the Diagnosis And Treatment Of Pulmonary Hypertension of the European Society of Cardiology (ESC) and the European Respiratory Society (ERS): endorsed by: Association for European Paediatric and Congenital Cardiology (AEPC), International Society for Heart and Lung Transplantation (ISHLT). Eur Respir J. 2015;46(4):903–75.
4. Seeger W, Adir Y, Barberà JA, Champion H, Coghlan JG, Cottin V, et al. Pulmonary hypertension in chronic lung diseases. J Am Coll Cardiol. 2013;62(25 Suppl):D109–16.
5. Weill D, Benden C, Corris PA, Dark JH, Davis RD, Keshavjee S, et al. A consensus document for the selection of lung transplant candidates: 2014–an update from the Pulmonary Transplantation Council of the International Society for Heart And Lung Transplantation. J Heart Lung Transplant. 2015;34(1):1–15.

6. Vogelmeier CF, Criner GJ, Martinez FJ, Anzueto A, Barnes PJ, Bourbeau J, et al. Global strategy for the diagnosis, management, and prevention of chronic obstructive lung disease 2017 report. GOLD executive summary. Am J Respir Crit Care Med. 2017;195(5):557–82.
7. Chaouat A, Naeije R, Weitzenblum E. Pulmonary hypertension in COPD. Eur Respir J. 2008;32(5):1371–85.
8. Continuous or nocturnal oxygen therapy in hypoxemic chronic obstructive lung disease: a clinical trial. Nocturnal Oxygen Therapy Trial Group. Ann Intern Med. 1980;93(3):391–8.
9. Timms RM, Khaja FU, Williams GW. Hemodynamic response to oxygen therapy in chronic obstructive pulmonary disease. Ann Intern Med. 1985;102(1):29–36.
10. Weitzenblum E, Sautegeau A, Ehrhart M, Mammosser M, Pelletier A. Long-term oxygen therapy can reverse the progression of pulmonary hypertension in patients with chronic obstructive pulmonary disease. Am Rev Respir Dis. 1985;131(4):493–8.
11. Chaouat A, Bugnet A-S, Kadaoui N, Schott R, Enache I, Ducoloné A, et al. Severe pulmonary hypertension and chronic obstructive pulmonary disease. Am J Respir Crit Care Med. 2005;172(2):189–94.
12. Kovacs G, Agusti A, Barberà JA, Celli B, Criner G, Humbert M, et al. Pulmonary vascular involvement in chronic obstructive pulmonary disease. Is there a pulmonary vascular phenotype? Am J Respir Crit Care Med. 2018;198(8):1000–11.
13. Boerrigter BG, Bogaard HJ, Trip P, Groepenhoff H, Rietema H, Holverda S, et al. Ventilatory and cardiocirculatory exercise profiles in COPD: the role of pulmonary hypertension. Chest. 2012;142(5):1166–74.
14. Girard A, Jouneau S, Chabanne C, Khouatra C, Lannes M, Traclet J, et al. Severe pulmonary hypertension associated with COPD: hemodynamic improvement with specific therapy. Respiration. 2015;90(3):220–8.
15. Calcaianu G, Canuet M, Schuller A, Enache I, Chaouat A, Kessler R. Pulmonary arterial hypertension-specific drug therapy in COPD patients with severe pulmonary hypertension and mild-to-moderate airflow limitation. Respiration. 2016;91(1):9–17.
16. Hurdman J, Condliffe R, Elliot CA, Swift A, Rajaram S, Davies C, et al. Pulmonary hypertension in COPD: results from the ASPIRE registry. Eur Respir J. 2013;41(6):1292–301.
17. Agostoni P, Doria E, Galli C, Tamborini G, Guazzi MD. Nifedipine reduces pulmonary pressure and vascular tone during short- but not long-term treatment of pulmonary hypertension in patients with chronic obstructive pulmonary disease. Am Rev Respir Dis. 1989;139(1):120–5.
18. Domenighetti GM, Saglini VG. Short- and long-term hemodynamic effects of oral nifedipine in patients with pulmonary hypertension secondary to COPD and lung fibrosis. Deleterious effects in patients with restrictive disease. Chest. 1992;102(3):708–14.
19. Kennedy TP, Michael JR, Huang CK, Kallman CH, Zahka K, Schlott W, et al. Nifedipine inhibits hypoxic pulmonary vasoconstriction during rest and exercise in patients with chronic obstructive pulmonary disease. A controlled double-blind study. Am Rev Respir Dis. 1984;129(4):544–51.
20. Barberà JA, Roger N, Roca J, Rovira I, Higenbottam TW, Rodriguez-Roisin R. Worsening of pulmonary gas exchange with nitric oxide inhalation in chronic obstructive pulmonary disease. Lancet. 1996;347(8999):436–40.
21. Vonbank K, Ziesche R, Higenbottam TW, Stiebellehner L, Petkov V, Schenk P, et al. Controlled prospective randomised trial on the effects on pulmonary haemodynamics of the ambulatory long term use of nitric oxide and oxygen in patients with severe COPD. Thorax. 2003;58(4):289–93.
22. Dernaika TA, Beavin M, Kinasewitz GT. Iloprost improves gas exchange and exercise tolerance in patients with pulmonary hypertension and chronic obstructive pulmonary disease. Respir Int Rev Thorac Dis. 2010;79(5):377–82.
23. Boeck L, Tamm M, Grendelmeier P, Stolz D. Acute effects of aerosolized iloprost in COPD related pulmonary hypertension – a randomized controlled crossover trial. PLoS One. 2012;7(12):e52248.

24. Blanco I, Gimeno E, Munoz PA, Pizarro S, Gistau C, Rodriguez-Roisin R, et al. Hemodynamic and gas exchange effects of sildenafil in patients with chronic obstructive pulmonary disease and pulmonary hypertension. Am J Respir Crit Care Med. 2010;181(3):270–8.
25. Rao RS, Singh S, Sharma BB, Agarwal VV, Singh V. Sildenafil improves six-minute walk distance in chronic obstructive pulmonary disease: a randomised, double-blind, placebo-controlled trial. Indian J Chest Dis Allied Sci. 2011;53(2):81–5.
26. Lederer DJ, Bartels MN, Schluger NW, Brogan F, Jellen P, Thomashow BM, et al. Sildenafil for chronic obstructive pulmonary disease: a randomized crossover trial. COPD. 2012;9(3):268–75.
27. Blanco I, Santos S, Gea J, Güell R, Torres F, Gimeno-Santos E, et al. Sildenafil to improve respiratory rehabilitation outcomes in COPD: a controlled trial. Eur Respir J. 2013;42(4):982–92.
28. Goudie AR, Lipworth BJ, Hopkinson PJ, Wei L, Struthers AD. Tadalafil in patients with chronic obstructive pulmonary disease: a randomised, double-blind, parallel-group, placebo-controlled trial. Lancet Respir Med. 2014;2(4):293–300.
29. Vitulo P, Stanziola A, Confalonieri M, Libertucci D, Oggionni T, Rottoli P, et al. Sildenafil in severe pulmonary hypertension associated with chronic obstructive pulmonary disease: a randomized controlled multicenter clinical trial. J Heart Lung Transplant. 2017;36(2):166–74.
30. Stolz D, Rasch H, Linka A, Di Valentino M, Meyer A, Brutsche M, et al. A randomised, controlled trial of bosentan in severe COPD. Eur Respir J. 2008;32(3):619–28.
31. Valerio G, Bracciale P, Grazia D'Agostino A. Effect of bosentan upon pulmonary hypertension in chronic obstructive pulmonary disease. Ther Adv Respir Dis. 2009;3(1):15–21.
32. Barst RJ, Rubin LJ, Long WA, McGoon MD, Rich S, Badesch DB, et al. A comparison of continuous intravenous epoprostenol (prostacyclin) with conventional therapy for primary pulmonary hypertension. N Engl J Med. 1996;334(5):296–301.
33. Archer SL, Mike D, Crow J, Long W, Weir EK. A placebo-controlled trial of prostacyclin in acute respiratory failure in COPD. Chest. 1996;109(3):750–5.
34. Jones K, Higenbottam T, Wallwork J. Pulmonary vasodilation with prostacyclin in primary and secondary pulmonary hypertension. Chest. 1989;96(4):784–9.
35. Ghofrani HA, Staehler G, Grünig E, Halank M, Mitrovic V, Unger S, et al. Acute effects of riociguat in borderline or manifest pulmonary hypertension associated with chronic obstructive pulmonary disease. Pulm Circ. 2015;5(2):296–304.
36. Sprunger DB, Olson AL, Huie TJ, Fernandez-Perez ER, Fischer A, Solomon JJ, et al. Pulmonary fibrosis is associated with an elevated risk of thromboembolic disease. Eur Respir J. 2012;39(1):125–32.
37. Lettieri CJ, Nathan SD, Barnett SD, Ahmad S, Shorr AF. Prevalence and outcomes of pulmonary arterial hypertension in advanced idiopathic pulmonary fibrosis. Chest. 2006;129(3):746–52.
38. Lancaster LH, Mason WR, Parnell JA, Rice TW, Loyd JE, Milstone AP, et al. Obstructive sleep apnea is common in idiopathic pulmonary fibrosis. Chest. 2009;136(3):772–8.
39. Ghigna MR, Mooi WJ, Grünberg K. Pulmonary hypertensive vasculopathy in parenchymal lung diseases and/or hypoxia: number 1 in the series "pathology for the clinician" edited by Peter Dorfmüller and Alberto Cavazza. Eur Respir Rev. 2017;26(144):170003.
40. Hoeper MM, Behr J, Held M, Grunig E, Vizza CD, Vonk-Noordegraaf A, et al. Pulmonary hypertension in patients with chronic Fibrosing idiopathic interstitial pneumonias. PLoS One. 2015;10(12):e0141911.
41. Launay D, Sobanski V, Hachulla E, Humbert M. Pulmonary hypertension in systemic sclerosis: different phenotypes. Eur Respir Rev. 2017;26(145):170056.
42. Lefèvre G, Dauchet L, Hachulla E, Montani D, Sobanski V, Lambert M, et al. Survival and prognostic factors in systemic sclerosis-associated pulmonary hypertension: a systematic review and meta-analysis. Arthritis Rheum. 2013;65(9):2412–23.
43. Launay D, Montani D, Hassoun PM, Cottin V, Le Pavec J, Clerson P, et al. Clinical phenotypes and survival of pre-capillary pulmonary hypertension in systemic sclerosis. PLoS One. 2018;13(5):e0197112.
44. Le Pavec J, Girgis RE, Lechtzin N, Mathai SC, Launay D, Hummers LK, et al. Systemic sclerosis-related pulmonary hypertension associated with interstitial lung disease: impact of pulmonary arterial hypertension therapies. Arthritis Rheum. 2011;63(8):2456–64.

45. King TE, Behr J, Brown KK, du Bois RM, Lancaster L, de Andrade JA, et al. BUILD-1: a randomized placebo-controlled trial of bosentan in idiopathic pulmonary fibrosis. Am J Respir Crit Care Med. 2008;177(1):75–81.
46. King TE, Brown KK, Raghu G, du Bois RM, Lynch DA, Martinez F, et al. BUILD-3: a randomized, controlled trial of bosentan in idiopathic pulmonary fibrosis. Am J Respir Crit Care Med. 2011;184(1):92–9.
47. Raghu G, Behr J, Brown KK, Egan JJ, Kawut SM, Flaherty KR, et al. Treatment of idiopathic pulmonary fibrosis with ambrisentan: a parallel, randomized trial. Ann Intern Med. 2013;158(9):641–9.
48. Raghu G, Million-Rousseau R, Morganti A, Perchenet L, Behr J, MUSIC Study Group. Macitentan for the treatment of idiopathic pulmonary fibrosis: the randomised controlled MUSIC trial. Eur Respir J. 2013;42(6):1622–32.
49. Idiopathic Pulmonary Fibrosis Clinical Research Network, Zisman DA, Schwarz M, Anstrom KJ, Collard HR, Flaherty KR, et al. A controlled trial of sildenafil in advanced idiopathic pulmonary fibrosis. N Engl J Med. 2010;363(7):620–8.
50. Han MK, Bach DS, Hagan PG, Yow E, Flaherty KR, Toews GB, et al. Sildenafil preserves exercise capacity in patients with idiopathic pulmonary fibrosis and right-sided ventricular dysfunction. Chest. 2013;143(6):1699–708.
51. Corte TJ, Keir GJ, Dimopoulos K, Howard L, Corris PA, Parfitt L, et al. Bosentan in pulmonary hypertension associated with fibrotic idiopathic interstitial pneumonia. Am J Respir Crit Care Med. 2014;190(2):208–17.
52. Raghu G, Rochwerg B, Zhang Y, Garcia CAC, Azuma A, Behr J, et al. An official ATS/ERS/JRS/ALAT clinical practice guideline: treatment of idiopathic pulmonary fibrosis. An update of the 2011 clinical practice guideline. Am J Respir Crit Care Med. 2015;192(2):e3–19.
53. Raghu G, Nathan SD, Behr J, Brown KK, Egan JJ, Kawut SM, et al. Pulmonary hypertension in idiopathic pulmonary fibrosis with mild-to-moderate restriction. Eur Respir J. 2015;46(5):1370–7.
54. Krowka MJ, Ahmad S, de Andrade JA, Frost A, Glassberg MK, Lancaster LH, et al. A randomized, double-blind, placebo-controlled study to evaluate the safety and efficacy of iloprost inhalation in adults with abnormal pulmonary arterial pressure and exercise limitation associated with idiopathic pulmonary fibrosis. Chest. 2007;132(4):633A.
55. Jackson RM, Glassberg MK, Ramos CF, Bejarano PA, Butrous G, Gómez-Marín O. Sildenafil therapy and exercise tolerance in idiopathic pulmonary fibrosis. Lung. 2010;188(2):115–23.
56. Seibold JR, Denton CP, Furst DE, Guillevin L, Rubin LJ, Wells A, et al. Randomized, prospective, placebo-controlled trial of bosentan in interstitial lung disease secondary to systemic sclerosis. Arthritis Rheum. 2010;62(7):2101–8.
57. Ghofrani HA, Wiedemann R, Rose F, Schermuly RT, Olschewski H, Weissmann N, et al. Sildenafil for treatment of lung fibrosis and pulmonary hypertension: a randomised controlled trial. Lancet. 2002;360(9337):895–900.
58. Saggar R, Khanna D, Vaidya A, Derhovanessian A, Maranian P, Duffy E, et al. Changes in right heart haemodynamics and echocardiographic function in an advanced phenotype of pulmonary hypertension and right heart dysfunction associated with pulmonary fibrosis. Thorax. 2014;69(2):123–9.
59. Hoeper MM, Halank M, Wilkens H, Günther A, Weimann G, Gebert I, et al. Riociguat for interstitial lung disease and pulmonary hypertension: a pilot trial. Eur Respir J. 2013;41(4):853–60.
60. Nathan S, Behr J, Collard HR, Cottin V, Hoeper MM, Martinez F, et al. RISE-IIP: Riociguat for the treatment of pulmonary hypertension associated with idiopathic interstitial pneumonia. Eur Respir J. 2017;50(suppl 61):OA1985.
61. Weatherald J, Savale L, Humbert M. Medical Management of Pulmonary Hypertension with unclear and/or multifactorial mechanisms (group 5): is there a role for pulmonary arterial hypertension medications? Curr Hypertens Rep. 2017;19(11):86.
62. Nunes H, Humbert M, Capron F, Brauner M, Sitbon O, Battesti J-P, et al. Pulmonary hypertension associated with sarcoidosis: mechanisms, haemodynamics and prognosis. Thorax. 2006;61(1):68–74.

63. Baughman RP, Engel PJ, Taylor L, Lower EE. Survival in sarcoidosis-associated pulmonary hypertension: the importance of hemodynamic evaluation. Chest. 2010;138(5):1078–85.
64. Boucly A, Cottin V, Nunes H, Jaïs X, Tazi A, Prévôt G, et al. Management and long-term outcomes of sarcoidosis-associated pulmonary hypertension. Eur Respir J. 2017;50(4):1700465.
65. Baughman RP, Culver DA, Cordova FC, Padilla M, Gibson KF, Lower EE, et al. Bosentan for sarcoidosis-associated pulmonary hypertension: a double-blind placebo controlled randomized trial. Chest. 2014;145(4):810–7.
66. Barnett CF, Bonura EJ, Nathan SD, Ahmad S, Shlobin OA, Osei K, et al. Treatment of sarcoidosis-associated pulmonary hypertension. A two-center experience. Chest. 2009;135(6):1455–61.
67. Bonham CA, Oldham JM, Gomberg-Maitland M, Vij R. Prostacyclin and oral vasodilator therapy in sarcoidosis-associated pulmonary hypertension: a retrospective case series. Chest. 2015;148(4):1055–62.
68. Seferian A, Steriade A, Jaïs X, Planché O, Savale L, Parent F, et al. Pulmonary hypertension complicating Fibrosing Mediastinitis. Medicine (Baltimore). 2015;94(44):e1800.
69. Condado JF, Babaliaros V, Henry TS, Kaebnick B, Kim D, Staton GW. Pulmonary stenting for the treatment of sarcoid induced pulmonary vascular stenosis. Sarcoidosis Vasc Diffuse Lung Dis. 2016;33(3):281–7.
70. Fartoukh M, Humbert M, Capron F, Maître S, Parent F, Le Gall C, et al. Severe pulmonary hypertension in histiocytosis X. Am J Respir Crit Care Med. 2000;161(1):216–23.
71. Lazor R, Etienne-Mastroianni B, Khouatra C, Tazi A, Cottin V, Cordier J-F. Progressive diffuse pulmonary Langerhans cell histiocytosis improved by cladribine chemotherapy. Thorax. 2009;64(3):274–5.
72. Lorillon G, Bergeron A, Detourmignies L, Jouneau S, Wallaert B, Frija J, et al. Cladribine is effective against cystic pulmonary Langerhans cell histiocytosis. Am J Respir Crit Care Med. 2012;186(9):930–2.
73. Le Pavec J, Lorillon G, Jaïs X, Tcherakian C, Feuillet S, Dorfmüller P, et al. Pulmonary Langerhans cell histiocytosis-associated pulmonary hypertension: clinical characteristics and impact of pulmonary arterial hypertension therapies. Chest. 2012;142(5):1150–7.
74. McCormack FX, Gupta N, Finlay GR, Young LR, Taveira-DaSilva AM, Glasgow CG, et al. Official American Thoracic Society/Japanese Respiratory Society clinical practice guidelines: Lymphangioleiomyomatosis diagnosis and management. Am J Respir Crit Care Med. 2016;194(6):748–61.
75. Cottin V, Harari S, Humbert M, Mal H, Dorfmüller P, Jaïs X, et al. Pulmonary hypertension in lymphangioleiomyomatosis: characteristics in 20 patients. Eur Respir J. 2012;40(3):630–40.
76. Reynaud-Gaubert M, Mornex J-F, Mal H, Treilhaud M, Dromer C, Quétant S, et al. Lung transplantation for lymphangioleiomyomatosis: the French experience. Transplantation. 2008;86(4):515–20.

Chapter 7
Imaging in Chronic Lung Disease: Cardiac Considerations

Firdaus A. A. Mohamed Hoesein

Pearls
- Echocardiography is the first-line imaging technique used, but is often less reliable in those with emphysema.
- Cardiac computed tomography (CT) is frequently used to assess coronary atherosclerosis which is increased in many chronic lung diseases, like COPD.
- Cardiac magnetic resonance imaging (MRI) provides detailed information on left and right ventricular (dys)function and morphology, valvular disease, and presence and extent of cardiac fibrosis.

Introduction to Imaging Techniques and State of the Art

Introduction

In this chapter, non-invasive imaging methods and their applications in cardiac imaging will be discussed including echocardiography, computed tomography, and magnetic resonance imaging. Further on, the role of cardiac imaging in chronic lung disease will be reviewed by cardiac disease entity: coronary artery disease, pulmonary hypertension, right ventricular dysfunction, left ventricular disease, and cerebrovascular and peripheral arterial disease.

F. A. A. Mohamed Hoesein (✉)
Department of Radiology, University Medical Center Utrecht, University Utrecht, Utrecht, The Netherlands

© Springer Nature Switzerland AG 2020
S. P. Bhatt (ed.), *Cardiac Considerations in Chronic Lung Disease*,
Respiratory Medicine, https://doi.org/10.1007/978-3-030-43435-9_7

Echocardiography

Echocardiography is frequently used as a first-step imaging modality in many cardiac diseases and for evaluation of cardiac function. One of the advantages of echocardiography is its non-invasiveness and that it is harmless to patients. It can be used for the diagnosis of cardiac diseases, but also for prognostication and for follow-up in patients with chronic disease. There are many indications for the use of echocardiography, but quantification of ventricular function and measuring atrial and ventricular dimensions probably is the most common indication. Echocardiography is also frequently used for cardiac valve evaluation. Valvular regurgitation can be diagnosed and graded. Recent advances in echocardiography include three-dimensional (3-D) echocardiography and deformation imaging which will extend the use of echocardiography in the near future. 3-D echocardiography is more accurate in determining left ventricular volumes and function compared to 2-D echocardiography. Deformation imaging provides quantitative information on regional cardiac (dys)function. One of its advantages is that it can provide quantitative information on function. Traditional echocardiography is based on visual assessment, which is more prone to operator subjectivity, but also is less sensitive for early changes and (mal-)adaptation of the left ventricle. In patients with chronic lung diseases, deformation imaging may be used to detect and follow up right and left ventricular function abnormalities. One of the drawbacks of echocardiography is the poor acoustic window in individuals with COPD, especially in those with emphysema and/or hyperinflation. This makes echocardiography a less reliable imaging tool in COPD patients.

Computed Tomography

Computed tomography (CT) is commonly used in the evaluation of coronary artery disease, cerebrovascular disease, and peripheral artery disease. In patients with chronic lung disease, a chest CT is commonly performed for evaluation of pulmonary disease. Improvements of CT techniques in the last decade have allowed radiologists to also evaluate the heart.

Cardiac CT is mainly used for the detection and quantification of coronary artery calcium (Fig. 7.1) and detection of coronary artery stenosis (Figs. 7.2 and 7.3). The Agatston score, which is a marker of cardiovascular disease and an independent risk marker of future cardiovascular events, is calculated from a non-contrast cardiac CT (Fig. 7.1). The amount of coronary calcium is dependent on age, sex, and race [1]. The Agatston score is a risk factor independent of known cardiovascular risk factors like age, sex, hypertension, cholesterol levels, family history, and smoking. Non-contrast non-ECG-gated chest CT can be used to reliably determine coronary artery calcification. This is important information because in most of the COPD patients and patients with other pulmonary diseases, a non-contrast non-ECG-gated chest

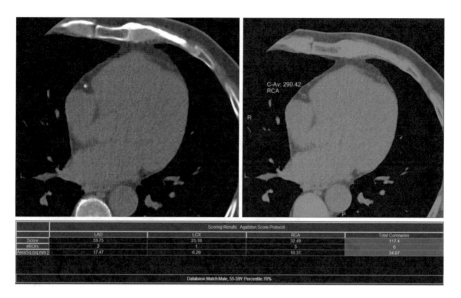

Scoring Results - Agatston Score Protocol			
	LAD	LCX	RCA	Total Coronaries
Score	59.75	25.16	32.49	117.4
#ROIs	2	1	3	6
AreaSq (sq.mm)	17.47	6.29	10.31	34.07

Database Match:Male, 55-59Y Percentile:70%

Fig. 7.1 Agatston score. Coronary artery calcifications scored by the Agatston method. Non-contrast CT scan and annotated scan. Table gives the score per coronary artery and in total

Fig. 7.2 Left anterior descending (LAD) artery with significant stenosis due to non-calcified plaque

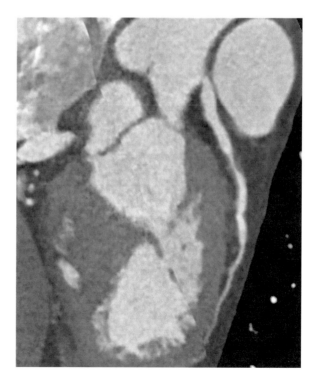

Fig. 7.3 Left anterior
descending artery with
multiple calcified plaques
with a significant stenosis

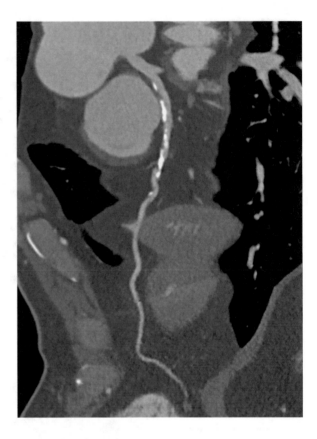

CT will be performed. The correlation between Agatston scores derived from non-contrast non-ECG-gated and ECG-gated scans is excellent [2].

In the last decade, technical advances in CT scanning equipment and acquisition techniques have led to high spatial and temporal resolution and a significant decrease of radiation dose for the imaging of the coronary arteries. Several factors are important to ensure adequate imaging quality including CT scanning equipment (low versus high number of detector rows; dual-energy imaging), patient characteristics (body mass index (BMI); heart rhythm; heart rate), and post-processing techniques (reconstruction algorithms). One of the most important patient-related factors for high-quality images is the heart rate. Ideally, heart rate should be 60 beats per minute or less, although some CT scanners allow a slight higher rate. Beta-blocker is used to ensure the desired heart rate; however, in chronic lung disease patients with bronchospasm, this is contraindicated. If a heart rate of 60 beats per minute cannot be achieved, so-called retrospective scanning can be done. In retrospective scanning, the heart and the coronaries are imaged during an entire heart cycle. This is in contrast to the standard scanning method (prospective scanning) in which the heart is imaged at one time-point at which the cardiac motion is least (end-diastole, 78% of the R-R interval). CT uses x-rays to produce images, and thus radiation dose control is an important factor. Recent advances have led to significant decreases in dose in such a way that dose is no longer an issue if the indication to perform cardiac CT is appropriate. However, retrospective scanning still has a relatively high radiation dose, and thus prospective scanning is preferred when possible.

In most of the cases, chest CT in COPD is performed to evaluate the pulmonary manifestations of COPD. However, information on cardiovascular manifestations of COPD can also be captured on chest CT. Body composition can be quantified on chest CT by measuring subcutaneous, mediastinal, and epicardial fat. The latter is associated with coronary artery disease [3]. COPD patients have more epicardial fat compared to controls, and it is associated with future cardiovascular events [4].

MRI

Cardiac magnetic resonance imaging (MRI) is widely used for evaluation of cardiac disease. It provides detailed high-quality information on left and right ventricular (dys)function and morphology, valvular disease, and presence and extent of cardiac fibrosis. Respiratory gating and ECG-triggering allow for high temporal and spatial resolution images (Fig. 7.4). Use of the intravenous contrast agent gadolinium gives information on the presence and extent of cardiac fibrosis (Fig. 7.5). Late gadolinium enhancement is good in the detection of focal areas of fibrosis, however is not suited to detect diffuse fibrosis of the left ventricle. Diffuse fibrosis is missed by late gadolinium enhancement because there is no normal non-diseased myocardial tissue to compare with. New mapping techniques and imaging sequences do provide information on diffuse fibrosis by measuring the extracellular volume and T1 values of the left ventricular myocardium (Fig. 7.6) [5]. In case of diffuse fibrosis, the interstitium and extracellular matrix are enlarged resulting in an increase in extracellular volume.

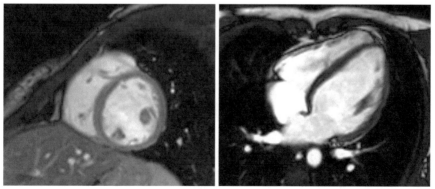

Fig. 7.4 MRI cine images of the heart. Left: 2-chamber view showing the left ventricle and the right ventricle. Right: 4-chamber view showing the ventricles and atria

Fig. 7.5 Delayed
enhancement MR image
showing mid-wall septal
delayed enhancement

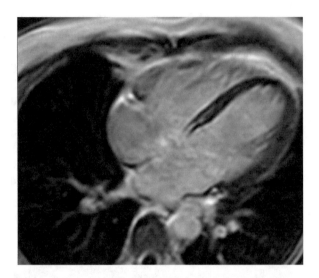

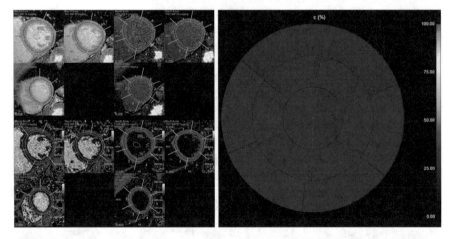

Fig. 7.6 T1 mapping at MRI of a patient with systemic sclerosis and a slightly lowered ejection fraction. T1 values were slightly increased, which could be a sign of diffuse cardiac fibrosis in a patient with systemic sclerosis. There were no abnormalities on delayed enhancement images

Role of Imaging

Coronary Artery Disease

Calcifications of the coronary artery and thoracic aorta are correlated with the severity of COPD and the presence of emphysema. COPD patients have more coronary artery calcium compared to non-COPD controls. These correlations remain even after extensive correction for known confounding risk factors for cardiovascular disease. Higher coronary artery calcium scores are associated with lower $FEV_1\%$

predicted values [6, 7]. In addition, in COPD patients coronary artery calcifications are associated with an increased morbidity and mortality compared to non-COPD controls [8]. Because COPD patients have a higher risk of cardiovascular disease, screening in this high-risk group by CT could be beneficial [9].

Pulmonary Hypertension

The gold standard for diagnosing pulmonary hypertension is right heart catheterization to directly measure the pulmonary artery pressure. However, in most patients suspected of pulmonary hypertension, non-invasive imaging techniques are performed first to assess the likelihood of the diagnosis. Pulmonary hypertension causes are classically classified into five groups, of which lung diseases and hypoxia (group 3) are an important group of causes of pulmonary hypertension [10]. Lung diseases known to cause pulmonary hypertension include COPD, sarcoid, interstitial lung disease, and sleep apnea. In fact, COPD is the second most common cause of pulmonary hypertension in the general population [11]. Prevalence of pulmonary hypertension varies from up to 60% in COPD patients to up to 84% in interstitial lung disease [12]. Echocardiography is frequently used as a first imaging step in pulmonary hypertension. Pulmonary artery pressure can be estimated by Doppler. However, in lung disease, echocardiography is suboptimal because parenchymal diseases and COPD limit the acoustic windows [13]. Echocardiography is mainly used to exclude significantly elevated pulmonary artery pressures. However, an estimated elevated pulmonary artery pressure by Doppler warrants additional diagnostic tests to confirm the diagnosis.

In patients with pulmonary hypertension but without a clear cause, a CT pulmonary angiogram is recommended in order to try to classify the cause into one of the five groups of pulmonary hypertension. Dual-energy CT can be used to create a perfusion map providing information beyond morphologic imaging (Fig. 7.7). In clinical practice, ventilation-perfusion scintigraphy still is the gold standard.

Pulmonary artery diameter can be used as a marker of pulmonary hypertension [14]. COPD subjects with pulmonary hypertension have a significantly larger pulmonary artery diameter compared to COPD subjects without pulmonary hypertension (Fig. 7.8) [15–18]. Pulmonary artery diameter can also be used as a prognostic marker in COPD patients. COPD patients with a pulmonary artery-to-aorta ratio of more than 1 have a significantly higher number of exacerbations [19]. In interstitial lung diseases, the ratio of the main pulmonary artery diameter to the ascending aorta diameter on chest CT is more reliable for the presence pulmonary hypertension than the diameter of the main pulmonary artery [14]. Combining echocardiography with the ratio of the main pulmonary artery diameter to the ascending aorta diameter on chest further improves the diagnostic value.

MRI can be used to assess pulmonary arterial stiffness non-invasively by measuring pulmonary arterial pulse wave velocity and pulsatility. It has been shown that pulmonary arterial stiffness is associated with COPD and emphysema [20].

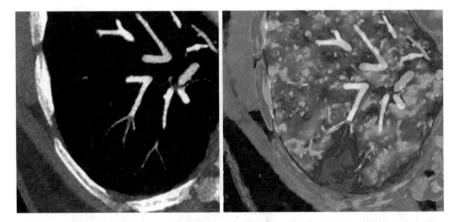

Fig. 7.7 Right: Normal CT pulmonary angiogram showing a pulmonary embolus in a right lower lobe artery. Left: Results from dual-energy CT showing a segmental subpleural iodine defect

Fig. 7.8 Contrast-enhanced CT scan. The pulmonary artery diameter is increased which is a sign of pulmonary hypertension

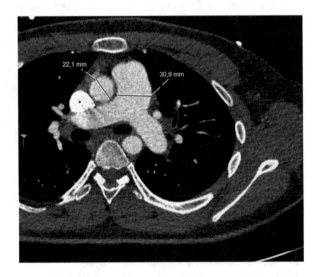

Pulmonary arterial stiffness is an early indicator for pulmonary vascular remodeling and is associated with measures of right ventricular dysfunction [21, 22].

Right Ventricular Dysfunction

COPD and its severity are associated with right ventricular function impairment. Cor pulmonale has traditionally been described as hypertrophy of the right ventricle resulting from diseases affecting the function and/or structure of the lungs including pulmonary hypertension. Right ventricular ejection fraction is significantly lower in

COPD subjects compared to controls, and subjects with more severe COPD have significantly lower right ventricular ejection fractions compared to those with mild COPD [23]. Right ventricular ejection fraction was measured on a retrospectively CT scan and on cardiac MRI. The measured ejection fraction on both techniques were highly correlated showing that both CT and MRI are capable of measuring ejection fraction in COPD subjects. MRI is preferred as CT uses a relatively high dose of radiation. In patients with both COPD and obstructive sleep apnea, signs of right ventricular dysfunction are more common compared to patients with COPD alone [24].

Left Ventricular Disease

COPD

COPD and heart failure are each important causes of death. In addition, concurrent COPD and heart failure are not uncommon [25]. In patients with heart failure and COPD, left ventricular ejection fraction measured by echocardiography is lower compared to patients with heart failure alone [26, 27]. Also left ventricular diastolic function is abnormal in COPD patients which can be evaluated with echocardiography [27]. In COPD patients, the quality of echocardiography may be hampered because of emphysema impeding acoustic windows. Estimations of unsatisfactory echocardiography in COPD patients range from 10% up to even 50% depending on disease severity. In case of poor-quality echocardiography, cardiac MIR can be performed to evaluate left ventricular function. A diagnosis of heart failure with preserved ejection fraction is even harder to establish in COPD patients as natriuretic peptides can be elevated in both heart failure and COPD [28].

Many patients with COPD and individuals at-risk of COPD undergo chest CT scanning. The chest CT includes information not only on the lungs but also on extra-pulmonary structures like the heart and the great vessels. COPD is associated with left ventricular dysfunction and with heart failure with preserved ejection fraction. Because in most patients with COPD non-contrast non-ECG-gated chest CTs will be performed, no reliable information on cardiac volumes and function can be attained [29].

Changes in the pulmonary vasculature are related to COPD. Pruning of distal pulmonary vessels is already present in smokers [30]. The area of small pulmonary vessels in COPD patients is associated with pulmonary hypertension [31]. Automatic segmentation and separation of pulmonary arteries and veins is possible, but more studies are needed to explore the clinical relevance. Pulmonary vein dimensions can be assessed by MRI and contrast-enhanced CT, and it has been shown that COPD and emphysema are associated with lower pulmonary vein dimensions [32]. Quantifying hyperinflation in COPD patients can be done by measuring total lung capacity at CT. Hyperinflation in COPD is a known cause of cardiovascular disease

[32, 33], and decreasing of the extent of hyperinflation is associated with an improvement of right ventricular filling indices on cardiac MRI [34]. Reducing hyperinflation is also associated with improvement in left ventricular filling [35]. Hyperinflation on CT in COPD patients is also associated with an increase in pulmonary artery diameter suggesting an association with pulmonary hypertension [36].

On cardiac MRI structural changes of the myocardium may be visualized, for instance, due to chronic hypoxia. Myocardial extracellular volume (ECV) and T1 mapping were increased in a small study comparing COPD patients with controls. ECV was associated with left ventricular remodeling and reduced left atrial function [37]. Although only a small number of subjects were included, the study showed that patients with COPD have evidence of diffuse myocardial fibrosis. Future research should show whether ECV can be used as an early marker for myocardial fibrosis in COPD and/or if it could be used to stratify COPD patients with a high and low risk for cardiac abnormalities.

Sarcoid

Cardiac involvement of sarcoid is not rare and can result in conduction abnormalities, heart failure, and even sudden cardiac death. Cardiac sarcoid may even occur in patients without pulmonary involvement [38]. In post-mortem studies up to 20–25% of sarcoid patients have cardiac involvement [39]. Morbidity and mortality of cardiac sarcoid are related to the site and extent of cardiac involvement. Mortality in most cases is related to conduction defects resulting in ventricular fibrillation. In patients with an unexplained AV block, cardiac sarcoid is the cause in almost a third of cases [40]. Morbidity is related to cardiomyopathy caused by infiltration of the myocardium by granulomas resulting in (progressive) heart failure and to conductional defects like atrioventricular blocks. Cardiac involvement can be imaged by echocardiography, MRI, and [18F]-fluorodeoxyglucose positron emitting tomography (18F-FDG-PET) (Fig. 7.9). Echocardiography is mainly used to evaluate ventricular function, dimensions, and hypertrophy, but is not suitable to diagnose cardiac sarcoid. A lowered left ventricular ejection fraction is associated with poorer prognosis [41]. Cardiac MRI with gadolinium can detect myocardial sarcoid involvement. Enhancement is seen both in fibrosis and in active cardiac disease in which delayed enhancement associates with inflammation. In case of cardiac involvement, focal patchy delayed enhancement of the epicardium and/or mid-myocardium can be seen, although cardiac sarcoid can also be associated with non-specific enhancement patterns. This is in contrast to ischemic enhancement which is sub-endocardial and mostly in a coronary territory [42]. The presence and extent of delayed enhancement in cardiac sarcoid may serve as a prognostic tool. Patients without delayed enhancement have a better prognosis, and the number of segments involved is associated with left ventricular dysfunction [43]. It is not possible to differentiate fibrosis from active disease with delayed enhancement

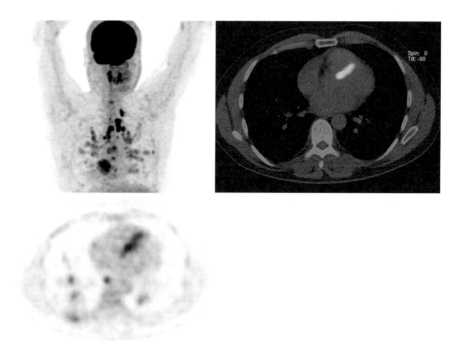

Fig. 7.9 18F-FDG-PET CT showing increased uptake in mediastinal and hilar lymph nodes in a patient with sarcoid. Cross-sectional sections through the heart show increased uptake in the septum indicating active cardiac sarcoid

MRI. 18F-FDG-PET is frequently used for diagnosing and staging of sarcoid. 18F-FDG-PET can detect active cardiac sarcoid, which is in contrast to delayed enhancement MRI. Key to a reliable evaluation of the myocardium on PET scan is adequate suppression of normal FDG uptake. To ensure this, a low-carbohydrate diet and prolonged fasting protocol are prescribed to switch to free fatty acid metabolism. In many centers, low doses of intravenous unfractionated heparin are administered before scanning. Heparin induces lipolysis resulting in higher serum free fatty acid levels which suppresses physiologic FDG uptake [44]. In most patients suspected of cardiac sarcoid, both cardiac MRI and 18F-FDG-PET are performed. Cardiac MRI is more sensitive for cardiac fibrosis and 18F-FDG-PET for inflammation without cardiac fibrosis. Combining the results of both studies increases the diagnostic value for cardiac sarcoid [42]. Follow-up PET scans can be used to evaluate response to therapy as increased FDG uptake is related to active disease [45]. Cardiac MRI is not suited for monitoring of disease severity as both fibrosis and inflammation cause similar delayed enhancement [46]. Currently, there are no guidelines regarding dosage and duration of corticosteroid therapy and the use of additional immunotherapies such as like infliximab. Deciding on the duration of treatment in patients without significant symptoms or complaints, but with cardiac abnormalities on initial 18F-FDG-PET, is challenging.

With 18F-FDG-PET, corticosteroid and new immunological therapies can be monitored and doses can be titrated.

Connective Tissue Disease

Lung involvement of connective tissue diseases (CTD), including rheumatoid arthritis, scleroderma, Sjogren's syndrome, systemic lupus erythematosus (SLE), and vasculitides, is not rare. Lung involvement in CTD most commonly includes interstitial lung disease. Cardiac involvement is also common in these conditions [47]. Peri-myocarditis and diastolic dysfunction are most commonly reported, but coronary artery disease is also common. Patients with rheumatoid arthritis and SLE have a high prevalence of coronary artery disease [48–49]. Cardiac MRI can detect cardiac involvement in early and acute stages. Late gadolinium enhancement may be used to diagnose (peri-)myocarditis which occurs in up to 15% of SLE patients [50]. New cardiac MRI techniques like T1 and T2 mapping may play a role in assessing myocardial involvement in CTD. A study in SLE patients suspected of cardiac involvement showed that T1 and T2 mapping values were higher compared to control patients [51]. After treatment, mapping values in SLE patients decreased.

Cardiac involvement in ANCA-associated small vessel vasculitides (eosinophilic granulomatosis with polyangiitis [EGPA] and granulomatosis with polyangiitis [GPA]) is not common, but if present has a poor prognostic outcome. Cardiac involvement is more common in EGPA than in GPA. Cardiomyopathy, myocarditis, pericarditis, and endomyocardial fibrosis are the most common patterns of involvement. Cardiac MR with late gadolinium is used for the evaluation of cardiac involvement. The cardiomyopathy is caused by microvascular ischemia. In endomyocardial fibrosis, there is sub-endocardial delayed enhancement with intraventricular thrombus. Signs of pericarditis on cardiac MRI are pericardial fluid in combination with pericardial thickening and pericardial late gadolinium enhancement. Also in ANCA-associated vasculitis, T1 and T2 mapping values are increased indicating that new mapping methods may play a role in detecting cardiac involvement [52].

Cardiac involvement of systemic sclerosis is not rare and if present has a poor prognosis [53–54]. Cardiac systemic sclerosis includes myocarditis, valvular regurgitation, cardiac fibrosis, and microvascular disease. Myocarditis and cardiac fibrosis can be detected by late gadolinium enhancement on MRI. In a study of 58 systemic sclerosis patients, almost half had late gadolinium enhancement on MRI [55]. Abnormalities in the coronary microcirculation are common in systemic sclerosis and are thought to be the main cause of cardiac fibrosis in systemic sclerosis. Microvascular disease can be detected by stress perfusion MRI and cardiac PET CT [53, 56]. A "cardiac" Raynaud's phenomenon has also been described in systemic sclerosis as patients with Raynaud's phenomenon more frequently have cardiac fibrosis. Epicardial coronary disease is not more common in systemic sclerosis. T1 mapping at cardiac MRI, a marker of diffuse cardiac fibrosis, was found to be significantly higher in systemic sclerosis compared to control patients [57].

Cerebrovascular Disease and Peripheral Arterial Disease

COPD patients have an increased prevalence of carotid atherosclerotic disease and an increased risk of stroke [58]. In COPD patients the prevalence of stroke is 6.9–9.9% [59]. There is a lot of knowledge on the use of carotid ultrasound to assess subclinical atherosclerosis. Carotid ultrasound can measure the intima-media thickness which is a marker for cardiovascular disease [60]. COPD is associated with greater intima-media thickness at carotid ultrasound [61], and in COPD patients, there is a correlation between intima-media thickness and lung function [62–63]. In elderly subjects with carotid artery wall thickening, COPD is an independent predictor for the evaluation of vulnerable plaques [64]. Carotid ultrasound thus may be a surrogate marker for (subclinical) atherosclerosis and cardiovascular risk assessment in COPD. However, future studies are needed how to incorporate carotid ultrasound in the optimal management strategy of COPD patients.

CT angiography (CTA) and MR angiography (MRA) are excellent in depicting cranial and extra-cranial vessels and can reliably detect stenosis and occlusions. CTA requires the use of intravenous contrast agents. MRA can be performed without and with administration of intravenous gadolinium. To my knowledge, there are no studies examining CTA and/or MRA of the carotids or peripheral arteries in COPD.

Next to carotid atherosclerotic disease, it is known that peripheral arterial disease (PAD) is also more prevalent in COPD patients (8.5% versus 1.8%) [65]. COPD patients with PAD have a significantly lower 6-minute walk distance after extensive correction for confounding factors.

Conclusion

Imaging plays a central role in the evaluation of cardiac involvement of chronic lung diseases. Echocardiography, cardiac CT, and cardiac MRI all have their own indications and pros and cons.

References

1. Agatston AS, Janowitz WR, Hildner FJ, Zusmer NR, Viamonte M Jr, Detrano R. Quantification of coronary artery calcium using ultrafast computed tomography. J Am Coll Cardiol. 1990;15:827–32.
2. Budoff MJ, Nasir K, Kinney GL, Hokanson JE, Barr RG, Steiner R, Nath H, Lopez-Garcia C, Black-Shinn J, Casaburi R. Coronary artery and thoracic calcium on noncontrast thoracic CT scans: comparison of ungated and gated examinations in patients from the COPD Gene cohort. J Cardiovasc Comput Tomogr. 2011;5(2):113–8.
3. Mancio J, Azevedo D, Saraiva F, Azevedo AI, Pires-Morais G, Leite-Moreira A, Falcao-Pires I, Lunet N, Bettencourt N. Epicardial adipose tissue volume assessed by computed tomography

and coronary artery disease: a systematic review and meta-analysis. Eur Heart J Cardiovasc Imaging. 2018;19(5):490–7.

4. Zagaceta J, Zulueta JJ, Bastarrika G, Colina I, Alcaide AB, Campo A, Celli BR, de Torres JP. Epicardial adipose tissue in patients with chronic obstructive pulmonary disease. PLoS One. 2013;8(6):e65593.

5. Haaf P, Garg P, Messroghli DR, Broadbent DA, Greenwood JP, Plein S. Cardiac T1 Mapping and Extracellular Volume (ECV) in clinical practice: a comprehensive review. J Cardiovasc Magn Reson. 2016;18(1):89.

6. Dransfield MT, Huang F, Nath H, Singh SP, Bailey WC, Washko GR. CT emphysema predicts thoracic aortic calcification in smokers with and without COPD. COPD. 2010;7(6): 404–10.

7. Rasmussen T, Køber L, Pedersen JH, Dirksen A, Thomsen LH, Stender S, Brodersen J, Groen J, Ashraf H, Kofoed KF. Relationship between chronic obstructive pulmonary disease and subclinical coronary artery disease in long-term smokers. Eur Heart J Cardiovasc Imaging. 2013;14(12):1159–66.

8. Williams MC, Murchison JT, Edwards LD, Agustí A, Bakke P, Calverley PM, Celli B, Coxson HO, Crim C, Lomas DA, Miller BE, Rennard S, Silverman EK, Tal-Singer R, Vestbo J, Wouters E, Yates JC, van Beek EJ, Newby DE, MacNee W, Evaluation of COPD Longitudinally to Identify Predictive Surrogate Endpoints (ECLIPSE) investigators. Coronary artery calcification is increased in patients with COPD and associated with increased morbidity and mortality. Thorax. 2014;69(8):718–23.

9. Chen W, Thomas J, Sadatsafavi M, FitzGerald JM. Risk of cardiovascular comorbidity in patients with chronic obstructive pulmonary disease: a systematic review and meta-analysis. Lancet Respir Med. 2015;3(8):631–9. https://doi.org/10.1016/S2213-2600(15)00241-6. Epub 2015 Jul 22.

10. Simonneau G, Gatzoulis MA, Adatia I, et al. Updated clinical classification of pulmonary hypertension. J Am Coll Cardiol. 2013;62(25 suppl):D34–41.

11. Hyduk A, Croft JB, Ayala C, Zheng K, Zheng ZJ, Mensah GA. Pulmonary hypertension surveillance--United States, 1980-2002. MMWR Surveill Summ. 2005;54(5):1–28.

12. Klinger JR. Group III pulmonary hypertension: pulmonary hypertension associated with lung disease: epidemiology, pathophysiology, and treatments. Cardiol Clin. 2016;34(3):413–33. https://doi.org/10.1016/j.ccl.2016.04.003.

13. Arcasoy SM, Christie JD, Ferrari VA, Sutton MS, Zisman DA, Blu-menthal NP, Pochettino A, Kotloff RM. Echocardiographic assessment of pulmonary hypertension in patients with advanced lung disease. Am J Respir Crit Care Med. 2003;167:735–40.

14. Devaraj A, Wells AU, Meister MG, Corte TJ, Wort SJ, Hansell DM. Detection of pulmonary hypertension with multidetector CT and echocardiography alone and in combination. Radiology. 2010;254(2):609–16.

15. Chen X, Liu K, Wang Z, Zhu Y, Zhao Y, Kong H, Xie W, Wang H. Computed tomography measurement of pulmonary artery for diagnosis of COPD and its comorbidity pulmonary hypertension. Int J Chron Obstruct Pulmon Dis. 2015;10:2525–33.

16. Iyer AS, Wells JM, Vishin S, Bhatt SP, Wille KM, Dransfield MT. CT scan-measured pulmonary artery to aorta ratio and echocardiography for detecting pulmonary hypertension in severe COPD. Chest. 2014;145(4):824–32.

17. Shin S, King CS, Brown AW, Albano MC, Atkins M, Sheridan MJ, Ahmad S, Newton KM, Weir N, Shlobin OA, Nathan SD. Pulmonary artery size as a predictor of pulmonary hypertension and outcomes in patients with chronic obstructive pulmonary disease. Respir Med. 2014;108(11):1626–32.

18. Mohamed Hoesein FA, Besselink T, Pompe E, Oudijk EJ, de Graaf EA, Kwakkel-van Erp JM, de Jong PA, Luijk B. Accuracy of CT pulmonary artery diameter for pulmonary hypertension in end-stage COPD. Lung. 2016;194(5):813–9.

19. Wells JM, Washko GR, Han MK, Abbas N, Nath H, Mamary AJ, Regan E, Bailey WC, Martinez FJ, Westfall E, Beaty TH, Curran-Everett D, Curtis JL, Hokanson JE, Lynch DA,

Make BJ, Crapo JD, Silverman EK, Bowler RP. Dransfield MT; COPDGene Investigators; ECLIPSE Study Investigators. Pulmonary arterial enlargement and acute exacerbations of COPD. N Engl J Med. 2012;367(10):913–21.

20. Liu CY, Parikh M, Bluemke DA, Balte P, Carr J, Dashnaw S, Poor HD, Gomes AS, Hoffman EA, Kawut SM, Lima JAC, McAllister DA, Prince MA, Vogel-Claussen J, Barr RG. Pulmonary artery stiffness in chronic obstructive pulmonary disease (COPD) and emphysema: the Multi-Ethnic Study of Atherosclerosis (MESA) COPD Study. J Magn Reson Imaging. 2018;47(1):262–71.

21. Weir-McCall JR, Struthers AD, Lipworth BJ, Houston JG. The role of pulmonary arterial stiffness in COPD. Respir Med. 2015;109(11):1381–90.

22. Mills NL, Miller JJ, Anand A, Robinson SD, Frazer GA, Anderson D, Breen L, Wilkinson IB, McEniery CM, Donaldson K, Newby DE, Macnee W. Increased arterial stiffness in patients with chronic obstructive pulmonary disease: a mechanism for increased cardiovascular risk. Thorax. 2008;63(4):306–11.

23. Gao Y, Du X, Liang L, Cao L, Yang Q, Li K. Evaluation of right ventricular function by 64-row CT in patients with chronic obstructive pulmonary disease and cor pulmonale. Eur J Radiol. 2012;81(2):345–53. https://doi.org/10.1016/j.ejrad.2010.11.004. Epub 2010 Nov 27.

24. Sharma B, Neilan TG, Kwong RY, Mandry D, Owens RL, McSharry D, Bakker JP, Malhotra A. Evaluation of right ventricular remodeling using cardiac magnetic resonance imaging in co-existent chronic obstructive pulmonary disease and obstructive sleep apnea. COPD. 2013;10(1):4–10.

25. Hawkins NM, Petrie MC, Jhund PS, Chalmers GW, Dunn FG, McMurray JJ. Heart failure and chronic obstructive pulmonary disease: diagnostic pitfalls and epidemiology. Eur J Heart Fail. 2009;11(2):130–9.

26. Rusinaru D, Saaidi I, Godard S, Mahjoub H, Battle C, Tribouilloy C. Impact of chronic obstructive pulmonary disease on long-term outcome of patients hospitalized for heart failure. Am J Cardiol. 2008;101(3):353–8.

27. Boussuges A, Pinet C, Molenat F, Burnet H, Ambrosi P, Badier M, Sainty JM, Orehek J. Left atrial and ventricular filling in chronic obstructive pulmonary disease. An echocardiographic and Doppler study. Am J Respir Crit Care Med. 2000;162(2 Pt 1):670–5.

28. Cabanes L, Richaud-Thiriez B, Fulla Y, Heloire F, Vuillemard C, Weber S, Dusser D. Brain natriuretic peptide blood levels in the differential diagnosis of dyspnea. Chest. 2001;120(6):2047–50.

29. Iversen K, Kjaergaard J, Akkan D, Kober L, Torp-Pedersen C, Hassager C, Vestbo J, Kjoller E, ECHOS-Lung Function Study Group. Chronic obstructive pulmonary disease in patients admitted with heart failure. J Intern Med. 2008;264(4):361–9. https://doi.org/10.1111/j.1365-2796.2008.01975.x. Epub 2008 Jun 5.

30. Estépar RS, Kinney GL, Black-Shinn JL, Bowler RP, Kindlmann GL, Ross JC, Kikinis R, Han MK, Come CE, Diaz AA, Cho MH, Hersh CP, Schroeder JD, Reilly JJ, Lynch DA, Crapo JD, Wells JM, Dransfield MT, Hokanson JE. Washko GR; COPDGene Study. Computed tomographic measures of pulmonary vascular morphology in smokers and their clinical implications. Am J Respir Crit Care Med. 2013;188(2):231–9.

31. Matsuoka S, Washko GR, Yamashiro T, Estepar RS, Diaz A, Silverman EK, Hoffman E, Fessler HE, Criner GJ, Marchetti N, Scharf SM, Martinez FJ, Reilly JJ, Hatabu H, National Emphysema Treatment Trial Research Group. Pulmonary hypertension and computed tomography measurement of small pulmonary vessels in severe emphysema. Am J Respir Crit Care Med. 2010;181(3):218–25.

32. Smith BM, Prince MR, Hoffman EA, Bluemke DA, Liu CY, Rabinowitz D, Hueper K, Parikh MA, Gomes AS, Michos ED, Lima JAC, Barr RG. Impaired left ventricular filling in COPD and emphysema: is it the heart or the lungs? The Multi-Ethnic Study of Atherosclerosis COPD Study. Chest. 2013;144(4):1143–51.

33. Barr RG, Bluemke DA, Ahmed FS, Carr JJ, Enright PL, Hoffman EA, Jiang R, Kawut SM, Kronmal RA, Lima JA, Shahar E, Smith LJ, Watson KE. Percent emphysema, air-

flow obstruction, and impaired left ventricular filling. N Engl J Med. 2010;362(3): 217–27.

34. Hohlfeld JM, Vogel-Claussen J, Biller H, Berliner D, Berschneider K, Tillmann HC, Hiltl S, Bauersachs J, Welte T. Effect of lung deflation with indacaterol plus glycopyrronium on ventricular filling in patients with hyperinflation and COPD (CLAIM): a double-blind, randomised, crossover, placebo-controlled, single-centre trial. Lancet Respir Med. 2018;6(5):368–78.

35. Jörgensen K, Houltz E, Westfelt U, Nilsson F, Scherstén H, Ricksten SE. Effects of lung volume reduction surgery on left ventricular diastolic filling and dimensions in patients with severe emphysema. Chest. 2003;124(5):1863–70.

36. Poor HD, Kawut SM, Liu C, Smith BM, Hoffman EA, Lima JA, Ambale-Venkatesh B, Michos ED, Prince MR, Barr RG. Pulmonary hyperinflation due to gas trapping and pulmonary artery size: the MESA COPD Study. PLoS One. 2017;12(5):e0176812.

37. Neilan TG, Bakker JP, Sharma B, Owens RL, Farhad H, Shah RV, Abbasi SA, Kohli P, Wilson J, DeMaria A, Jerosch-Herold M, Kwong RY, Malhotra A. T1 measurements for detection of expansion of the myocardial extracellular volume in chronic obstructive pulmonary disease. Can J Cardiol. 2014;30(12):1668–75.

38. Tavora F, Cresswell N, Li L, Ripple M, Solomon C, Burke A. Comparison of necropsy findings in patients with sarcoidosis dying suddenly from cardiac sarcoidosis versus dying suddenly from other causes. Am J Cardiol. 2009;104(4):571–7.

39. Silverman KJ, Hutchins GM, Bulkley BH. Cardiac sarcoid: a clinicopathologic study of 84 unselected patients with systemic sarcoidosis. Circulation. 1978;58(6):1204–11.

40. Nery PB, Mc Ardle BA, Redpath CJ, Leung E, Lemery R, Dekemp R, Yang J, Keren A, Beanlands RS, Birnie DH. Prevalence of cardiac sarcoidosis in patients presenting with monomorphic ventricular tachycardia. Pacing Clin Electrophysiol. 2014;37(3):364–74.

41. Chiu CZ, Nakatani S, Zhang G, Tachibana T, Ohmori F, Yamagishi M, Kitakaze M, Tomoike H, Miyatake K. Prevention of left ventricular remodeling by long-term corticosteroid therapy in patients with cardiac sarcoidosis. Am J Cardiol. 2005;95(1):143–6.

42. Vita T, Okada DR, Veillet-Chowdhury M, Bravo PE, Mullins E, Hulten E, Agrawal M, Madan R, Taqueti VR, Steigner M, Skali H, Kwong RY, Stewart GC, Dorbala S, Di Carli MF, Blankstein R. Complementary value of cardiac magnetic resonance imaging and positron emission tomography/computed tomography in the assessment of cardiac sarcoidosis. Circ Cardiovasc Imaging. 2018;11(1):e007030. d.

43. Watanabe E, Kimura F, Nakajima T, Hiroe M, Kasai Y, Nagata M, Kawana M, Hagiwara N. Late gadolinium enhancement in cardiac sarcoidosis: characteristic magnetic resonance findings and relationship with left ventricular function. J Thorac Imaging. 2013;28(1):60–6.

44. Manabe O, Yoshinaga K, Ohira H, Masuda A, Sato T, Tsujino I, Yamada A, Oyama-Manabe N, Hirata K, Nishimura M, Tamaki N. The effects of 18-h fasting with low-carbohydrate diet preparation on suppressed physiological myocardial (18)F-fluorodeoxyglucose (FDG) uptake and possible minimal effects of unfractionated heparin use in patients with suspected cardiac involvement sarcoidosis. J Nucl Cardiol. 2016;23(2):244–52.

45. Teirstein AS, Machac J, Almeida O, Lu P, Padilla ML, Iannuzzi MC. Results of 188 whole-body fluorodeoxyglucose positron emission tomography scans in 137 patients with sarcoidosis. Chest. 2007;132(6):1949–53.

46. Chareonthaitawee P, Beanlands RS, Chen W, Dorbala S, Miller EJ, Murthy VL, Birnie DH, Chen ES, Cooper LT, Tung RH, White ES, Borges-Neto S, Di Carli MF, Gropler RJ, Ruddy TD, Schindler TH, Blankstein R. Joint SNMMI-ASNC expert consensus document on the role of 18F-FDG PET/CT in cardiac sarcoid detection and therapy monitoring. J Nucl Cardiol. 2017;24(5):1741–58.

47. Ungprasert P, Wannarong T, Panichsillapakit T, Cheungpasitporn W, Thongprayoon C, Ahmed S, Raddatz DA. Cardiac involvement in mixed connective tissue disease: a systematic review. Int J Cardiol. 2014;171(3):326–30.

48. Maradit-Kremers H, Crowson CS, Nicola PJ, Ballman KV, Roger VL, Jacobsen SJ, Gabriel SE. Increased unrecognized coronary heart disease and sudden deaths in rheumatoid arthritis: a population-based cohort study. Arthritis Rheum. 2005;52(2):402–11.
49. Ishimori ML, Martin R, Berman DS, Goykhman P, Shaw LJ, Shufelt C, Slomka PJ, Thomson LE, Schapira J, Yang Y, Wallace DJ, Weisman MH, Bairey Merz CN. Myocardial ischemia in the absence of obstructive coronary artery disease in systemic lupus erythematosus. JACC Cardiovasc Imaging. 2011;4(1):27–33.
50. O'Neill SG, Woldman S, Bailliard F, Norman W, McEwan J, Isenberg DA, Taylor AM, Rahman A. Cardiac magnetic resonance imaging in patients with systemic lupus erythematosus. Ann Rheum Dis. 2009;68(9):1478–81.
51. Hinojar R, Foote L, Sangle S, Marber M, Mayr M, Carr-White G, D'Cruz D, Nagel E, Puntmann VO. Native T1 and T2 mapping by CMR in lupus myocarditis: disease recognition and response to treatment. Int J Cardiol. 2016;222:717–26.
52. Greulich S, Mayr A, Kitterer D, Latus J, Henes J, Steubing H, Kaesemann P, Patrascu A, Greiser A, Groeninger S, Braun N, Alscher MD, Sechtem U, Mahrholdt H. T1 and T2 mapping for evaluation of myocardial involvement in patients with ANCA-associated vasculitides. J Cardiovasc Magn Reson. 2017;19(1):6.
53. Rodríguez-Reyna TS, Morelos-Guzman M, Hernández-Reyes P, Montero-Duarte K, Martínez-Reyes C, Reyes-Utrera C, Vazquez-La Madrid J, Morales-Blanhir J, Núñez-Álvarez C, Cabiedes-Contreras J. Assessment of myocardial fibrosis and microvascular damage in systemic sclerosis by magnetic resonance imaging and coronary angiotomography. Rheumatology (Oxford). 2015;54(4):647–54.
54. Ioannidis JP, Vlachoyiannopoulos PG, Haidich AB, Medsger TA Jr, Lucas M, Michet CJ, Kuwana M, Yasuoka H, van den Hoogen F, Te Boome L, van Laar JM, Verbeet NL, Matucci-Cerinic M, Georgountzos A, Moutsopoulos HM. Mortality in systemic sclerosis: an international meta-analysis of individual patient data. Am J Med. 2005;118(1):2–10.
55. Di Cesare E, Battisti S, Di Sibio A, Cipriani P, Giacomelli R, Liakouli V, Ruscitti P, Masciocchi C. Early assessment of sub-clinical cardiac involvement in systemic sclerosis (SSc) using delayed enhancement cardiac magnetic resonance (CE-MRI). Eur J Radiol. 2013;82(6):e268–73.
56. Schindler TH, Schelbert HR, Quercioli A, Dilsizian V. Cardiac PET imaging for the detection and monitoring of coronary artery disease and microvascular health. JACC Cardiovasc Imaging. 2010;3(6):623–40.
57. Lee DC, Hinchcliff ME, Sarnari R, Stark MM, Lee J, Koloms K, Hoffmann A, Carns M, Thakrar A, Aren K, Varga J, Aquino A, Carr JC, Benefield BC, Shah SJ. Diffuse cardiac fibrosis quantification in early systemic sclerosis by magnetic resonance imaging and correlation with skin fibrosis. J Scleroderma Relat Disord. 2018;3(2):159–169. 12.
58. Portegies ML, Lahousse L, Joos GF, Hofman A, Koudstaal PJ, Stricker BH, Brusselle GG, Ikram MA. Chronic obstructive pulmonary disease and the risk of stroke. The Rotterdam Study. Am J Respir Crit Care Med. 2016;193(3):251–8.
59. Müllerova H, Agusti A, Erqou S, Mapel DW. Cardiovascular comorbidity in COPD: systematic literature review. Chest. 2013;144:1163–78.
60. Stein JH, Korcarz CE, Hurst RT, Lonn E, Kendall CB, Mohler ER, Najjar SS, Rembold CM, Post WS, American Society of Echocardiography Carotid Intima-Media Thickness Task Force. Use of carotid ultrasound to identify subclinical vascular disease and evaluate cardiovascular disease risk: a consensus statement from the American Society of Echocardiography Carotid Intima-Media Thickness Task Force. Endorsed by the Society for Vascular Medicine. J Am Soc Echocardiogr. 2008;21(2):93–111; quiz 189-90.
61. Fisk M, McEniery CM, Gale N, Mäki-Petäjä K, Forman JR, Munnery M, Woodcock-Smith J, Cheriyan J, Mohan D, Fuld J, Tal-Singer R, Polkey MI, Cockcroft JR, Wilkinson IB, ERICA Consortium and ACCT Investigators. Surrogate markers of cardiovascular risk and chronic obstructive pulmonary disease: a large case-controlled study. Hypertension. 2018;71(3):499–506.

62. Schroeder EB, Welch VL, Evans GW, Heiss G. Impaired lung function and subclinical athero-sclerosis. The ARIC study. Atherosclerosis. 2005;180:367–73.
63. Ambrosino P, Lupoli R, Cafaro G, Iervolino S, Carone M, Pappone N, Di Minno MND. Subclinical carotid atherosclerosis in patients with chronic obstructive pulmonary dis-ease: a meta-analysis of literature studies. Ann Med. 2017;49(6):513–24.
64. Lahousse L, van den Bouwhuijsen QJ, Loth DW, Joos GF, Hofman A, Witteman JC, van der Lugt A, Brusselle GG, Stricker BH. Chronic obstructive pulmonary disease and lipid core carotid artery plaques in the elderly: the Rotterdam Study. Am J Respir Crit Care Med. 2013;187(1):58–64. https://doi.org/10.1164/rccm.201206-1046OC. Epub 2012 Nov 9.
65. Houben-Wilke S, Jörres RA, Bals R, Franssen FM, Gläser S, Holle R, Karch A, Koch A, Magnussen H, Obst A, Schulz H, Spruit MA, Wacker ME, Welte T, Wouters EF, Vogelmeier C, Watz H. Peripheral artery disease and its clinical relevance in patients with chronic obstructive pulmonary disease in the COPD and systemic consequences-comorbidities network study. Am J Respir Crit Care Med. 2017;195(2):189–97.

Chapter 8
Cardiovascular Comorbidity in Chronic Lung Disease: The Role of Cardiopulmonary Exercise Testing

J. Alberto Neder, Alcides Rocha, Flavio F. Arbex, Mayron Oliveira, Maria Clara N. Alencar, and Denis E. O'Donnell

Clinical Pearls
- Cardiopulmonary exercise testing (CPET) provides unique insights into the sensory and physiological determinants of exercise intolerance in patients with chronic lung disease (e.g., COPD and ILD) and associated cardiovascular disease.
- Poor muscle O_2 delivery, impaired stroke volume, and increased ventilatory demands (i.e., "out of proportion" to emphysema burden in COPD and hypoxemia in ILD) suggest a relevant role for impaired cardiocirculatory responses to decrease exercise tolerance.
- In overlapping COPD-heart failure, CPET can determine if symptomatic patients are primarily limited by critical mechanical-ventilatory constraints (suggesting a greater role for COPD) or, alternatively, exercise is interrupted due to poor muscle O_2 delivery but preserved mechanical reserves (suggesting a dominant contribution of heart failure).
- In COPD or ILD patients with suspected or proven pulmonary hypertension at rest, severe ventilatory inefficiency, impaired intra-pulmonary gas exchange efficiency, and preserved mechanical reserves at peak exercise provide evidence that pulmonary vascular disease contributes to exercise intolerance.

J. A. Neder (✉) · D. E. O'Donnell
Laboratory of Clinical Exercise Physiology (LACEP), Queen's University & Kingston General Hospital, Kingston, ON, Canada

Respiratory Investigation UniT (RIU), Queen's University & Kingston General Hospital, Kingston, ON, Canada
e-mail: alberto.neder@queensu.ca

A. Rocha · F. F. Arbex · M. Oliveira · M. C. N. Alencar
Pulmonary Function and Clinical Exercise Physiology Unit (SEFICE), Division of Respirology, Federal University of Sao Paulo, Sao Paulo, Brazil

© Springer Nature Switzerland AG 2020
S. P. Bhatt (ed.), *Cardiac Considerations in Chronic Lung Disease*,
Respiratory Medicine, https://doi.org/10.1007/978-3-030-43435-9_8

Symbols and Abbreviations

Ca	Arterial content
Cv	Venous content
CO	Cardiac output
COPD	Chronic obstructive pulmonary disease
CPET	Cardiopulmonary exercise test
EELV	End-expiratory lung volume
EILV	End-inspiratory lung volume
f or RR	Respiratory frequency or respiratory rate
FEV_1	Forced expiratory volume in one second
HR	Heart rate
IC	Inspiratory capacity
ILD	Interstitial lung disease
IRV	Inspiratory reserve volume
LT	Lactate threshold
LVEF	Left ventricular ejection fraction
mPAP	Mean pulmonary artery pressure
MVV	Maximal voluntary ventilation
Pa	Arterial partial pressure
PA	Alveolar partial pressure
$P\bar{A}$	Mean alveolar pressure
PH	Pulmonary a hypertension
Pc	Capillary (arterialized) pressure
PE	Expiratory partial pressure
PET	End-tidal partial pressure
PFT	Pulmonary function test
RER	Respiratory exchange ratio
RV	Residual volume
Sa	Arterial saturation
Sp	Saturation by pulse oximetry
SV	Stroke volume
TLC	Total lung capacity
TL_{CO}	Transfer factor for carbon monoxide
$\dot{V}_E$	Minute ventilation
VC	Vital capacity
$\dot{V}_{CO_2}$	Carbon dioxide output
V_D	Dead space
$\dot{V}_{O_2}$	Oxygen uptake
V_T	Tidal volume
WR	Work rate

...it does not seem that all movement is exercise, but only when it is vigorous...The criterion of vigorousness is change of respiration; those movements which do not alter the respiration are not called exercise. But if anyone is compelled by any movement to breathe more or less faster, that movement becomes exercise for him.

In: Galen. A translation of Galen's hygiene (De Sanitate Tuenda) by Green RM. Charles C Thomas, Springfield, IL; 1951

Introduction

Exercise intolerance is a hallmark of chronic lung and heart disease. Effort-related symptoms, particularly dyspnea, are key clinical outcomes leading to impaired quality of life and poor survival in these patients [1]. Cardiopulmonary exercise testing (CPET) integrates a range of mechanical-ventilatory, cardiovascular, metabolic, and perceptual measurements to unravel the causes and consequences of exercise intolerance in cardiorespiratory diseases [2–5]. In symptomatic patients with chronic respiratory diseases, particularly chronic obstructive pulmonary disease (COPD) and interstitial lung disease (ILD), CPET is frequently useful to elucidate the underlying mechanisms and to quantify functional impairment [6]. The usual pattern of CPET responses in these diseases, however, can be substantially modified by comorbid cardiac and pulmonary vascular conditions. Thus, abnormalities in cardiac performance, central hemodynamics, and blood flow distribution compound with mechanical-ventilatory and gas exchange disturbances to worsen symptom burden and severely impair exercise tolerance in lung-heart disease [7].

This chapter succinctly presents how CPET interpretation in chronic lung diseases is impacted by coexistent cardiocirculatory disease. Special attention is given to translate pathophysiological concepts into clinical outcomes; thus, we critically discuss the key clinical scenarios wherein CPET might (or not) provide relevant information in these patients. We start by summarizing the normal cardiorespiratory responses to exercise. We then focus on overlapping COPD-heart failure to illustrate the devastating clinical consequences of abnormal lung mechanics and gas exchange associated with a failing heart. After briefly presenting what should be expected in a CPET performed in "isolated" COPD or heart failure, we highlight emerging concepts from recent CPET-based investigations which shed new light on the complex cardiopulmonary interactions in COPD-heart failure. We then explore the consequences of pulmonary hypertension on ventilatory control and pulmonary gas exchange efficiency during exercise in COPD and ILD. We finalize outlining some extant clinical gaps which might benefit from future CPET-based investigations.

Cardiopulmonary Adjustments to Incremental Exercise: The Basics

A rapidly incremental CPET (i.e., continuous increase in work rate (ramp) or discrete increase every 1 or 2 min) performed in cycle ergometer is the more common test format in clinical laboratories [2–5]. Thus, we will restrain our discussion to the findings observed in this testing modality, usually accompanied by serial measurements of inspiratory capacity and symptoms (Borg category-ratio scale) [8].

Respiratory Responses

The respiratory system adapts to the increased muscle metabolism by closely following its key by-product, i.e., CO_2. Thus, ventilation ($\dot{V}_E$) required to wash out a given rate of CO_2 production ($\dot{V}_{CO_2}$) is higher the lower the arterial CO_2 ($PaCO_2$) (as more $\dot{V}_E$ is needed to keep $PaCO_2$ at a low compared to a high value) and the larger the ventilation "wasted" in the dead space (V_D), i.e., [2]

$$\dot{V}_E / \dot{V}_{CO_2} \sim 1 / PaCO_2 \times \left(1 - V_D / V_T\right) \tag{8.1}$$

where $\dot{V}_E / \dot{V}_{CO_2}$ ratio is the ventilatory equivalent for CO_2 and V_D/V_T is the physiological (anatomic plus alveolar) dead space fraction of tidal volume. Efficiency of gas exchange (i.e., lower V_D/V_T) is optimized by higher V_T, enhanced ventilation/perfusion matching, and higher lung perfusion pressures due to higher cardiac output (CO) and lower pulmonary vascular resistance [9]. As discussed in Section "Cardiovascular Responses," the development of anaerobioses further stimulates $\dot{V}_E$ at higher exercise intensities [2].

Increases in $\dot{V}_E$ during exercise depend on changes in V_T and respiratory frequency (*f*). Although both V_T and *f* change almost simultaneously with activity onset, V_T expansion predominates over *f* up to the mid-stages of incremental exercise. V_T expands to about 50–60% of the vital capacity (VC) [10] by encroaching on both the inspiratory and expiratory reserve volumes [11]. Assuming that total lung capacity (TLC) does not change appreciably [12], higher inspiratory capacity (IC) on exercise means that end-expiratory lung volume (EELV) decreases due to expiratory muscle recruitment [13]. The decrease in EELV is crucial to avoid breathing too close to TLC where compliance is low and the work of breathing is high [14]. At the point of exhaustion in a normal subject, $V_T/IC < 0.7$, end-inspiratory lung volume (EILV)/TLC < 0.9, large flow reserves at a given lung volume and dyspnea scores lower than muscle effort scores indicate that the ventilatory pump is not the proximate source of exercise limitation [15]. Arterial blood typically remains well-saturated with O_2 throughout exercise in healthy subjects. Thus, exertional hypoxemia and hypercapnia are not normal features in non-trained to moderately trained younger humans.

Cardiovascular Responses

Muscle O_2 utilization during exercise increases through higher O_2 delivery (DO_2) and O_2 extraction, i.e., a wider difference between arterial and venous capacity for O_2 (CaO_2–CvO_2). The main determinant of DO_2 in non-hypoxemic subjects is cardiac output, i.e., stroke volume (SV) and heart rate (HR). Thus,

$$\dot{V}_{O_2} = \left(HR \times SV\right) \times \left(CaO_2 - CvO_2\right) \tag{8.2}$$

where $\dot{V}_{O_2}$ is the O_2 uptake. CO increases by early SV augmentation and a continuous acceleration of HR throughout exercise. Despite four- to fivefold increase in cardiac output at peak exercise, pulmonary intra-vascular pressures increase only modestly due to lower vascular resistance secondary to capillary recruitment and dilatation [3]. A large fraction of the cardiac output is redirected to the contracting peripheral muscles and, to a lesser extent, to the respiratory muscles. Extraction is maximized by decreases in hemoglobin affinity for O_2 due to lower pH and higher temperature within the exercising muscle. It follows that if the work rate increases continuously during exercise, $\dot{V}_{O_2}$ also increases linearly (Fig. 8.1).

Rearranging (Eq. 8.2) gives how much O_2 is consumed per beat:

$$\dot{V}_{O_2} / HR = SV \times \left(CaO_2 - CvO_2\right) \tag{8.3}$$

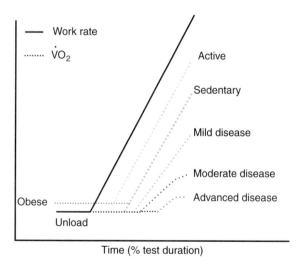

Fig. 8.1 Expected changes in oxygen uptake ($\dot{V}_{O_2}$) in response to a rapid and continuous increase in work rate ("ramp") in normal subjects and in patients with cardiocirculatory disease. Note the continuum of longer $\dot{V}_{O_2}$ delay and shallower $\dot{V}_{O_2}$ responses as disease progresses from mild to advanced stages. Although obesity is associated with increased O costs, the incremental cost of work ($\Delta \dot{V}_{O_2} / \Delta$work rate) remains unaltered. (Reproduced with permission of the publisher, from Neder et al. [80])

Thus, a low $\dot{V}_{O_2}$/HR ratio (O_2 pulse) might be secondary to central hemodynamic abnormality (low SV) and/or poor muscle ability to extract O_2 (low CaO_2–CvO_2) [4]. As exercise progresses, the rate of O_2 offered due to either low O_2 content or low blood flow might be insufficient to muscle O_2 needs. At this point, there is a shift toward anaerobic metabolism leading to lactate accumulating in arterial blood. This is called the "lactate (anaerobic) threshold," a physiological phenomenon which decreases the tolerance to further exercise [16].

CPET in Combvined COPD-Heart Failure

Key CPET Findings in COPD

In a patient with COPD, the most noticeable CPET abnormalities reflect *reduced ventilatory reserves*, *increased ventilatory demands*, *critical mechanical constraints*, and *disturbed pulmonary gas exchange* in variable combinations (Fig. 8.2) [8, 15]. These derangements may coexist with secondary evidence of impaired skeletal muscle strength and function (e.g., an early "anaerobic threshold") [17].

Reduced ventilatory reserve has been traditionally indicated by a low breathing reserve, usually expressed as an increased peak $\dot{V}_E$/maximal voluntary ventilation (MVV) ratio (>0.8) [18]. However, the proximate limitation of exercise tolerance in chronic lung disease is very often intolerable symptoms, particularly dyspnea [13]; thus, low peak $\dot{V}_E$ and apparently preserved breathing reserve may merely reflect early symptom limitation before the physiological limits of the respiratory system are reached. It follows that peak $\dot{V}_E$/MVV may underestimate the role of ventilation in limiting patients' exercise tolerance (Fig. 8.2, *panel 4*).

Increased ventilatory demand is expressed by a high submaximal $\dot{V}_E$/$\dot{V}_{CO_2}$ ratio usually due to a high physiological dead space (wasted ventilation) (Eq. 8.1). It should be emphasized, however, that increased dead space is readily translated into high $\dot{V}_E$/$\dot{V}_{CO_2}$ in patients with only mild to moderate ventilatory constraints. As the disease progresses, inspiratory constraints and higher $PaCO_2$ preclude large increases in $\dot{V}_E$/$\dot{V}_{CO_2}$ (Fig. 8.2, *panel 4*); in fact, "normal" or even low $\dot{V}_E$/$\dot{V}_{CO_2}$ might be seen in end-stage COPD (Fig. 8.2, *panel 5* and Fig. 8.3) [19].

Critical mechanical constraints (Fig. 8.2, *third row*) stem from expiratory flow limitation and the curtailing of expiratory time when *f* increases; thus, expiratory time becomes too short to allow full exhalation if airflow is slowed by airway disease and/or loss of lung elastic recoil [20]. The resulting gas trapping leads to a temporary increase in EELV above the resting value, i.e., dynamic hyperinflation [21]. As a consequence, IC decreases (Fig. 8.2, *panel 7*), and V_T happens at higher volumes, where compliance is decreased and the inspiratory muscles are functionally weakened. Thus, EILV encroaches on TLC leading to a critically reduced IRV and dynamic mechanical constraints (Fig. 8.2, *panel 8*) [22]. The high physiological and perceptual (dyspnea) "price" to further decrease IRV explains why V_T cannot further increase (note V_T plateau in Fig. 8.2, *third row*). Increased respiratory motor

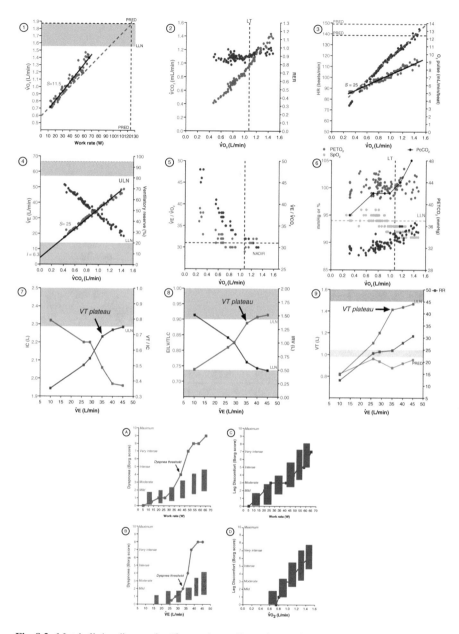

Fig. 8.2 Metabolic/cardiovascular (*first row*), ventilatory/gas exchange (*second row*), mechanical/breathing pattern (*third row*), and perceptual (*bottom graphs*) responses to incremental exercise in a 68-year-old male with COPD (FEV$_1$ = 56% predicted). See text for detailed discussion. *Definition of abbreviations and symbols*: pred predicted, LLN lower limit of normal, ULN upper limit of normal, *S* slope, *I* intercept, $\dot{V}_{O_2}$ oxygen uptake, WR work rate, $\dot{V}_{CO_2}$ carbon dioxide output, RER respiratory exchange ratio, LT estimated lactate threshold, HR heart rate, $\dot{V}_E$ minute ventilation, Pc capillary (arterialized) pressure, PET end-tidal pressure, SpO$_2$ oxyhemoglobin saturation by pulse oximetry, IC inspiratory capacity, V_T tidal volume, IRV inspiratory reserve volume, EILV end-inspiratory lung volume, TLC total lung capacity, RR respiratory rate

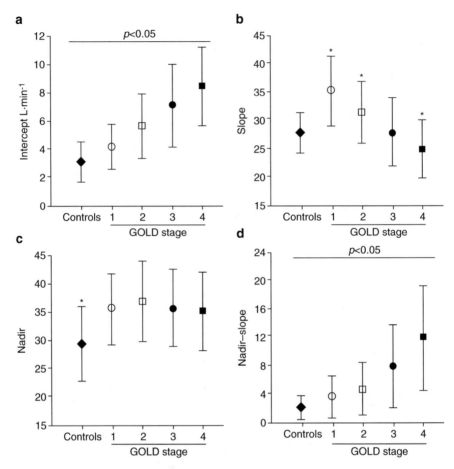

Fig. 8.3 Effects of COPD severity on markers of ventilatory efficiency during incremental exercise, i.e., ventilation ($\dot{V}_E$)-carbon dioxide output ($\dot{V}_{CO_2}$) relationship. Note that the intercept of the linear $\dot{V}_E - \dot{V}_{CO_2}$ relationship (i.e., its starting point in the $\dot{V}_E$ axis) increases as COPD progresses (**a**); in contrast, the slope decreases from GOLD 1 to GOLD 4 (**b**) (i.e., the difference between both parameters increases, (**d**)). Considering that both slope and intercept influence the $\dot{V}_E / \dot{V}_{CO_2}$ ratio at its lowest point, the latter tends to diminish from GOLD 1 to GOLD 4. See text for the practical implications of these findings. (Reproduced with permission of the publisher, from Neder et al. [19])

drive and inspiratory muscle effort which are not rewarded with chest-lung expansion explain why dyspnea increases as a function of WR and $\dot{V}_E$ at the so-called dyspnea threshold (Fig. 8.2, *bottom panels*) [23].

Disturbed pulmonary gas exchange might be demonstrated by variable degrees of (usually mild to moderate) hypoxemia and, in more severe patients, hypercapnia [8]. An estimate of mean alveolar PCO_2 (end-tidal PCO_2, $PETCO_2$) can increase (Fig. 8.2, *panel 6*) as a result of alveolar hypoventilation or late emptying of poorly ventilated units with higher PCO_2 (Fig. 8.4, *panels b, e*). Conversely, some patients

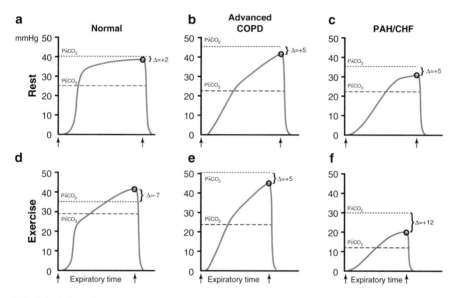

Fig. 8.4 Schematic representation of expiratory partial pressure for CO_2 ($PECO_2$) over a single breath at rest and exercise. "Δ" is the difference between mean alveolar ($\bar{A}$) and end-tidal (ET)($\circ$) partial pressures. At very early expiration, $PECO_2$ remains near zero as the first exhaled air comes from the anatomical dead space (with very low CO_2 concentration). Subsequently, $PECO_2$ increases faster: (a) the better CO_2 is washed out from mixed venous blood to the alveoli (better ventilation/perfusion matching) and (b) the more homogeneous the lungs empty. The last part of the exhaled tidal volume is less "contaminated" with the air from dead space; thus, it is biased to reflect alveolar gas which has the highest CO_2 concentration ($PETCO_2$). Resting $PETCO_2$, however, is slightly *lower* than $PaCO_2$ (and $P\bar{A}CO_2$) with their difference correlating well with wasted ventilation in both health and disease (*panels*, (**a, b, c**)). During exercise, $PETCO_2$ becomes *greater* than $PaCO_2$ in health (i.e., the $PaCO_2$-$PETCO_2$ difference becomes negative) due to the effects of (a) pulsatile increases in pulmonary perfusion with CO_2-enriched mixed venous blood, (b) faster and more homogenous lung emptying, and, importantly, (c) a larger V_T leading to greater sampling of alveolar gas (*panel* (**d**)). Less ventilated units (with high $PECO_2$) are the last to empty in COPD: this further increases $PETCO_2$ in more advanced disease (*panels* **b, e**). In the presence of impaired pulmonary blood flow (i.e., high ventilation/perfusion due to low perfusion), $PECO_2$ increases slowly, thereby leading to a lower $PETCO_2$; thus, $PaCO_2$-$PETCO_2$ difference fails to turn negative during exercise (PAH/CHF) (*panel* (**f**)). As expected, this abnormal response is worsened if a patient develops a shallow and faster breathing pattern as a relatively lesser amount of alveolar gas is sampled and expiratory time becomes too short. Additional decrements in $PETCO_2$ may occur if a patient with PAH or CHF presents with alveolar hyperventilation (*panel* (**f**))

may show normal-low $PETCO_2$ because impaired pulmonary perfusion relative to ventilation (e.g., emphysema) decreases the amount of CO_2 washed out in each breath (Fig. 8.4, *panels c, f*). Low V_T due to mechanical constraints, leading to less alveolar air sampling, may also contribute to decrease $PETCO_2$ in some patients [24].

Key CPET Findings in Heart Failure

In a non-treated patient with overt heart failure with reduced left ventricular ejection fraction, the most noticeable CPET abnormalities reflect *poor O_2 delivery, impaired SV*, and *increased ventilatory demands* (Fig. 8.5) [7].

Poor O_2 delivery secondary to low CO might lead to a downward inflection on $\dot{V}_{O_2}$ at an abnormally low work rate (Fig. 8.1 and Fig. 8.5, *panel a*). Thus, the slower rate of increase in $\dot{V}_{O_2}$ for a given change in work rate (shallow $\Delta \dot{V}_{O_2}$ / ΔWR) and a low peak WR contribute to a low peak $\dot{V}_{O_2}$ [25]. An early shift to a predominantly anaerobic metabolism is reflected by an early lactate threshold. $\dot{V}_{O_2}$ may also struggle to increase at exercise onset due to poor muscle oxidative capacity and a long circulatory delay. Similarly, $\dot{V}_{O_2}$ may take long to decrease on recovery (Fig. 8.5, *panel (g)*) [26].

Impaired SV means that HR should increase faster to increase O_2 delivery, leading to a steep ΔHR/$\Delta \dot{V}_{O_2}$ (note that this applies only to patients whose HR is not under pharmacological or external control, e.g., β-blocker (Fig. 8.5, *panels b, c*) and pacemaker, respectively). If $C(a-v)O_2$ is unable to fully compensate the low SV, low submaximal and maximal O_2 pulse can be expected. A plateau in O_2 pulse, in particular, has been associated with severe impairment in SV [27]. Some patients, however, do develop chronotropic insufficiency which indicate that CPET variables based on HR should be viewed with caution in these patients [28].

Increased ventilatory demands are not uncommon in patients with heart failure [29]. For instance, steep $\dot{V}_E - \dot{V}_{CO_2}$ slope (Fig. 8.5, *panel e*) has been related to reflex mechanisms (central and peripheral chemoreflexes, muscle metaboreflex, Bainbridge reflex) associated with sympathetic activation leading to a downward shift of the CO_2 set point. Higher V_D/V_T with a shallow breathing pattern may reflect the combined effects of impaired pulmonary perfusion, increased areas of ventilation/perfusion, and the restrictive effects of heart failure [30]. These abnormalities may jointly explain why $PETCO_2$ decreases as the disease evolves (Figure 8.4, *panels c, f*). A minority of patients with heart failure present with decrements in IC during exercise which might represent true dynamic hyperinflation or exercise-induced respiratory muscle weakness [31]. Another important CPET finding with ominous prognostic implications is exercise oscillatory ventilation (Fig. 8.5, *panels d, h, i*), a pattern of cyclic variations in $\dot{V}_E$, due to elevated left heart filling pressures, increased CO_2 chemosensitivity, and prolonged circulatory time [32].

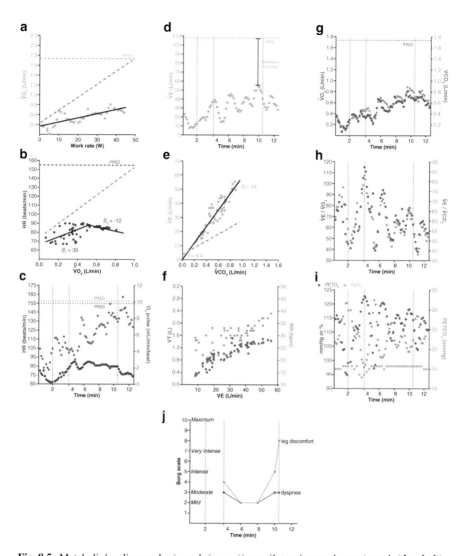

Fig. 8.5 Metabolic/cardiovascular (*panels* (**a–c**, **g**)), ventilatory/gas exchange (*panels* (**d**, **e**, **h**, **i**)), breathing pattern (*panel* (**f**)), and perceptual (*bottom graph*) responses to incremental exercise in a 68-year-old male with heart failure with reduced left ventricular ejection fraction (LVEF = 26% predicted). Note the presence of exertional oscillatory ventilation (EOV) (*panel* (**d**)) leading to cyclic fluctuations in expired gas tensions (*panel* (**i**)). Inspiratory capacity was not measured during exercise precluding assessment of non-invasive mechanics. See text for detailed discussion. *Definition of abbreviations and symbols*: pred predicted, *S* slope, *I* intercept, $\dot{V}_{O_2}$ oxygen uptake, WR work rate, $\dot{V}_{CO_2}$ carbon dioxide output, HR heart rate, $\dot{V}_E$ minute ventilation, PET end-tidal pressure, SpO$_2$ oxyhemoglobin saturation by pulse oximetry, V_T tidal volume, RR respiratory rate

Conflating Cardiopulmonary Abnormalities in COPD-Heart Failure

Among the cardiovascular comorbidities of COPD, there is growing interest in heart failure with reduced left ventricular ejection fraction (LVEF). The prevalence of overlapping COPD-heart failure varies from 9% to 33% [33–37] depending on the availability of pulmonary function tests, local practices regarding heart failure screening by trans-thoracic echocardiography in advanced COPD, definition criteria for each disease, and, in particular, whether the patients have been primarily seen by pulmonologists or cardiologists. Regardless of the actual prevalence, it is out of debate that incident heart failure carries a dismal prognosis in patients with COPD [33, 35]. The opposite, i.e., the impact of a "new" diagnosis of COPD in a patient with established heart failure, remains controversial – particularly in patients with less severe heart failure [38].

Nevertheless, it is now well-established that COPD-heart failure patients present with higher symptom burden, lower exercise tolerance, and poorer quality of life than their counterparts with COPD or heart failure with similar resting functional impairment [33–39]. In this context, there is a strong appeal for CPET in overlapping COPD-heart failure as, by definition, it carries the highest risk for negative cardiopulmonary interactions under the stress of exercise. Unfortunately, however, we are only starting to understand those complex interactions and their systemic consequences. It follows that much needs to be discovered, an enterprise that might greatly benefit from clinical physiology investigations (see 6 "Unanswered Questions").

Ventilatory Control and Gas Exchange

There is mounting evidence that the coexistence of heart failure in patients with COPD is associated with $\dot{V}_E - \dot{V}_{CO_2}$ values that are significantly higher than expected by the severity of resting ventilatory abnormalities (Fig. 8.6 for a representative patient and Fig. 8.7) [40–42]. Notably, however, there is a large variability in the $\dot{V}_E - \dot{V}_{CO_2}$ relationship regardless of the chosen metrics (i.e., $\dot{V}_E - \dot{V}_{CO_2}$ slope or $\dot{V}_E / \dot{V}_{CO_2}$ nadir) (Fig. 8.8) [40, 41]. In order to uncover the underlying mechanisms, we measured PCO_2 in arterialized (capillary, c) blood allowing V_D/V_T calculation. Our results demonstrated that the key abnormality leading to higher $\dot{V}_E - \dot{V}_{CO_2}$ values in a subset of patients (Fig. 8.9, *panel b*) was *not* a particularly high V_D/V_T (Fig. 8.9, *panel c*) but a low $PcCO_2$ set point (Fig. 8.9, *panel e*) [43]. This suggests a chronically increased drive to breathe which led to a ventilatory response beyond that required to wash out metabolically produced CO_2 and overcome an enlarged physiological dead space. Strictly from the gas exchange perspective, this strategy was beneficial as patients maintained better arterial oxygenation (Fig. 8.9, *panel e*) than their counterparts despite similar (in)efficiency in intra-pulmonary oxygenation. Thus, it is conceivable that the heightened ventilatory drive which led

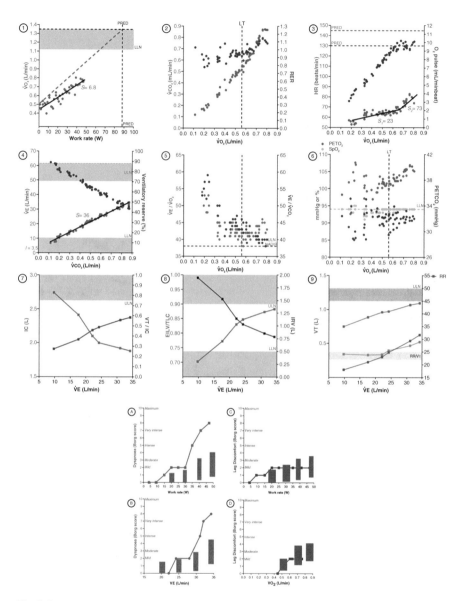

Fig. 8.6 Metabolic/cardiovascular (*first row*), ventilatory/gas exchange (*second row*), mechanical/breathing pattern (*third row*), and perceptual (*bottom graphs*) responses to incremental exercise in a 74-year-old male with COPD (FEV$_1$ = 58% predicted)-heart failure (LVEF = 34%). See text for detailed discussion. *Definition of abbreviations and symbols*: pred predicted, LLN lower limit of normal, ULN upper limit of normal, S slope, I intercept, $\dot{V}_{O_2}$ oxygen uptake, WR work rate, $\dot{V}_{CO_2}$ carbon dioxide output, RER respiratory exchange ratio, LT estimated lactate threshold, HR heart rate, $\dot{V}_E$ minute ventilation, Pc capillary (arterialized) pressure, PET end-tidal pressure, SpO$_2$ oxyhemoglobin saturation by pulse oximetry, IC inspiratory capacity, V_T tidal volume, IRV inspiratory reserve volume, EILV end-inspiratory lung volume, TLC total lung capacity, RR respiratory rate

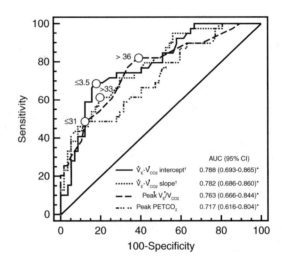

Fig. 8.7 Receiver operating characteristic (ROC) curve analysis showing the best CPET variables able to discriminate patients with combined COPD-heart failure from those with COPD alone. Circles depict the optimal thresholds according to individual variables. Note that these variables reflect poor ventilatory and gas exchange efficiency. * $P < 0.05$. † $P < 0.05$ vs. peak PETCO$_2$. *Abbreviations*: AUC area under the curve, CI confidence interval, $\dot{V}_E$ ventilation, $\dot{V}_{CO_2}$ carbon dioxide output, PET end-tidal partial pressure. (Reproduced with permission of the publisher, from Arbex et al. [41])

to alveolar hyperventilation and better arterial oxygenation is part of a concerted systemic response to improve tissue O$_2$ delivery in the face of a failing heart [44]. PETCO$_2$ frequently does not increase with exercise progression in COPD-heart failure (compare PETCO$_2$ trajectory in *panel 6*, Fig. 8.6 (COPD-heart failure) versus *panel 6*, Fig. 8.2 (COPD)) due to the combining effects of low PaCO$_2$ set point and worse pulmonary perfusion (Fig. 8.4, *panels c, f*).

Heart failure-related sympathetic overstimulation, lactic acidosis, and increased stimulation or enhanced sensitivity of central chemoreceptors and peripheral muscle ergoreceptors might be involved in the exacerbated ventilatory response shown by the hypocapnic group in Fig. 8.9 [45]. Higher resting tricuspid annular plane systolic excursion/pulmonary artery systolic pressure ratio suggests worse right ventricle-pulmonary circulation uncoupling [46] due to higher afferent stimulation from cardiopulmonary receptors in patients with higher exertional pulmonary arterial pressures [47]. Greater emphysema burden may have also contributed to higher pulmonary vascular resistance [48] and overstimulation of stretch receptors in the right heart chambers (Bainbridge reflex) leading to hyperventilation. Low transfer factor for carbon monoxide in patients with higher $\dot{V}_E - \dot{V}_{CO_2}$ and hypocapnia are consistent with those hypotheses [49]. The former, in particular, may decline with even moderate lung congestion (Fig. 8.10), being associated with poorer prognosis in heart failure [50]. It remains to be explored whether the association of COPD and heart failure decreases transfer factor beyond the expected values for underlying emphysema burden. If so, this might enhance its prognostic role in this specific sub-population of patients with COPD [33].

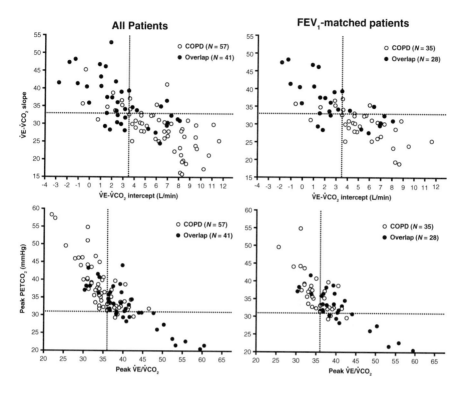

Fig. 8.8 Ventilation ($\dot{V}_E$)-CO_2 output ($\dot{V}_{CO_2}$) slope versus intercept (upper *panels*) and end-tidal partial pressure for CO_2 (PETCO$_2$) versus peak $\dot{V}_E / \dot{V}_{CO_2}$ ratio in COPD and combined COPD-heart failure ("overlap"). Dotted lines indicate the optimal thresholds for "overlap" discrimination as established by the ROC curve analysis (Fig. 8.7). (Reproduced with permission of the publisher, from Arbex et al. [41])

Lung Mechanics

The effects of heart failure on resting pulmonary function have been extensively investigated and recently reviewed in ref. [51]. Although patients with decompensated heart failure commonly present with airflow limitation, the disease tends to reduce the "static" lung volumes in COPD, particularly TLC and functional residual capacity (FRC) [52]. In a stable patient, those decrements are roughly similar which tends to somewhat "preserve" IC (Fig. 8.11) [53]. Of note, residual volume (RV) remains elevated in COPD-heart failure [54]; in fact, RV > 120% predicted has been found the most consistent finding in patients with COPD-heart failure [55] (Fig. 8.12). It follows that expiratory reserve volume is severely reduced. In practice, however, it is not uncommon to find patients with low RV (and TLC) due to associated morbid obesity [56]. Particularly low TLC values are seen in the presence of severe cardiomegaly and long-term lung congestion, leading to pronounced decrements in VC and IC (Fig. 8.10) [57]. Low (F)VC and increased lung elastic recoil may result in reduction in both FEV$_1$ and FVC leading to a pseudo-normal

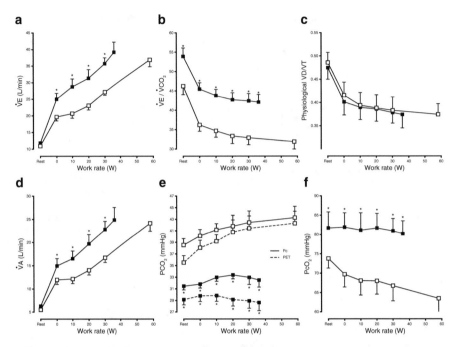

Fig. 8.9 Ventilatory (*panels* (**a–d**)) and pulmonary gas exchange (*panels* (**e, f**)) responses to incremental cardiopulmonary exercise testing in COPD-heart failure patients separated by presence ($N = 10$) or not ($N = 12$) of exercise hypocapnia (*closed symbols* and *open symbols*, respectively). * $P < 0.05$ for between-group comparisons at rest, standardized work rates, and the highest work rate attained by all subjects in a given group. Values are means ± SEM. *Abbreviations*: V_D/V_T dead space/tidal volume ratio, $\dot{V}_A$ alveolar ventilation, Pc capillary (arterialized) partial pressure, PET end-tidal partial pressure. (Reproduced with permission of the publisher, from Rocha et al. [43])

FEV$_1$/FVC ratio, i.e., the non-specific pattern of ventilatory dysfunction [58]. Thus, FEV$_1$ alone may overestimate the functional severity of COPD in some patients with combined COPD-heart failure [55].

Evaluation of operating lung volumes by serial exercise IC maneuvers is fraught with complexities in COPD-heart failure. It remains unclear, for instance, whether TLC actually remains stable during exercise in these patients [12]. For instance, TLC might decrease in some patients who develop exercise-induced pulmonary congestion. Patients with COPD-heart failure might present with greater inspiratory muscle weakness than their counterparts with either disease on isolation [59]. This casts doubt on whether they are able to fully activate their inspiratory muscles as exercise progresses. Despite those concerns, limited evidence demonstrates that IC either remains unaltered or decreases (Fig. 8.6, *panel 7*, and Fig. 8.13, *panel d*), thereby reducing the limits for V_T expansion [43]. Earlier attainment of critical mechanical constraints (higher V_T/IC ratio and low IRV) was found in patients with higher $\dot{V}_E / \dot{V}_{CO_2}$ (Fig. 8.13) [43] and exertional oscillatory ventilation (Fig. 8.14) [94]. Under this unfavorable combination of circumstances (high neural drive and

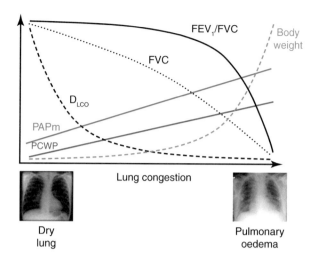

Fig. 8.10 Schematic representation of potential trajectories of lung function, hemodynamics, and body weight with lung congestion in heart failure. DL_{CO} diffusing capacity for carbon monoxide, FEV_1 forced expiratory volume in the first second, FVC forced vital capacity, PAPm mean pulmonary artery pressure, PCWP pulmonary capillary wedge pressure. (Reproduced with permission of the publisher, from Magnussen et al. [51])

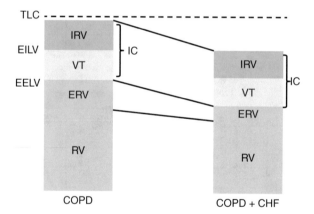

Fig. 8.11 Lung volumes and capacities expressed as absolute values (**a**) and corrected for differences in total lung capacity (**b**) in patients with COPD only and in those with combined COPD and chronic heart failure (CHF). TLC total lung capacity, RV residual volume, ERV expiratory reserve volume, V_T tidal volume, IRV inspiratory reserve volume, FRC functional residual capacity, EILV end-inspiratory lung volume, IC inspiratory capacity. (Modified with permission of the publisher, from de Souza et al. [53])

neuromechanical dissociation) [1], it is not surprising that these patients reported higher dyspnea for a given work rate and $\dot{V}_E$ (Fig. 8.6, *bottom panels*). It follows that therapeutic attempts to increase the "ceiling" for V_T expansion (e.g., increasing TLC by improving lung congestion and inspiratory muscle weakness) and/or to

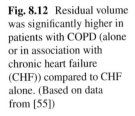

Fig. 8.12 Residual volume was significantly higher in patients with COPD (alone or in association with chronic heart failure (CHF)) compared to CHF alone. (Based on data from [55])

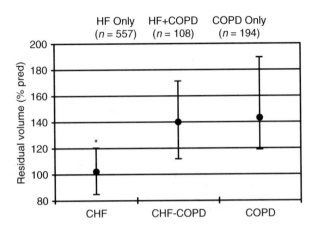

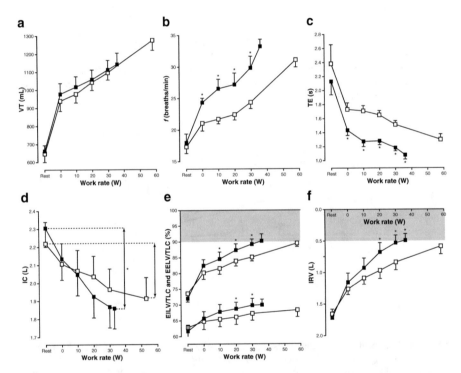

Fig. 8.13 Pattern and timing of breathing (*panels* (**a–c**)) and operating lung volume (*panels* (**d–f**)) during incremental exercise in cardiopulmonary exercise testing in COPD-heart failure patients separated by presence ($N = 10$) or not ($N = 12$) of exercise hypocapnia (*closed symbols* and *open symbols*, respectively). Shadowed areas in *panels* (**e**) and (**f**) represent the volumes typically associated with critical inspiratory constraints in COPD [30, 45]. * $P < 0.05$ for between-group comparisons at rest, standardized work rates, and the highest work rate attained by all subjects in a given group. Values are means ± SEM. *Abbreviations*: V_T tidal volume, f respiratory rate, IC inspiratory capacity, EILV end-inspiratory lung volume, EELV end-expiratory lung volume, TLC total lung capacity, IRV inspiratory reserve volume. (Reproduced with permission of the publisher, from Rocha et al. [43])

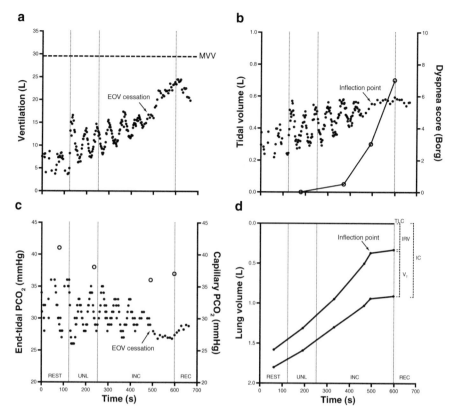

Fig. 8.14 Physiological and perceptual responses to incremental exercise in a representative patient with heart failure-COPD (female, age = 63 yrs, height = 146 cm) presenting with exercise oscillatory ventilation (EOV). *Abbreviations*: MVV maximal voluntary ventilation, TLC total lung capacity, IRV inspiratory reserve volume, V_T tidal volume, IC inspiratory capacity. (Reproduced with permission of the publisher, from Rocha et al. [94])

decrease its "floor" (i.e., decreasing EELV by reducing expiratory flow limitation and *f*) in association with less afferent ventilatory stimuli (e.g., heart failure treatment optimization) might positively impact on patient's activity–related dyspnea.

Central and Peripheral Hemodynamics

Non-invasive CPET (i.e., without concomitant cardiac catheterization) is ill-suited to expose the potential hemodynamic consequences of negative cardiopulmonary interactions in COPD-heart failure (Fig. 8.15) [60]. For instance, crude estimates of SV behavior (i.e., O_2 pulse) are likely invalid if HR is under pharmacological modulation (β-blockers) (Figure 8.5, *panels b* and *c*) and/or suffering the consequences of loss or desensitization of cardiac $β_1$ receptors (heart failure-related chronotropic incompetence [28]). In fact, SV alone may not provide the complete picture of underlying

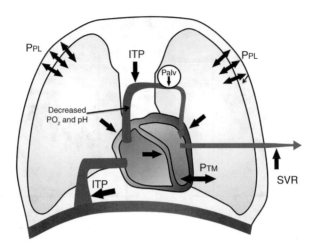

Fig. 8.15 Schematic representation of potential negative cardiopulmonary interactions in moderate to severe COPD which could be further worsened by the coexisted with heart failure with reduced left ventricular ejection fraction. Increases in mean intra-thoracic pressure (ITP) and large swings in pleural pressure (P_{PL}) may reduce venous return and right ventricular (RV) preload. High P_{PL} swings, compression of juxta-alveolar capillaries, and hypoxic vasoconstriction increase RV afterload and intra-cavitary pressures. The latter occurrence, in association with extrinsic compression of the right heart by the overdistended lungs, can impair RV relaxation and displace the inter-ventricular septum to the left. Reduced left heart filling pressures and dimensions may contribute to further impairments in stroke volume (SV). Large P_{PL} swings can also increase left ventricular (LV) afterload secondary to high transmural pressures (P_{TM}). Moreover, decreased aortic impedance and augmented systemic vascular resistance (SVR) further increase LV afterload, thus compromising cardiac output. Of note, the relative contribution of each of the above factors is likely to vary according to different phases of respiratory and cardiac cycles. (Reproduced with permission of the publisher, from Oliveira et al. [77])

abnormalities. For instance, patient's dyspnea might still be influenced by heart failure if a "normal" SV is maintained at expenses of high left ventricular filling pressures [61].

Under the light of those important limitations, a non-invasive CPET study which measured SV by signal-morphology cardio-impedance found lower $\Delta CO/\Delta \dot{V}_{O_2}$ relationship in COPD-heart failure compared with isolated heart failure despite similar resting LVEF (Fig. 8.16, *panels a, b*) [62]. These data suggest that some of negative cardiopulmonary interactions outlined in Fig. 8.15 contributed to further impair cardiac output in the former group. Of note, low leg muscle oxygenation [63, 64] and excessive lactate production (Fig. 8.17, *panels c, d, e,f*) worsened in tandem with dynamic abnormalities in cardiac output and peripheral blood flow (Fig. 8.16. *panels c, d, e, f*) leading to higher ratings of leg effort on exercise in COPD-heart failure compared to COPD alone [62]. Considering the lack of hypoxemia [62], these data lend support to the notion that central hemodynamic abnormalities in COPD-heart failure are instrumental to further decrease muscle blood flow under the stress of exercise [63, 64]. Interestingly, inspiratory muscles overloading also decreased leg muscle perfusion in these patients [65], likely a consequence of heightened sympathetic over-excitation [59] (Fig. 8.18). Peripheral arterial disease

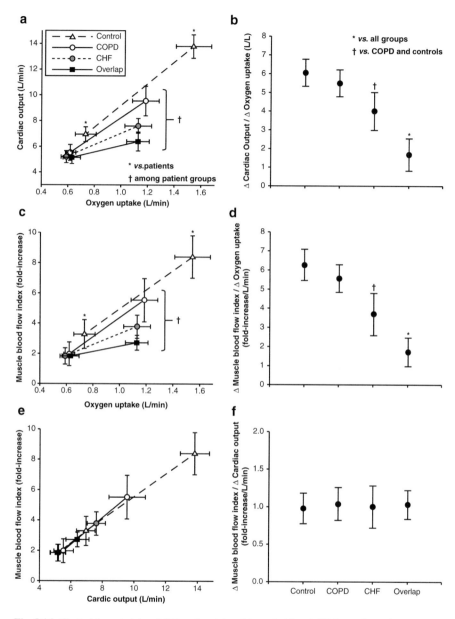

Fig. 8.16 Central (*panels* (**a**) and (**b**)) and peripheral (*panels* (**c**) and (**d**)) hemodynamic responses as a function of exercise intensity and their relationship (*panels* (**e**) and (**f**)) in healthy controls and patients with chronic obstructive pulmonary disease (COPD), chronic heart failure (CHF), and COPD-CHF (overlap). "Δ"is the difference between 20% and 80% peak work rate. (Reproduced with permission of the publisher, from Oliveira et al. [62])

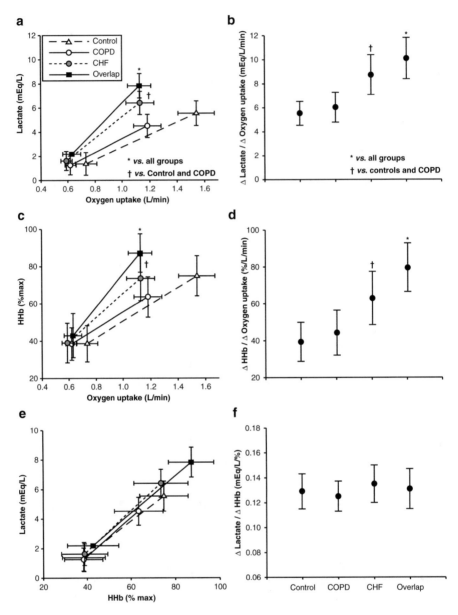

Fig. 8.17 Blood lactate concentration (*panels* (**a**), (**b**), (**e**) and (**f**)), and muscle deoxygenation (HHb) (*panels* (**c**) and (**d**)) as a function of exercise intensity in healthy controls and patients with chronic obstructive pulmonary disease (COPD), chronic heart failure (CHF), and COPD-CHF (overlap). "Δ"is the difference between 20% and 80% peak work rate. (Reproduced with permission of the publisher, from Oliveira et al. [62])

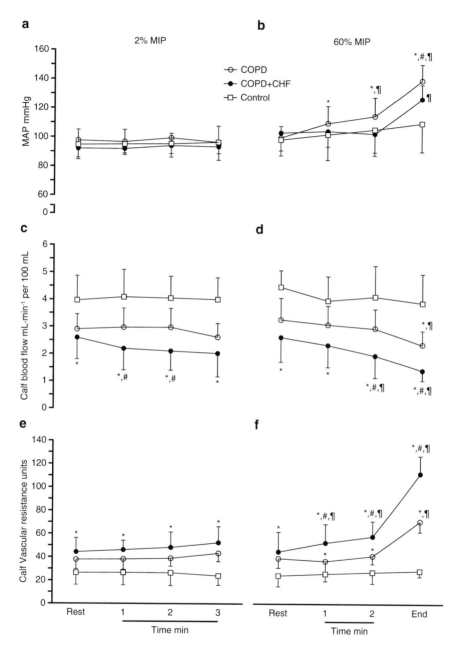

Fig. 8.18 Central (*panels* (**a**) and (**b**)) and peripheral (*panels* (**c**), (**d**), (**e**) and (**f**)) hemodynamic responses to inspiratory resistive loading set at 2% (sham) and 60% maximal inspiratory pressure (MIP) in patients with chronic obstructive pulmonary disease (COPD) or COPD plus chronic heart failure (CHF) and healthy controls. The 2% MIP trials lasted 3 min in all participants. Compared with controls, however, the 60% trials were significantly shorter in the COPD plus CHF group compared with COPD alone and controls, respectively (see main text for actual values). Data are presented as mean ± sd. MAP: mean arterial blood pressure. *: $p < 0.05$, COPD plus CHF or COPD versus controls; #: $p < 0.05$, COPD plus CHF versus COPD; ¶: $p < 0.05$, within-group difference from rest. (Reproduced with permission from the publisher, from: Chiappa et al. [65])

(including diabetes related) [66], which is more common in COPD-heart failure than COPD or heart failure alone [67], might worsen those abnormalities. It follows that rehabilitation strategies aimed at improving peripheral muscle capillarization and bioenergetics might be particularly valuable to improve exercise tolerance in these patients [44].

Cerebral Blood Flow

Cerebral muscle perfusion and oxygenation are paramount to normal muscle activation during exercise [68]. Despite the presence of powerful autoregulation mechanisms, brain blood flow (particularly through the small arterioles) is frequently impaired in heart failure [69]. In COPD-heart failure, Oliveira et al. [70] found that despite better preserved arterial oxygenation compared with COPD alone (Fig. 8.19, panel b)), the former group had poorer pre-frontal cortical oxygenation (Fig. 8.19, panel a)). As expected, this was associated with impaired central hemodynamics (low CO and low mean arterial pressure) (Fig. 8.19, panels c, d)); surprisingly, however, the closest correlate of poorer microvascular cerebral blood flow [71] (Fig. 8.20, panels c, d) was a low $PaCO_2$ (CO_2 is a potent cerebral vasodilator) (Fig. 8.20, panel b).

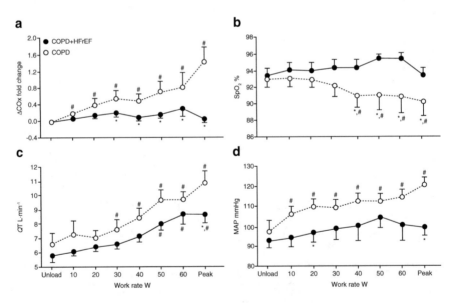

Fig. 8.19 Changes in (**a**) pre-frontal cerebral oxygenation (ΔCOx), (**b**) arterial oxygen saturation measured by pulse oximetry (S_{pO2}), (**c**) cardiac output (Q_T), and (**d**) mean arterial pressure (MAP) as a function of exercise intensity in chronic obstructive pulmonary disease (COPD) patients with or without heart failure with reduced ejection fraction (HFrEF) as comorbidity. Data are presented as mean ± se. *: $p < 0.05$ for between-group comparisons; #: $p < 0.05$ for intragroup comparisons against unloaded cycling. (Reproduced with permission from the publisher, from: Oliveira et al. [70])

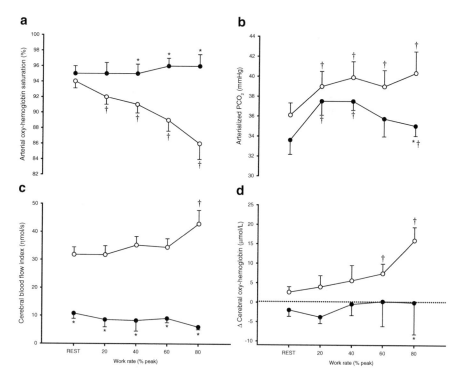

Fig. 8.20 Arterial oxygen saturation (**a**), arterialized partial pressure of carbon dioxide (**b**), and cerebral blood flow (**c**) and oxygenation (**d**) as a function of exercise intensity in COPD (*open symbols*) and COPD-heart failure (*closed symbols*). *Between-group differences at a given time point; † intragroup differences versus rest. (Reproduced with permission from the publisher, from: Oliveira et al. [71])

In this context, chronic hypocapnia has been found to impair cerebrovascular reactivity to CO_2 which is crucial to main pH relatively constant near the central chemoreceptors [72]. It follows that a blunted cerebrovascular reactivity to CO_2 might add to the stimulation of the central chemoreflex by avoiding adequate CO_2 washout [68]. This might constitute a self-perpetuating mechanism that contributes to the chronic hyperventilation effects of a low CO_2 set point [73]. The results of Oliveira et al. [71] indicating impaired cerebral perfusion and hypocapnia (Fig. 8.20) in conjunction with the findings of Rocha et al. [43] showing a strong association between low $PcCO_2$ and high $\dot{V}_E / \dot{V}_{CO_2}$ (Fig. 8.9) raise the prospect of a putative link between hypocapnia, impaired cerebrovascular reactivity to CO_2 [74], and excess exercise ventilation in COPD-heart failure [41]. Of note, poor cerebral oxygenation has been associated with low exercise tolerance in heart failure [69] and pulmonary arterial hypertension [75]. The potential contribution of reduced motor activation due to cerebral hypoxia ("central fatigue") [76] remains open to investigation in COPD-heart failure. A comprehensive discussion of the topic is provided in Ref. [77].

CPET in Pulmonary Hypertension Secondary to Chronic Respiratory Diseases

High pulmonary arterial pressures might develop on exercise in patients with COPD and ILD due to the combined effects of alveolar hypoxia (worse in ILD), microvascular destruction (or compression in COPD), and lower V_T [78]. Pulmonary hypertension secondary to hypoxemia is more likely to be seen in patients who present with exertional SaO_2 below 88% [78]. Due to the sigmoid shape of the O_2 dissociation curve, however, appreciable decrements in PaO_2 (a closer correlate of pulmonary arterial pressures than SaO_2) [78] may be occasionally missed by the isolated measurement of SaO_2 or SpO_2.

Patients with combined pulmonary fibrosis and emphysema (CPFE) are particularly prone to develop pulmonary hypertension (PH) [79]. Impaired pulmonary perfusion and larger areas of high alveolar ventilation ($\dot{V}_A$)/lung capillary perfusion (Qc) are expected to increase the amount of ventilation wasted in the physiological V_D leading to high $\dot{V}_E / \dot{V}_{CO_2}$ and low PETCO$_2$ (Fig. 8.4, *panels e, f*) [80]. Increased neural drive due to heightened afferent stimulation from pulmonary artery or cardiopulmonary receptors may also contribute as well as higher sympathetic drive and increased ergoreceptor stimulation [81]. In line with these considerations, there is growing evidence that a subset of patients with COPD who present with higher $\dot{V}_E / \dot{V}_{CO_2}$ and lower PETCO$_2$ develop higher pulmonary arterial pressures on exercise [81, 82]. If pulmonary hypertension (PH) is not yet apparent at rest, these patients are at greater risk of developing those abnormalities even without the stress of exercise. There is a trend of COPD patients with severe PH (resting mean mPAP ≥ 40 mm Hg) to stop exercise with more preserved ventilatory reserves (at least when estimated by the $\dot{V}_E$/MVV ratio) and "exhausted" cardiocirculatory reserves [78].

Clinical Application of CPET in Combined Lung-Heart Disease

Currently, the most obvious application of CPET in chronic lung disease at risk of cardiovascular complications relates to the search for physiological abnormalities suggestive of poor muscle O_2 delivery, impaired SV, and increased ventilatory demands which are deemed "out of proportion" to the severity of underlying respiratory disease, e.g., emphysema burden in COPD and hypoxemia in ILD. It should be recognized, however, the lack of unequivocal cutoffs to define what can be considered "out of proportion" in individual patients.

In COPD-heart failure, CPET is valuable to determine if symptomatic patients are primarily limited by critical mechanical-ventilatory constraints and hypoxemia (suggesting a greater role for COPD) or, alternatively, exercise is interrupted due to complaints of severe leg discomfort and preserved mechanical reserves (suggesting a dominant contribution of heart failure). This might impact on clinical decision-making vis-à-vis optimization and step-up of COPD or heart failure treatment. CPET results indicating excess exercise ventilation (high $\dot{V}_E / \dot{V}_{CO_2}$, low PETCO$_2$) when accompanied by hypocapnia and low transfer factor are associated with severe exertional dyspnea leading to poorer exercise tolerance [43]. Accordingly, it seems advisable that these patients are prioritized to closer follow-up and early rehabilitation. In fact, high $\dot{V}_E / \dot{V}_{CO_2}$ and low PETCO$_2$ emerged as useful predictors (in association with resting echocardiographic evidences of right ventricular strain) of poor prognosis in these patients (Fig. 8.21) [42]. In COPD or ILD patients with suspected or established PH at rest, severe ventilatory inefficiency, low PETCO$_2$ with positive P(a-ET)CO$_2$, low SpO$_2$, and preserved mechanical reserves at peak exercise provide objective evidence that pulmonary vascular disease is contributing to patient's exercise intolerance.

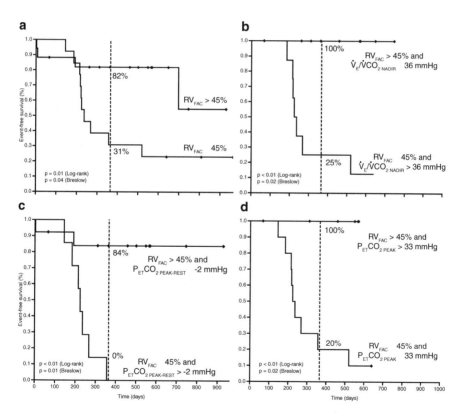

Fig. 8.21 Kaplan-Meier survival curves for (**a**) resting right ventricular fractional area change (RV$_{FAC}$) by echocardiography, (**b**) RV$_{FAC}$ plus exercise ventilation ($\dot{V}_E / \dot{V}_{CO_2}$) ratio at its lowest point during incremental CPET (nadir), (**c**) RV FAC plus peak exercise rest differences (Δ) in end-tidal partial pressure for CO$_2$ (PETCO$_2$), and (**d**) RV$_{FAC}$ plus PETCO$_2$ at peak exercise. Optimal thresholds were established by receiver-operating characteristics (ROC) curve analyses. (Reproduced with permission from the publisher, from: Alencar [42])

Unanswered Questions

We are only beginning to appreciate the potential clinical usefulness of CPET in combined lung-heart disease. Thus, the unanswered questions largely outnumber what has been learned in the past decade. Obviously, the individual contribution of COPD or heart failure to their combination varies markedly between subjects and so their impact on the mechanisms of exercise intolerance. For instance, we do not know if dyspnea and exercise intolerance parallel the progression of each disease in the same fashion. Based on available data from each disease in isolation, this seems unlikely. In this context, CPET might provide important clues regarding to those at greater risk of progressing to disabling dyspnea. Despite almost a century of interest in cardiopulmonary interactions, very little is known of how heart failure modulates the potential central hemodynamic consequences of COPD (Fig. 8.15). For instance, are the negative consequences of COPD on RV afterload particularly critical in combined COPD-heart failure? In fact, the combination of a left-shifted septum, disturbed ventricular interdependence, and low RV stroke volume might dynamically change the LV pre-load on exercise – with marked deleterious effects on the cardiac output.

It is important to develop milder, submaximal (constant load) tests in uncovering abnormalities in such severely disabled patients [83–85]. At least in those with COPD alone, poor ventilatory efficiency and low $PETCO_2$ are also seen during minimal, unloaded exercise and, occasionally, at rest [86]. Thus, if these variables also prove useful in these tests, we might not need to expose such frail patients to the discomfort and risks of progressive exercise. They might also prove helpful to indicate increased ventilatory drive secondary to high pulmonary venous pressures in COPD patients with (moderate to severe) diastolic dysfunction, left atrial enlargement, or atrial fibrillation.

Alone atrial fibrillation, in particular, has been associated with sympathetic over-excitation leading to high afferent ventilatory stimuli and dyspnea, likely from an hyper-activated ergoreflex [87]; interestingly, this remained true even when HR is "controlled" [87]. Does it mean that decreasing HR with atrial fibrillation might not be sufficient to substantially improve exertional dyspnea in COPD patients, i.e., should cardioversion or ablation be used more liberally in these patients? Assuming that persistent atrial fibrillation may also lead to lung congestion on exertion [88], it is conceivable that the retrograde transmission of increased left atrial filling pressures is higher in patients with more extensive destruction of the lung (micro)vasculature [89]. This might also apply to heart failure with preserved LVEF where marked elevations in LV filling pressures on exercise [90] coexist with high $\dot{V}_E / \dot{V}_{CO_2}$ [91]. If so, COPD patients presenting with the emphysema phenotype might be particularly sensitive to relatively modest increases in pulmonary venous pressures [89]. It is conceivable that most of these questions could only be satisfactorily answered by combining CPET with minimally invasive (e.g., arterialized capillary blood) [92] or non-invasive (exercise echocardiography) [93] techniques in large, multi-centric studies, i.e., an epi-physiologic approach to interrogate those highly variable biological phenomena.

References

1. Mahler DA, O'Donnell DE. Recent advances in dyspnea. Chest. 2015;147(1):232–41.
2. Whipp BJ. The bioenergetic and gas exchange basis of exercise testing. Clin Chest Med. 1994;15(2):173–92.
3. American Thoracic Society, American College of Chest Physicians. ATS/ACCP statement on cardiopulmonary exercise testing. Am J Respir Crit Care Med. 2003;167(2):211–77.
4. ERS Task Force, Palange P, Ward SA, Carlsen K-H, Casaburi R, Gallagher CG, et al. Recommendations on the use of exercise testing in clinical practice. Eur Respir J. 2007;29(1):185–209.
5. Guazzi M, Arena R, Halle M, Piepoli MF, Myers J, Lavie CJ. 2016 focused update: clinical recommendations for cardiopulmonary exercise testing data assessment in specific patient populations. Circulation. 2016;133(24):e694–711.
6. O'Donnell DE, Elbehairy AF, Berton DC, Domnik NJ, Neder JA. Advances in the evaluation of respiratory pathophysiology during exercise in chronic lung diseases. Front Physiol. 2017;8:82.
7. Arena R, Sietsema KE. Cardiopulmonary exercise testing in the clinical evaluation of patients with heart and lung disease. Circulation. 2011;123(6):668–80.
8. O'Donnell DE, Laveneziana P, Webb K, Neder JA. Chronic obstructive pulmonary disease: clinical integrative physiology. Clin Chest Med. 2014;35(1):51–69.
9. Neder J, Nery L. Clinical exercise physiology: theory and practice [in Portuguese]. Sao Paulo: Artes Medicas; 2002. 404 p.
10. Neder JA, Dal Corso S, Malaguti C, Reis S, De Fuccio MB, Schmidt H, et al. The pattern and timing of breathing during incremental exercise: a normative study. Eur Respir J. 2003;21(3):530–8.
11. Johnson BD, Weisman IM, Zeballos RJ, Beck KC. Emerging concepts in the evaluation of ventilatory limitation during exercise: the exercise tidal flow-volume loop. Chest. 1999;116(2):488–503.
12. Stubbing DG, Pengelly LD, Morse JL, Jones NL. Pulmonary mechanics during exercise in subjects with chronic airflow obstruction. J Appl Physiol. 1980;49(3):511–5.
13. O'Donnell DE, Hamilton AL, Webb KA. Sensory-mechanical relationships during high-intensity, constant-work-rate exercise in COPD. J Appl Physiol Bethesda Md 1985. 2006;101(4):1025–35.
14. Potter WA, Olafsson S, Hyatt RE. Ventilatory mechanics and expiratory flow limitation during exercise in patients with obstructive lung disease. J Clin Invest. 1971;50(4):910–9.
15. O'Donnell DE, Elbehairy AF, Faisal A, Webb KA, Neder JA, Mahler DA. Exertional dyspnoea in COPD: the clinical utility of cardiopulmonary exercise testing. Eur Respir Rev. 2016;25(141):333–47.
16. Wasserman K, Whipp BJ, Koyl SN, Beaver WL. Anaerobic threshold and respiratory gas exchange during exercise. J Appl Physiol. 1973;35(2):236–43.
17. Maltais F, Decramer M, Casaburi R, Barreiro E, Burelle Y, Debigaré R, et al. An official American Thoracic Society/European Respiratory Society statement: update on limb muscle dysfunction in chronic obstructive pulmonary disease. Am J Respir Crit Care Med. 2014;189(9):e15–62.
18. Wasserman K, Whipp BJ. Exercise physiology in health and disease. Am Rev Respir Dis. 1975;112(2):219–49.
19. Neder JA, Arbex FF, Alencar MCN, O'Donnell CDJ, Cory J, Webb KA, et al. Exercise ventilatory inefficiency in mild to end-stage COPD. Eur Respir J. 2015;45(2):377–87.
20. Milic-Emili J. Expiratory flow limitation: Roger S. Mitchell Lecture. Chest. 2000;117(5 Suppl 1):219S–23S.
21. Calverley PMA. Dynamic hyperinflation: is it worth measuring? Proc Am Thorac Soc. 2006;3(3):239–44.

22. O'Donnell DE, Webb KA. The major limitation to exercise performance in COPD is dynamic hyperinflation. J Appl Physiol Bethesda Md 1985. 2008;105(2):753–755; discussion 755-757.
23. O'Donnell DE, Guenette JA, Maltais F, Webb KA. Decline of resting inspiratory capacity in COPD: the impact on breathing pattern, dyspnea, and ventilatory capacity during exercise. Chest. 2012;141(3):753–62.
24. Hansen JE, Ulubay G, Chow BF, Sun X-G, Wasserman K. Mixed-expired and end-tidal CO2 distinguish between ventilation and perfusion defects during exercise testing in patients with lung and heart diseases. Chest. 2007;132(3):977–83.
25. Belardinelli R, Lacalaprice F, Carle F, Minnucci A, Cianci G, Perna G, et al. Exercise-induced myocardial ischaemia detected by cardiopulmonary exercise testing. Eur Heart J. 2003;24(14):1304–13.
26. Belardinelli R, Barstow TJ, Nguyen P, Wasserman K. Skeletal muscle oxygenation and oxygen uptake kinetics following constant work rate exercise in chronic congestive heart failure. Am J Cardiol. 1997;80(10):1319–24.
27. Whipp BJ, Higgenbotham MB, Cobb FC. Estimating exercise stroke volume from asymptotic oxygen pulse in humans. J Appl Physiol Bethesda Md 1985. 1996;81(6):2674–9.
28. Brubaker PH, Kitzman DW. Chronotropic incompetence: causes, consequences, and management. Circulation. 2011;123(9):1010–20.
29. Guazzi M, Arena R, Ascione A, Piepoli M, Guazzi MD. Gruppo di Studio Fisiologia dell'Esercizio, Cardiologia dello Sport e Riabilitazione Cardiovascolare of the Italian Society of Cardiology. Exercise oscillatory breathing and increased ventilation to carbon dioxide production slope in heart failure: an unfavorable combination with high prognostic value. Am Heart J. 2007;153(5):859–67.
30. Dubé B-P, Agostoni P, Laveneziana P. Exertional dyspnoea in chronic heart failure: the role of the lung and respiratory mechanical factors. Eur Respir Rev. 2016;25(141):317–32.
31. Laveneziana P, O'Donnell DE, Ofir D, Agostoni P, Padeletti L, Ricciardi G, et al. Effect of biventricular pacing on ventilatory and perceptual responses to exercise in patients with stable chronic heart failure. J Appl Physiol Bethesda Md 1985. 2009;106(5):1574–83.
32. Leite JJ, Mansur AJ, de Freitas HFG, Chizola PR, Bocchi EA, Terra-Filho M, et al. Periodic breathing during incremental exercise predicts mortality in patients with chronic heart failure evaluated for cardiac transplantation. J Am Coll Cardiol. 2003;41(12):2175–81.
33. Boudestein LCM, Rutten FH, Cramer MJ, Lammers JWJ, Hoes AW. The impact of concurrent heart failure on prognosis in patients with chronic obstructive pulmonary disease. Eur J Heart Fail. 2009;11(12):1182–8.
34. van Mourik Y, Bertens LCM, Cramer MJM, Lammers J-WJ, Reitsma JB, Moons KGM, et al. Unrecognized heart failure and chronic obstructive pulmonary disease (COPD) in frail elderly detected through a near-home targeted screening strategy. J Am Board Fam Med. 2014;27(6):811–21.
35. Divo M, Cote C, de Torres JP, Casanova C, Marin JM, Pinto-Plata V, et al. Comorbidities and risk of mortality in patients with chronic obstructive pulmonary disease. Am J Respir Crit Care Med. 2012;186(2):155–61.
36. Güder G, Brenner S, Störk S, Hoes A, Rutten FH. Chronic obstructive pulmonary disease in heart failure: accurate diagnosis and treatment. Eur J Heart Fail. 2014;16(12):1273–82.
37. van Riet EES, Hoes AW, Wagenaar KP, Limburg A, Landman MAJ, Rutten FH. Epidemiology of heart failure: the prevalence of heart failure and ventricular dysfunction in older adults over time. A systematic review. Eur J Heart Fail. 2016;18(3):242–52.
38. Triposkiadis F, Giamouzis G, Parissis J, Starling RC, Boudoulas H, Skoularigis J, et al. Reframing the association and significance of co-morbidities in heart failure. Eur J Heart Fail. 2016;18(7):744–58.
39. Evans RA, Singh SJ, Collier R, Loke I, Steiner MC, Morgan MDL. Generic, symptom based, exercise rehabilitation; integrating patients with COPD and heart failure. Respir Med. 2010;104(10):1473–81.

40. Apostolo A, Laveneziana P, Palange P, Agalbato C, Molle R, Popovic D, et al. Impact of chronic obstructive pulmonary disease on exercise ventilatory efficiency in heart failure. Int J Cardiol. 2015;189:134–40.
41. Arbex FF, Alencar MC, Souza A, Mazzuco A, Sperandio PA, Rocha A, et al. Exercise ventilation in COPD: influence of systolic heart failure. COPD. 2016;12:1–8.
42. Alencar MC, Arbex F, Souza A, Mazzuco A, Sperandio PA, Rocha A, et al. Does exercise ventilatory inefficiency predict poor outcome in heart failure patients with COPD? J Cardiopulm Rehabil Prev. 2016;36(6):454–9.
43. Rocha A, Arbex FF, Sperandio PA, Souza A, Biazzim L, Mancuso F, et al. Excess ventilation in COPD-heart failure overlap: implications for dyspnea and exercise intolerance. Am J Respir Crit Care Med. 2017;196:1264–74.
44. Poole DC, Hirai DM, Copp SW, Musch TI. Muscle oxygen transport and utilization in heart failure: implications for exercise (in)tolerance. Am J Physiol Heart Circ Physiol. 2012;302(5):H1050–63.
45. Sue DY. Excess ventilation during exercise and prognosis in chronic heart failure. Am J Respir Crit Care Med. 2011;183(10):1302–10.
46. Guazzi M, Naeije R, Arena R, Corrà U, Ghio S, Forfia P, et al. Echocardiography of right ventriculoarterial coupling combined with cardiopulmonary exercise testing to predict outcome in heart failure. Chest. 2015;148(1):226–34.
47. Naeije R, Manes A. The right ventricle in pulmonary arterial hypertension. Eur Respir Rev. 2014;23(134):476–87.
48. Jones JH, Zelt JT, Hirai DM, Diniz CV, Zaza A, O'Donnell DE, et al. Emphysema on thoracic CT and exercise ventilatory inefficiency in mild-to-moderate COPD. COPD. 2016;20:0.
49. Aaron CP, Hoffman EA, Lima JAC, Kawut SM, Bertoni AG, Vogel-Claussen J, et al. Pulmonary vascular volume, impaired left ventricular filling and dyspnea: the MESA lung study. PLoS One. 2017;12(4):e0176180.
50. Melenovsky V, Andersen MJ, Andress K, Reddy YN, Borlaug BA. Lung congestion in chronic heart failure: haemodynamic, clinical, and prognostic implications. Eur J Heart Fail. 2015;17(11):1161–71.
51. Magnussen H, Canepa M, Zambito PE, Brusasco V, Meinertz T, Rosenkranz S. What can we learn from pulmonary function testing in heart failure? Eur J Heart Fail. 2017;19(10):1222–9.
52. Johnson BD, Beck KC, Olson LJ, O'Malley KA, Allison TG, Squires RW, et al. Pulmonary function in patients with reduced left ventricular function: influence of smoking and cardiac surgery. Chest. 2001;120(6):1869–76.
53. de Souza AS, Sperandio PA, Mazzuco A, Alencar MC, Arbex FF, de Oliveira MF, et al. Influence of heart failure on resting lung volumes in patients with COPD. J Bras Pneumol. 2016;42(4):273–8.
54. Brenner S, Güder G, Berliner D, Deubner N, Fröhlich K, Ertl G, et al. Airway obstruction in systolic heart failure--COPD or congestion? Int J Cardiol. 2013;168(3):1910–6.
55. Güder G, Rutten FH, Brenner S, Angermann CE, Berliner D, Ertl G, et al. The impact of heart failure on the classification of COPD severity. J Card Fail. 2012;18(8):637–44.
56. Ray CS, Sue DY, Bray G, Hansen JE, Wasserman K. Effects of obesity on respiratory function. Am Rev Respir Dis. 1983;128(3):501–6.
57. Apostolo A, Giusti G, Gargiulo P, Bussotti M, Agostoni P. Lungs in heart failure. Pulm Med. 2012;2012:952741.
58. Pellegrino R, Viegi G, Brusasco V, Crapo RO, Burgos F, Casaburi R, et al. Interpretative strategies for lung function tests. Eur Respir J. 2005;26(5):948–68.
59. Ribeiro JP, Chiappa GR, Neder JA, Frankenstein L. Respiratory muscle function and exercise intolerance in heart failure. Curr Heart Fail Rep. 2009;6(2):95–101.
60. Huang W, Resch S, Oliveira RK, Cockrill BA, Systrom DM, Waxman AB. Invasive cardiopulmonary exercise testing in the evaluation of unexplained dyspnea: insights from a multidisciplinary dyspnea center. Eur J Prev Cardiol. 2017;24(11):1190–9.

61. Borlaug BA, Kass DA. Invasive hemodynamic assessment in heart failure. Heart Fail Clin. 2009;5(2):217–28.
62. Oliveira MF, Arbex F, Alencar MC, Souza A, Sperandio PA, Medeiros WM, et al. Heart failure impairs muscle blood flow and endurance exercise tolerance in COPD. COPD. 2016;20:1–9.
63. Borghi-Silva A, Oliveira CC, Carrascosa C, Maia J, Berton DC, Queiroga F, et al. Respiratory muscle unloading improves leg muscle oxygenation during exercise in patients with COPD. Thorax. 2008;63(10):910–5.
64. Barroco AC, Sperandio PA, Reis M, Almeida DR, Neder JA. A practical approach to assess leg muscle oxygenation during ramp-incremental cycle ergometry in heart failure. Braz J Med Biol Res Rev Bras Pesqui Medicas E Biol. 2017;50(12):e6327.
65. Chiappa GR, Vieira PJC, Umpierre D, Corrêa APS, Berton DC, Ribeiro JP, et al. Inspiratory resistance decreases limb blood flow in COPD patients with heart failure. Eur Respir J. 2014;43(5):1507–10.
66. Roseguini BT, Hirai DM, Alencar MC, Ramos RP, Silva BM, Wolosker N, et al. Sildenafil improves skeletal muscle oxygenation during exercise in men with intermittent claudication. Am J Physiol Regul Integr Comp Physiol. 2014;307(4):R396–404.
67. Mentz RJ, Kelly JP, von Lueder TG, Voors AA, Lam CSP, Cowie MR, et al. Noncardiac comorbidities in heart failure with reduced versus preserved ejection fraction. J Am Coll Cardiol. 2014;64(21):2281–93.
68. Ogoh S, Ainslie PN. Cerebral blood flow during exercise: mechanisms of regulation. J Appl Physiol Bethesda Md 1985. 2009;107(5):1370–80.
69. Koike A, Itoh H, Oohara R, Hoshimoto M, Tajima A, Aizawa T, et al. Cerebral oxygenation during exercise in cardiac patients. Chest. 2004;125(1):182–90.
70. Oliveira MF, Arbex F, Alencar MC, Soares A, Borghi-Silva A, Almeida D, Neder JA. Heart failure impairs cerebral oxygenation during exercise in patients with COPD. Eur Respir J. 2013;42(5):1423–6.
71. Oliveira MF, Alencar MC, Arbex F, Souza A, Sperandio P, Medina L, et al. Effects of heart failure on cerebral blood flow in COPD: rest and exercise. Respir Physiol Neurobiol. 2016;221:41–8.
72. Vicenzi M, Deboeck G, Faoro V, Loison J, Vachiery J-L, Naeije R. Exercise oscillatory ventilation in heart failure and in pulmonary arterial hypertension. Int J Cardiol. 2016;202:736–40.
73. Oren A, Wasserman K, Davis JA, Whipp BJ. Effect of CO2 set point on ventilatory response to exercise. J Appl Physiol. 1981;51(1):185–9.
74. Treptow E, Oliveira MF, Soares A, Ramos RP, Medina L, Lima R, et al. Cerebral microvascular blood flow and CO2 reactivity in pulmonary arterial hypertension. Respir Physiol Neurobiol. 2016;233:60–5.
75. Ulrich S, Hasler ED, Saxer S, Furian M, Müller-Mottet S, Keusch S, et al. Effect of breathing oxygen-enriched air on exercise performance in patients with precapillary pulmonary hypertension: randomized, sham-controlled cross-over trial. Eur Heart J. 2017;38(15):1159–68.
76. Verges S, Rupp T, Jubeau M, Wuyam B, Esteve F, Levy P, et al. Cerebral perturbations during exercise in hypoxia. Am J Physiol Regul Integr Comp Physiol. 2012;302(8):R903–16.
77. Oliveira MF, Zelt JTJ, Jones JH, Hirai DM, O'Donnell DE, Verges S, et al. Does impaired O_2 delivery during exercise accentuate central and peripheral fatigue in patients with coexistent COPD-CHF? Front Physiol. 2014;5:514.
78. Seeger W, Adir Y, Barberà JA, Champion H, Coghlan JG, Cottin V, et al. Pulmonary hypertension in chronic lung diseases. J Am Coll Cardiol. 2013;62(25 Suppl):D109–16.
79. Cottin V, Le Pavec J, Prévot G, Mal H, Humbert M, Simonneau G, et al. Pulmonary hypertension in patients with combined pulmonary fibrosis and emphysema syndrome. Eur Respir J. 2010;35(1):105–11.
80. Neder JA, Ramos RP, Ota-Arakaki JS, Hirai DM, D'Arsigny CL, O'Donnell D. Exercise intolerance in pulmonary arterial hypertension. The role of cardiopulmonary exercise testing. Ann Am Thorac Soc. 2015;12(4):604–12.

81. Boerrigter BG, Bogaard HJ, Trip P, Groepenhoff H, Rietema H, Holverda S, et al. Ventilatory and cardiocirculatory exercise profiles in COPD: the role of pulmonary hypertension. Chest. 2012;142(5):1166–74.
82. Thirapatarapong W, Armstrong HF, Bartels MN. Comparing cardiopulmonary exercise testing in severe COPD patients with and without pulmonary hypertension. Heart Lung Circ. 2014;23(9):833–40.
83. Bhatt DV, Kocheril AG. Submaximal cardiopulmonary exercise testing for the evaluation of unexplained dyspnea. South Med J. 2014;107(3):144–9.
84. Koike A, Yajima T, Adachi H, Shimizu N, Kano H, Sugimoto K, et al. Evaluation of exercise capacity using submaximal exercise at a constant work rate in patients with cardiovascular disease. Circulation. 1995;91(6):1719–24.
85. Kim C-H, Hansen JE, MacCarter DJ, Johnson BD. Algorithm for predicting disease likelihood from a submaximal exercise test. Clin Med Insights Circ Respir Pulm Med. 2017;11:1179548417719248.
86. Neder JA, Berton DC, Arbex FF, Alencar MCN, Rocha A, Sperandio PA, et al. Physiological and clinical relevance of exercise ventilatory efficiency in COPD. Eur Respir J. 2017;49(3):pii 1602036.
87. Guazzi M, Belletti S, Tumminello G, Fiorentini C, Guazzi MD. Exercise hyperventilation, dyspnea sensation, and ergoreflex activation in lone atrial fibrillation. Am J Physiol Heart Circ Physiol. 2004;287(6):H2899–905.
88. Ariansen I, Edvardsen E, Borchsenius F, Abdelnoor M, Tveit A, Gjesdal K. Lung function and dyspnea in patients with permanent atrial fibrillation. Eur J Intern Med. 2011;22(5):466–70.
89. Barr RG. The epidemiology of vascular dysfunction relating to chronic obstructive pulmonary disease and emphysema. Proc Am Thorac Soc. 2011;8(6):522–7.
90. Abudiab MM, Redfield MM, Melenovsky V, Olson TP, Kass DA, Johnson BD, et al. Cardiac output response to exercise in relation to metabolic demand in heart failure with preserved ejection fraction. Eur J Heart Fail. 2013;15(7):776–85.
91. Nedeljkovic I, Banovic M, Stepanovic J, Giga V, Djordjevic-Dikic A, Trifunovic D, et al. The combined exercise stress echocardiography and cardiopulmonary exercise test for identification of masked heart failure with preserved ejection fraction in patients with hypertension. Eur J Prev Cardiol. 2016;23(1):71–7.
92. Neder JA, Ramos RP, Ota-Arakaki JS, Ferreira EMV, Hirai DM, Sperandio PA, et al. Insights into ventilation-gas exchange coupling in chronic thromboembolic pulmonary hypertension. Eur Respir J. 2016;48(1):252–4.
93. Guazzi M, Bandera F, Ozemek C, Systrom D, Arena R. Cardiopulmonary exercise testing: what is its value? J Am Coll Cardiol. 2017;70(13):1618–36.
94. Rocha A, Arbex FF, Alencar MC, Sperandio PA, Hirai DM, Berton DC, et al. Physiological and sensory consequences of exercise oscillatory ventilation in heart failure-COPD. Int J Cardiol. 2016;224:447–53.

Chapter 9
Physiology of Heart-Lung Interactions

Alicia K. Gerke and Gregory A. Schmidt

Chapter Pearls
1. The effects of heart and lung interactions differ by spontaneous and mechanical ventilation and depend upon intrathoracic pressure and volume changes.
2. Hemodynamic changes related to the heart-lung interaction are most often dominated by right ventricular preload changes. Occasionally, effects on ventricular afterload, pulmonary vascular resistance, or gas exchange become important.
3. The interaction between the lungs and the heart is complex and unpredictable; the ultimate outcome is affected by volume status, metabolic demand, mode of ventilation, and underlying chronic heart or lung disease.

The Importance of Heart-Lung Interaction

The goal of the cardiopulmonary system is to supply oxygen and other nutrients to body tissues while eliminating carbon dioxide, and the heart and lung work closely together to achieve these ends. Because the heart and lung share volume and pressures within the thorax, each system tends to alter the other, especially when there is preexisting heart or lung disease, or when challenged by rising demand. Cardiopulmonary interactions are mediated by changes in pleural pressure (P_{pl}), lung volume, and gas exchange, all explored in the sections to follow. The complexity of their interactions is further magnified by comorbidities, such as heart failure, COPD, interstitial lung disease, and acute respiratory distress syndrome (ARDS), and by intravascular volume state. Finally, drug therapy, mechanical ventilation, and

A. K. Gerke · G. A. Schmidt (✉)
University of Iowa, Department of Internal Medicine, Division of Pulmonary Diseases,
Critical Care, and Occupational Medicine, Iowa City, IA, USA
e-mail: alicia-gerke@uiowa.edu; gregory-a-schmidt@uiowa.edu

© Springer Nature Switzerland AG 2020
S. P. Bhatt (ed.), *Cardiac Considerations in Chronic Lung Disease*,
Respiratory Medicine, https://doi.org/10.1007/978-3-030-43435-9_9

Table 9.1 Considerations in heart-lung interactions	Considerations in heart-lung interactions
	Intravascular volume
	Cardiac function
	Lung compliance
	Pulmonary vascular resistance
	Gas exchange abnormalities (hypoxia, hypercarbia, acidemia)
	Overall oxygen demand

extracorporeal circulatory devices may dramatically impact how the heart and lungs interact. For the clinician managing patients with heart or lung failure, understanding cardiopulmonary physiology is essential for guiding therapy and avoiding unintended harms. In this chapter, we first focus on the heart-lung interaction in both the normal physiologic state and with mechanical ventilation and then discuss the complexities of predicting heart-lung interactions in different clinical scenarios (Table 9.1).

Impact of Respiration on the Circulation

Respiration has cyclical effects on the circulation, as witnessed by respiratory variation in stroke volume, pulse pressure, and heart rate. These overt circulatory changes are the consequence of varying right and left ventricular preload and afterload, autonomic output, and ventricular interdependence. In health, most of this variation is due to the impact of P_{pl} on right ventricular (RV) preload. In the presence of disease, however, other factors may predominate.

Cardiovascular effects of changing pleural pressure As described by Guyton, blood returns to the heart under the influence of the pressure difference between upstream venous reservoirs (at the mean systemic pressure, not varying significantly with respiration) and the right atrium [1, 2]. Because the right atrial pressure (P_{ra}) is directly altered by respiration, instantaneous venous return varies cyclically and this preload effect represents the largest contributor to normal heart-lung interaction. At the same time, breathing also affects RV afterload and the left ventricle (both preload and afterload), as well as abdominal pressure; in certain circumstances, these effects become magnified (Fig. 9.1).

(i) Spontaneous breathing During spontaneous inspiration, the P_{pl} drops by roughly 5 cmH$_2$O. Although there are complex regional differences in pleural pressure, especially in the presence of lung disease, a reasonable approximation is that inspiration causes the juxtacardiac pressure ($P_{juxtacardiac}$) to fall by a similar value. As a consequence, right atrial transmural pressure (P_{ra} minus $P_{juxtacardiac}$) rises, tending to transiently augment venous return (Fig. 9.2). Right heart volume increases so that, through ventricular interdependence, left heart filling is impeded. At the same time, left ventricular (LV) systolic transmural pressure (systolic LV pressure minus

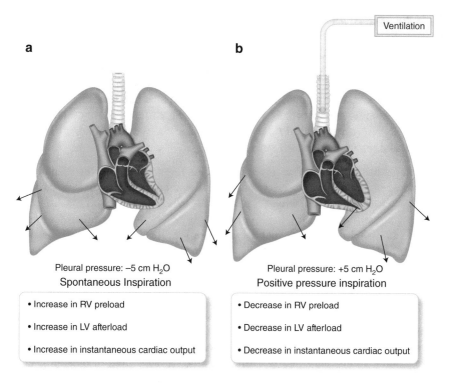

a Pleural pressure: –5 cm H$_2$O
Spontaneous Inspiration

- Increase in RV preload
- Increase in LV afterload
- Increase in instantaneous cardiac output

b Pleural pressure: +5 cm H$_2$O
Positive pressure inspiration

- Decrease in RV preload
- Decrease in LV afterload
- Decrease in instantaneous cardiac output

Fig. 9.1 Hemodynamic effects of inspiration in normal lungs with (**a**) spontaneous inspiration and (**b**) mechanical ventilation (RV = right ventricular, LV = left ventricular)

Fig. 9.2 Increase in right ventricular inflow at the tricuspid valve with deep inspiration in a normal healthy patient (sweep speed 25 mm/s)

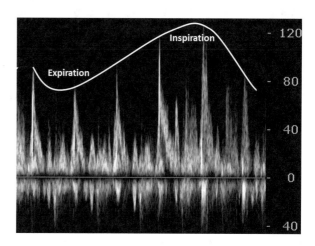

left ventricular $P_{\text{juxtacardiac}}$) rises, increasing LV afterload and tending to transiently depress LV stroke volume. Overall, the effect of inspiration is to briefly increase preload to the right heart, raising its stroke volume, while depressing LV ejection. Expiration reverses these effects, producing the classic respiratory variation in blood pressure and pulse pressure (a surrogate for LV stroke volume).

(ii) Spontaneous breathing in pathological states Respirophasic variation in stroke volume is amplified by conditions that cause pleural pressure to abnormally vary. Even breathing at high tidal volumes intensifies these cardiovascular changes [3], but they are particularly notable in the presence of lung disease. A common example is status asthmaticus, in which dramatic swings in pleural pressure produce pulsus paradoxus, a finding which is not truly paradoxical but, instead, an exaggerated manifestation of the normal heart-lung interaction. Similar findings, albeit less striking, accompany the raised P_{pl} swings in chronic obstructive pulmonary disease (COPD) and interstitial lung disease (ILD).

Spontaneous inspiration raises intra-abdominal pressure as the diaphragm descends, reducing the unstressed volume of the abdominal vasculature, pushing blood flow towards the thoracic cavity. This acts synergistically with the fall in P_{ra} to further boost venous return, but is generally very modest in magnitude. Its role is revealed in pathological states that demonstrate Kussmaul respiration (an inspiratory rise in P_{ra}), such as severe RV dysfunction, restrictive cardiomyopathy, constrictive pericarditis, or tricuspid stenosis. Abdominal venous congestion and an inability of the right heart to accommodate increased flow from the abdomen combine so that inspiration causes P_{ra} to rise, despite the fall in $P_{juxtacardiac}$ [4, 5].

Inspiration also raises LV afterload as transmural pressure rises [6]. This effect is normally modest, since the left ventricle is not usually afterload-sensitive, but can be very detrimental in patients with LV systolic dysfunction. The onset of cardiogenic pulmonary edema is poorly tolerated as the elevated work of breathing, and attendant supranormal swings in P_{pl} combine with reduced lung compliance to seriously compromise cardiac output. The LV afterload effect of spontaneous inspiration may be an important mechanism of weaning failure [7, 8]. Moreover, this could explain the efficacy of noninvasive ventilation to reduce reintubation risk in patients extubated following acute respiratory decompensation due to cardiac failure [9].

(iii) Passive ventilation During mechanical ventilation of the passive patient, P_{pl} rises in proportion to tidal volume and chest wall compliance, causing P_{ra} also to rise. This reduces the pressure gradient for venous return; as a result, intrathoracic blood volume, transmural P_{ra}, and cardiac output fall [6]. Positive end-expiratory pressure (PEEP) has similar consequences. For these reasons, significant hypotension can occur upon initiation of mechanical ventilation, especially in the hypovolemic patient, which can be mitigated by volume loading. Compensatory autonomic reflexes raise mean systemic pressure, tending to reestablish the pressure gradient, defending cardiac output [10]. Similarly, the increase in lung volume and lowering of the diaphragm can augment the venous return to minimize the effect of increased right atrial pressure.

The rise in P_{pl} due to PEEP and passive ventilation also reduces LV afterload, an effect that is usually small, but in the setting of LV systolic dysfunction can become meaningful. Because these patients often operate on the flat portion of the cardiac function curve (i.e., cardiac output is not sensitive to changes in preload), PEEP may even increase cardiac output [11]. In addition, increases in PEEP and mean airway pressures can compress the congested pulmonary venous bed and increase LV end-diastolic volume so that stroke volume increases on both a preload and afterload basis.

Cardiovascular effects of changing lung volume The pulmonary vasculature bed normally is characterized by low resistance (and low transpulmonary pressure gradient) which allows increased blood flow with minimal pressure changes. Pulmonary vascular resistance (PVR) can be viewed as a U-shape relationship with lung volumes, with higher resistance at very low or very high lung volumes and lowest resistance around functional residual capacity (FRC). At markedly low volumes below FRC (as can be seen with forced expiration or in ARDS), the larger extra-alveolar vessels collapse which increases PVR. With large tidal volumes, the hyperinflation seen in obstructive lung disease, or tidal overdistention of the "baby lung" of ARDS, pulmonary vascular resistance rises due to increased alveolar pressure and compression of the intra-alveolar vasculature [12–14]. Due to the effect of gravity, this compression varies between dependent and nondependent lung zones and is affected by intravascular volume status [15]. Large tidal volumes (with zero PEEP), causing large variations in P_{pl} and alveolar pressure, have been shown to produce acute cor pulmonale in healthy animals [16]. Perhaps not coincidentally, the era of low tidal volume ventilation for patients with ARDS has led to a substantial reduction in the incidence of clinical cor pulmonale [17].

In contrast to the LV, the RV is more sensitive to changing afterload. Acutely, the RV responds to increased afterload through homeometric adaptation in which contractility is augmented to match afterload (the Anrep effect). When the limits of this mechanism are exceeded, the RV dilates to preserve flow (heterometric adaptation or Starling mechanism), but at the cost of venous congestion. The lung volume effect on PVR takes on special significance when the RV is in a compensated, but precarious, state. In these settings, the added impact of excessive (or even normal tidal) lung expansion can precipitate RV decompensation [18, 19].

Recent data on the effect of PEEP in patients with RV dysfunction due to ARDS show the relevance of this effect. Increasing PEEP (while limiting tidal volume and plateau airway pressure) caused cardiac output to fall, a finding that was not surprising [20, 21]. However, this was not the result of reduced preload since end-diastolic volume rose instead of falling (Table 9.2). Rather, the fall in cardiac output was attributed to increased RV afterload, as revealed by a rise in end-systolic RV volume. An additional complexity is that volume state can also determine which effect (preload vs. afterload) will predominate, and increasing PEEP to a preload-depleted

Table 9.2 Comparative effects of increased positive end-expiratory pressure (PEEP) in mechanically ventilated patients with acute respiratory distress syndrome (ARDS) versus mechanical ventilation in normal lungs showing that afterload effects predominate in ARDS compared to preload effects in the normal lung

Hemodynamic parameter	ARDS + PEEP	Normal lung + PEEP
Pulmonary vascular resistance	Increases	Increases
RV end-diastolic area	Increases	Decreases
Transmural right atrial pressure	Increases	Decreases
End-diastolic RV/LV area ratio	Increases	Unchanged

Adapted from Fougeres et al. [20]

heart may further diminish cardiac output [22]. These results have been documented in patients with ARDS, but likely pertain also to those ventilated with acute-on-chronic pulmonary hypertension [23].

Gas exchange and heart-lung interaction Blood gas tensions have important circulatory consequences. In addition, overall body gas exchange, such as the total body oxygen consumption, can challenge hemodynamic homeostasis, especially in the presence of disease.

(i) Blood gas tensions Blood values of partial pressure of oxygen (PO2), carbon dioxide (PCO2) and pH modulate vascular tone, myocardial function, and the autonomic nervous system. Acute and chronic lung disease can induce hypoxemia, hypercarbia, and acidemia, altering PVR and contributing to pulmonary heart dysfunction [24]. Hypoxia impairs contractility of the heart and induces hypoxic pulmonary vasoconstriction (HPV), especially at partial pressures less than 60 mmHg [25]. Hypoxic vasoconstriction improves ventilation/perfusion (VQ) matching by reducing blood flow to poorly ventilated regions, but also raises overall PVR. However, the response to hypoxia and HPV is not uniform across individuals, thereby patient responses to hypoxia are difficult to predict [26, 27]. Similarly, hypercarbia and acidemia cause increased PVR and can induce increased RV afterload, RV dilation, and subsequent cor pulmonale [21].

These gas exchange effects can produce a spiral of decompensation. For example, worsening pulmonary dead space can raise PCO2, provoking RV deterioration which, in turn, compromises cardiac output, lowering venous PO2, amplifying HPV, causing more RV dysfunction, and culminating in circulatory failure. For mechanically ventilated patients, gas exchange and mechanical effects can be intertwined in complex ways, making it hard to predict the consequences of changing ventilator settings. For example, if a patient ventilated for severe ILD becomes hypoxemic, the impact of raising PEEP is complex. If the dominant effect of PEEP is to recruit lung and raise PO2, the circulatory impact may be salutary. On the other hand, if PEEP raises dead space fraction, impedes RV filling, or presents an overwhelming afterload challenge to the RV, the patient may become unstable. Even the amount of PEEP transmitted to the pleural space is highly variable, ranging from more than 50% to less than 25% [28], and may be distributed quite heterogeneously [29]. These effects may not be apparent immediately, but may play out over many minutes, making it very difficult for the clinician to disentangle the many potential threads of decompensation.

(ii) Overall oxygen consumption and carbon dioxide production The total body demand for gas exchange will rise with exercise, fever, seizure, and many other causes, testing the limits of both respiration and circulation. Three clinical scenarios are particularly germane. The first is seen in patients with severe airflow obstruction, in whom increasing minute ventilation causes dynamic hyperinflation, raising the juxtacardiac and alveolar pressures. At times, this can produce shock (largely due to impaired right heart filling), especially in the setting of mechanical or bag-

mask ventilation. A second example is that of cardiogenic pulmonary edema, in which heart failure leads to reduced lung compliance, increased airway resistance, and failing gas exchange, precipitating respiratory failure on top of circulatory failure. A third illustration is of weaning failure in patients with circulatory compromise: the work of spontaneous breathing for many patients with lung disease is severalfold that of normal individuals [30], overloading the circulation and precipitating weaning failure [31].

Example Clinical Scenarios: Why Are Heart-Lung Interactions Relevant?

1. Pulmonary function alterations in heart disease Just as lung disease can cause alterations in the vasculature and cardiac performance due to hyperinflation and dynamic air trapping, disease of the vasculature and heart has been shown to conversely affect lung function. Hypertrophy and dilation of the muscular and elastic arteries such as those seen in idiopathic pulmonary hypertension have been associated with peripheral airway obstruction and increased residual volume, in addition to the expected decrease in diffusing capacity [32, 33]. These obstructive changes are presumably due to the close proximity of the vasculature to the airway, but other causes related to the effects of vasoconstrictors on bronchial epithelium have been postulated. More remote studies have shown mild restrictive ventilatory defects in patients with precapillary pulmonary hypertension with decrease total lung capacity and vital capacity [34, 35]. Similarly, patients with left heart failure and an elevated wedge pressure have restrictive defects on pulmonary function testing with reduced vital capacity and total lung capacity [36]. Obstructive defects are less common, but can occur with bronchial wall congestion in patients with decompensated heart failure. Pulmonary function abnormalities in patients with chronic heart failure have been associated with poorer survival [37, 38].

2. Nocturnal noninvasive ventilation: heart-lung consequences In patients with obstructive sleep apnea, high levels of negative inspiratory force against a closed glottis lead to high amounts of venous return. A shift in the interventricular septum in response to this volume leads to a reduction in LV compliance and stroke volume with increased LV afterload. Nighttime hypoventilation and chronic hypoxemia lead to HPV with elevated sympathetic activation related to frequent arousals and gas exchange abnormalities. These factors contribute to high pulmonary pressures, increased RV afterload, and eventual cor pulmonale in a proportion of patients, particularly those with concurrent COPD or obesity. Positive pressure decreases the work of the heart and oxygen consumption by opening the airways and alleviating severe negative swings of inspiratory effort. Further, positive pressure can decrease pulmonary vascular resistance by raising FRC as described earlier, improving hemodynamics in these patients.

In chronic heart failure patients, obstructive sleep apnea is common and associated with poor outcomes [39]. Use of noninvasive ventilation in heart failure patients diminishes intrathoracic swings in pressure, lowers LV afterload, and improves cardiovascular performance. Positive pressure maintains alveolar patency, improving oxygenation, and shifts fluid from the lung interstitium into the pulmonary vasculature [40]. There may also be humoral effects of CPAP on the heart, as positive pressure ventilation induces pressure on the heart and diminishes atrial stretch with consequent improved blood flow. Likely because of these mechanisms, use of CPAP has been associated with decreased atrial peptides, decreased sympathetic catecholamines, improved LV contractility, improved symptoms, and increased survival in patients with congestive heart failure [41–46]. However, these benefits of NIV may not translate to patients with low ejection fraction with prominent central sleep apnea, as treatment with adaptive servo-ventilation did not improve outcome in these patients; rather this group of patients appears to have higher all-cause and cardiovascular mortality and no improvement in quality of life when treated with adaptive servo-ventilation [47]. It is unclear whether varying effects of nocturnal ventilation are due to disruption of the compensatory mechanisms for heart failure or a reflection of the ventilator settings or pressures trialed.

3. Hypotension on initiating mechanical ventilation There are many issues to consider upon initiating mechanical ventilation in the critically ill patient, including the patient's volume status, induction medications, and underlying cardiac function. Upon intubation itself, hypotension can be marked if a patient is hypovolemic, in combination with medications that diminish mean systemic pressure and sympathetic drive, synergistically reducing venous return. Since most patients are therapeutically paralyzed at the time of intubation, ventilation raises $P_{juxtacardiac}$, impeding RV filling. This effect can be even greater when PEEP or recruitment maneuvers are added [48]. In patients with COPD or asthma, close attention to minute volume and best PEEP are important to limit dynamic hyperinflation and unnecessary cardiac compression, which could produce shock. At the same time, mechanical ventilation can lessen the work of breathing and sympathetic tone, as well as ameliorating hypoxemia or respiratory acidosis. These beneficial effects could outweigh any negative impact on cardiac preload or afterload.

4. Predicting fluid responsiveness The interaction of the lungs and heart allows prediction of fluid responsiveness in critically ill patients by examining the impact of positive pressure ventilation on the circulation. For example, respiratory variations in pulse pressure, stroke volume, superior and inferior vena cava diameters, LV outflow tract velocity time integral, and other cardiovascular parameters predict accurately the ability of a fluid bolus to raise cardiac output [49–51]. Significant respiratory change in these parameters indicates a preload-responsive state that might hemodynamically benefit from volume resuscitation. These predictors rely on the RV preload effect and can be confounded in the presence of significant RV systolic dysfunction (in which case respiratory variation may be due to RV afterload changes, rather than preload reserve) or abdominal hypertension [52, 53]. Especially important is the input signal: if tidal volume is insufficient (<8 mL/kg ideal body weight), so too will be the cardiovascular impact, potentially causing a false-negative assessment [7, 54]. Finally, patients must be passively ventilated – active effort makes these predictors unreliable [55, 56]. These functional assessments are attractive, as traditional static measures of volume status such as central venous pressure, pulmonary artery occlusion pressure, or ventricular end-diastolic volumes do not correlate well with fluid responsiveness [57, 58]. The accuracy of functional hemodynamic monitoring may be limited to specific patient subgroups in the clinical setting [59, 60].

Conclusions

Heart-lung interactions are complex, however, and multiple conflicting interactions can occur simultaneously, making it more difficult to predict actual outcome of the combined forces in any one individual patient. Many of these above-described effects differ based on volume status, the underlying disease process, medications, and baseline cardiac function. In ill patients with high work of breathing necessitating increased oxygen delivery and cardiac output, the intervention of mechanical ventilation can improve some of these parameters by decreasing demand and energy consumption, which may predominate over the potential negative effects on the cardiopulmonary circulation. Although this concept is clearly exemplified by the critically ill patient, this may also contribute to the mechanism by which noninvasive ventilatory interventions improve cardiopulmonary performance in patients with obstructive sleep apnea or other sleep-disordered breathing on an outpatient basis. It is important for the clinician to understand the normal cardiopulmonary interaction, as both diagnostic and therapeutic strategies depend on how the homeostasis is altered in the disease state.

References

1. Guyton AC. Determination of cardiac output by equating venous return curves with cardiac response curves. Physiol Rev. 1955;35(1):123–9.
2. Guyton AC, Lindsey AW, Abernathy B, Richardson T. Venous return at various right atrial pressures and the normal venous return curve. Am J Phys. 1957;189(3):609–15.
3. Guz A, Innes JA, Murphy K. Respiratory modulation of left ventricular stroke volume in man measured using pulsed Doppler ultrasound. J Physiol. 1987;393:499–512.
4. Takata M, Beloucif S, Shimada M, Robotham JL. Superior and inferior vena caval flows during respiration: pathogenesis of Kussmaul's sign. Am J Phys. 1992;262(3 Pt 2):H763–70.
5. Meyer TE, Sareli P, Marcus RH, Pocock W, Berk MR, McGregor M. Mechanism underlying Kussmaul's sign in chronic constrictive pericarditis. Am J Cardiol. 1989;64(16):1069–72.
6. Buda AJ, Pinsky MR, Ingels NB Jr, Daughters GT 2nd, Stinson EB, Alderman EL. Effect of intrathoracic pressure on left ventricular performance. N Engl J Med. 1979;301(9):453–9.

7. Pinsky MR. Heart lung interactions during mechanical ventilation. Curr Opin Crit Care. 2012;18(3):256–60.
8. Jubran A, Mathru M, Dries D, Tobin MJ. Continuous recordings of mixed venous oxygen saturation during weaning from mechanical ventilation and the ramifications thereof. Am J Respir Crit Care Med. 1998;158(6):1763–9.
9. Ferrer M, Valencia M, Nicolas JM, Bernadich O, Badia JR, Torres A. Early noninvasive ventilation averts extubation failure in patients at risk: a randomized trial. Am J Respir Crit Care Med. 2006;173(2):164–70.
10. Fessler HE, Brower RG, Wise RA, Permutt S. Effects of positive end-expiratory pressure on the gradient for venous return. Am Rev Respir Dis. 1991;143(1):19–24.
11. Bradley TD, Holloway RM, McLaughlin PR, Ross BL, Walters J, Liu PP. Cardiac output response to continuous positive airway pressure in congestive heart failure. Am Rev Respir Dis. 1992;145(2 Pt 1):377–82.
12. Dawson CA, Grimm DJ, Linehan JH. Effects of lung inflation on longitudinal distribution of pulmonary vascular resistance. J Appl Physiol Respir Environ Exerc Physiol. 1977;43(6):1089–92.
13. Murray J. The normal lung. 2nd ed. Philadelphia: W.B. Saunders Company; 1986.
14. Pinsky MR. Cardiovascular issues in respiratory care. Chest. 2005;128(5 Suppl 2):592S–7S.
15. Permutt S, Bromberger-Barnea B, Bane HN. Alveolar pressure, pulmonary venous pressure, and the vascular waterfall. Med Thorac. 1962;19:239–60.
16. Katira BH, Giesinger RE, Engelberts D, Zabini D, Kornecki A, Otulakowski G, et al. Adverse heart-lung interactions in ventilator-induced lung injury. Am J Respir Crit Care Med. 2017;196(11):1411–21.
17. Mekontso Dessap A, Boissier F, Charron C, Begot E, Repesse X, Legras A, et al. Acute cor pulmonale during protective ventilation for acute respiratory distress syndrome: prevalence, predictors, and clinical impact. Intensive Care Med. 2016;42(5):862–70.
18. Schmitt JM, Vieillard-Baron A, Augarde R, Prin S, Page B, Jardin F. Positive end-expiratory pressure titration in acute respiratory distress syndrome patients: impact on right ventricular outflow impedance evaluated by pulmonary artery Doppler flow velocity measurements. Crit Care Med. 2001;29(6):1154–8.
19. Vieillard-Baron A, Prin S, Chergui K, Dubourg O, Jardin F. Echo-Doppler demonstration of acute cor pulmonale at the bedside in the medical intensive care unit. Am J Respir Crit Care Med. 2002;166(10):1310–9.
20. Fougeres E, Teboul JL, Richard C, Osman D, Chemla D, Monnet X. Hemodynamic impact of a positive end-expiratory pressure setting in acute respiratory distress syndrome: importance of the volume status. Crit Care Med. 2010;38(3):802–7.
21. Mekontso Dessap A, Charron C, Devaquet J, Aboab J, Jardin F, Brochard L, et al. Impact of acute hypercapnia and augmented positive end-expiratory pressure on right ventricle function in severe acute respiratory distress syndrome. Intensive Care Med. 2009;35(11):1850–8.
22. Schreuder JJ, Jansen JR, Versprille A. Hemodynamic effects of PEEP applied as a ramp in normo-, hyper-, and hypovolemia. J Appl Physiol (1985). 1985;59(4):1178–84.
23. Ventetuolo CE, Klinger JR. Management of acute right ventricular failure in the intensive care unit. Ann Am Thorac Soc. 2014;11(5):811–22.
24. Forfia PR, Vaidya A, Wiegers SE. Pulmonary heart disease: the heart-lung interaction and its impact on patient phenotypes. Pulm Circ. 2013;3(1):5–19.
25. Madden JA, Dawson CA, Harder DR. Hypoxia-induced activation in small isolated pulmonary arteries from the cat. J Appl Physiol (1985). 1985;59(1):113–8.
26. Naito T, Miyahara Y, Ikeda S. Ventilatory and pulmonary vascular responses to acute hypoxia are nonuniform in healthy man. Respiration. 1995;62(4):185–9.
27. Fishman AP, Mc CJ, Himmelstein A, Cournand A. Effects of acute anoxia on the circulation and respiration in patients with chronic pulmonary disease studied during the steady state. J Clin Invest. 1952;31(8):770–81.

28. Jardin F, Genevray B, Brun-Ney D, Bourdarias JP. Influence of lung and chest wall compliances on transmission of airway pressure to the pleural space in critically ill patients. Chest. 1985;88(5):653–8.

29. Silva PL, Gama de Abreu M. Regional distribution of transpulmonary pressure. Ann Transl Med. 2018;6(19):385.

30. Coussa ML, Guerin C, Eissa NT, Corbeil C, Chasse M, Braidy J, et al. Partitioning of work of breathing in mechanically ventilated COPD patients. J Appl Physiol (1985). 1993;75(4):1711–9.

31. Jubran A, Tobin MJ. Pathophysiologic basis of acute respiratory distress in patients who fail a trial of weaning from mechanical ventilation. Am J Respir Crit Care Med. 1997;155(3):906–15.

32. Jing ZC, Xu XQ, Badesch DB, Jiang X, Wu Y, Liu JM, et al. Pulmonary function testing in patients with pulmonary arterial hypertension. Respir Med. 2009;103(8):1136–42.

33. Meyer FJ, Ewert R, Hoeper MM, Olschewski H, Behr J, Winkler J, et al. Peripheral airway obstruction in primary pulmonary hypertension. Thorax. 2002;57(6):473–6.

34. Horn M, Ries A, Neveu C, Moser K. Restrictive ventilatory pattern in precapillary pulmonary hypertension. Am Rev Respir Dis. 1983;128(1):163–5.

35. Rich S, Dantzker DR, Ayres SM, Bergofsky EH, Brundage BH, Detre KM, et al. Primary pulmonary hypertension. A national prospective study. Ann Intern Med. 1987;107(2):216–23.

36. Ries AL, Gregoratos G, Friedman PJ, Clausen JL. Pulmonary function tests in the detection of left heart failure: correlation with pulmonary artery wedge pressure. Respiration. 1986;49(4):241–50.

37. Melenovsky V, Andersen MJ, Andress K, Reddy YN, Borlaug BA. Lung congestion in chronic heart failure: haemodynamic, clinical, and prognostic implications. Eur J Heart Fail. 2015;17(11):1161–71.

38. Iversen KK, Kjaergaard J, Akkan D, Kober L, Torp-Pedersen C, Hassager C, et al. The prognostic importance of lung function in patients admitted with heart failure. Eur J Heart Fail. 2010;12(7):685–91.

39. Wang H, Parker JD, Newton GE, Floras JS, Mak S, Chiu KL, et al. Influence of obstructive sleep apnea on mortality in patients with heart failure. J Am Coll Cardiol. 2007;49(15):1625–31.

40. Malo J, Ali J, Wood LD. How does positive end-expiratory pressure reduce intrapulmonary shunt in canine pulmonary edema? J Appl Physiol Respir Environ Exerc Physiol. 1984;57(4):1002–10.

41. Frass M, Watschinger B, Traindl O, Popovic R, Podolsky A, Gisslinger H, et al. Atrial natriuretic peptide release in response to different positive end-expiratory pressure levels. Crit Care Med. 1993;21(3):343–7.

42. Wilkins MA, Su XL, Palayew MD, Yamashiro Y, Rolli P, McKenzie JK, et al. The effects of posture change and continuous positive airway pressure on cardiac natriuretic peptides in congestive heart failure. Chest. 1995;107(4):909–15.

43. Shirakami G, Magaribuchi T, Shingu K, Suga S, Tamai S, Nakao K, et al. Positive end-expiratory pressure ventilation decreases plasma atrial and brain natriuretic peptide levels in humans. Anesth Analg. 1993;77(6):1116–21.

44. Kaneko Y, Floras JS, Usui K, Plante J, Tkacova R, Kubo T, et al. Cardiovascular effects of continuous positive airway pressure in patients with heart failure and obstructive sleep apnea. N Engl J Med. 2003;348(13):1233–41.

45. Naughton MT, Benard DC, Liu PP, Rutherford R, Rankin F, Bradley TD. Effects of nasal CPAP on sympathetic activity in patients with heart failure and central sleep apnea. Am J Respir Crit Care Med. 1995;152(2):473–9.

46. Javaheri S, Caref EB, Chen E, Tong KB, Abraham WT. Sleep apnea testing and outcomes in a large cohort of Medicare beneficiaries with newly diagnosed heart failure. Am J Respir Crit Care Med. 2011;183(4):539–46.

47. Cowie MR, Woehrle H, Wegscheider K, Angermann C, d'Ortho MP, Erdmann E, et al. Adaptive servo-ventilation for central sleep apnea in systolic heart failure. N Engl J Med. 2015;373(12):1095–105.

48. Nielsen J, Nilsson M, Freden F, Hultman J, Alstrom U, Kjaergaard J, et al. Central hemody-namics during lung recruitment maneuvers at hypovolemia, normovolemia and hypervolemia. A study by echocardiography and continuous pulmonary artery flow measurements in lung-injured pigs. Intensive Care Med. 2006;32(4):585–94.
49. Blanco P, Aguiar FM, Blaivas M. Rapid ultrasound in shock (RUSH) velocity-time integral: a proposal to expand the RUSH protocol. J Ultrasound Med. 2015;34(9):1691–700.
50. Pinsky MR. Functional haemodynamic monitoring. Curr Opin Crit Care. 2014;20(3):288–93.
51. Monnet X, Marik PE, Teboul JL. Prediction of fluid responsiveness: an update. Ann Intensive Care. 2016;6(1):111.
52. Wyler von Ballmoos M, Takala J, Roeck M, Porta F, Tueller D, Ganter CC, et al. Pulse-pressure variation and hemodynamic response in patients with elevated pulmonary artery pressure: a clinical study. Crit Care. 2010;14(3):R111.
53. Royer P, Bendjelid K, Valentino R, Resiere D, Chabartier C, Mehdaoui H. Influence of intra-abdominal pressure on the specificity of pulse pressure variations to predict fluid responsive-ness. J Trauma Acute Care Surg. 2015;78(5):994–9.
54. De Backer D, Heenen S, Piagnerelli M, Koch M, Vincent JL. Pulse pressure variations to pre-dict fluid responsiveness: influence of tidal volume. Intensive Care Med. 2005;31(4):517–23.
55. Perner A, Faber T. Stroke volume variation does not predict fluid responsiveness in patients with septic shock on pressure support ventilation. Acta Anaesthesiol Scand. 2006;50(9):1068–73.
56. Heenen S, De Backer D, Vincent JL. How can the response to volume expansion in patients with spontaneous respiratory movements be predicted? Crit Care. 2006;10(4):R102.
57. Michard F, Teboul JL. Predicting fluid responsiveness in ICU patients: a critical analysis of the evidence. Chest. 2002;121(6):2000–8.
58. Mesquida J, Kim HK, Pinsky MR. Effect of tidal volume, intrathoracic pressure, and cardiac contractility on variations in pulse pressure, stroke volume, and intrathoracic blood volume. Intensive Care Med. 2011;37(10):1672–9.
59. Marik PE. Techniques for assessment of intravascular volume in critically ill patients. J Intensive Care Med. 2009;24(5):329–37.
60. Marik PE, Cavallazzi R, Vasu T, Hirani A. Dynamic changes in arterial waveform derived variables and fluid responsiveness in mechanically ventilated patients: a systematic review of the literature. Crit Care Med. 2009;37(9):2642–7.

Chapter 10
Medication Safety in Chronic Lung Disease with Cardiac Comorbidity

Roy Pleasants (ID)

Clinical Pearls
1. Although not often considered by clinicians, significant alterations in the pharmacokinetics of inhaled agents because of renal or hepatic disease or interacting drugs may lead to higher systemic exposure and should be considered in patients, particularly those at high risk of adverse effects.
2. At recommended doses, the CV risks of inhaled long-acting β2-agonists and antimuscarinics as well as chronic azithromycin in COPD appear to be low.
3. Corticosteroids, particularly systemic therapies, can directly affect heart disease through worsening heart failure and also augmentation of cardiac effects of β2-agonists leading to increased adverse effects such as tachyarrhythmias.
4. Cardioselective β-blockers provide significant clinical and mortality benefits in COPD and are unlikely to worsen lung function.

Introduction

In 2015, CVD and COPD together accounted for nearly 780,000 deaths in the United States [1] and 12 million worldwide [2]; likely many of these patients had both types of diseases. COPD-related mortality is common, and in one US state COPD was listed as the primary or secondary cause of death among 1 in 6 adults [3]. Because drug therapies play such a vital role in managing chronic obstructive

R. Pleasants (✉)
Division of Pulmonary Diseases and Critical Care Medicine,
University of North Carolina at Chapel Hill, Chapel Hill, NC, USA

Pulmonary Department, Durham VA Medical Center, Durham, NC, USA
e-mail: roy.pleasants@unchealth.unc.edu

© Springer Nature Switzerland AG 2020
S. P. Bhatt (ed.), *Cardiac Considerations in Chronic Lung Disease*,
Respiratory Medicine, https://doi.org/10.1007/978-3-030-43435-9_10

pulmonary and cardiac diseases, ensuring optimal medication efficacy and safety has significant implications at many levels. Drug regimens are often complex in the typical elderly patient with pulmonary and cardiac diseases because of polypharmacy, other diseases, reliance upon inhalational therapies, and alterations in drug disposition. As the diseases progress, drug regimens change and often become more challenging, further increasing the risk of adverse drug effects. The elderly patient with lung and heart disease is at particularly high risk of adverse effects.

The Institute of Medicine report "To Err is Human" highlights the tremendous burden of adverse drug effects, which are responsible for many deaths each year [4]. Adverse drug effects can be directly from the individual agent, as the result of an interaction between medications, and/or as a consequence of the underlying pathophysiology. Further, some would define nonadherence as a side effect of medications when efficacy is not achieved. Whereas oral therapies are the first-line maintenance treatments for CVD, inhalational therapies constitute the bulk of medications for COPD. Both CV side effects of drugs used for COPD treatment and respiratory-related side effects of cardiac drugs are important factors that can influence patient outcomes. To best minimize risks associated with drug therapies, an understanding of the pharmacokinetics and pharmacodynamics is necessary. The purpose of this chapter is to discuss clinical pharmacology, drug interactions, and adverse effects of medications used in COPD and heart disease that can affect the pulmonary and/or cardiovascular systems.

Drug Disposition in the COPD Patient with Heart Disease

For patients with concurrent COPD and CV diseases, the key factors influencing drug disposition are 1) the unique pharmacokinetics of drugs administered by the aerosol route 2) the effect of impaired cardiac function on drug pharmacokinetics, and 3) age-related changes in drug disposition. Whereas there is substantial evidence of altered pharmacokinetics with heart failure [5, 6], there is little such evidence that COPD can directly alter drug disposition. Although inhaled medications are targeted delivery, the drug primarily reaches the systemic circulation through the pulmonary vasculature and to a lesser extent gastrointestinal (GI) absorption of swallowed drug; thus, clinically relevant extrapulmonary effects may occur [7]. Polypharmacy and aging also affect drug disposition, but are not unique to patients with COPD and/or CVD.

Disposition of Drugs Administered by the Systemic Route

After a drug is ingested orally, it is typically absorbed in the upper intestine and then enters the enterohepatic circulation where liver metabolism can occur; it then enters the systemic circulation to reach target tissues and receptors. Although dissolution of solid dosage forms occurs in the stomach, the vast majority of drugs are primarily absorbed in the jejunum [8]. If a significant portion of the drug is removed when initially delivered to the liver, it is considered to have a high first-pass effect and lower systemic bioavailability. Sublingual, parenteral, inhalational, and to some extent rectal administration of drugs bypass the initial hepatic first-pass metabolism.

In various organs including the liver, lungs, and intestine, cytochrome (CYP) P450 metabolizes drugs, largely to increase the water solubility of lipophilic compounds by oxidative metabolism (Phase I metabolism) to facilitate renal or GI elimination [9]. Some parent drugs and metabolites undergo Phase I and Phase II conjugative metabolism (e.g., UDP-glucuronosyltransferases and sulfotransferases). The nomenclature of CYP enzymes is based on their amino acid sequence where the number represents the family based on amino acid identity (CYP2), a letter represents the subfamily (CYP2D), and the last number represents the specific isoenzyme [10, 11]. In humans, among ~30 CYP isoforms, less than ten are responsible for the metabolism of the majority of drugs – CYP1, 2, and 3 families [12]. Overall, CYP3A4 and CYP2D6 are the most important drug-metabolizing enzymes, whereas a smaller number of drugs metabolized are by CYP2C9, CYP2C19, CYP1A2, and CYP2E1 [10–12].

Pharmacogenomics (or pharmacogenetics) is the study of the effects of genetic differences on a human's response to a drug or on disposition [11, 14]. Genetic makeup determines inherent pharmacokinetics and may affect interperson differences in drug absorption, distribution, metabolism, and excretion as well as drug responses. Pharmacogenomics is relevant to drug metabolism and response in the COPD patient with comorbid CVD, mostly from the perspective of cardiac-related agents, but also to some extent for pulmonary medications. Some of these differences can be explained by genetic variations in the presence and/or function of Phase I or Phase II drug-metabolizing enzymes and/or membrane transport proteins (e.g., P-glycoprotein [P-gp]) and drug targets (e.g., adrenergic receptors).

Drug metabolism via CYP450 enzymes exhibits significant genetic polymorphism for isoenzymes such as CYP2D6, whereas CYP3A4 polymorphisms either are rare or lack phenotypic effect and are thus unable to explain a sizeable fraction of heritable variation [14]. The polymorphic enzymes CYP2C9, CYP2C19, and CYP2D6 mediate 40% of CYP-mediated drug metabolism, which can make drug dosing problematic because of genetic differences for these isoenzymes. In general, there are four phenotypes of metabolism with these isoenzymes: (1) poor metabolizers that lack the functional enzyme; (2) intermediary metabolizers who are heterozygous for one deficient allele or carry two alleles that have reduced activity; (3) extensive metabolizers, who have two normal alleles; and (4) ultrarapid metabolizers, who have multiple gene copies [13]. Genetic polymorphisms relevant to pulmonary and cardiac diseases can greatly affect the activity of some of the CYP450 enzymes, e.g., CYP2C19 and CYP2D6, such as occurs with the metabolism of formoterol, isoniazid, warfarin, and clopidogrel.

Also important in drug disposition are efflux membrane transporters, such as P-gp and organic anion transporting polypeptide (OATP) [15]. Found in the liver, small and large intestine, and kidney among other tissues, P-gp serves a protective role by influencing the transmembrane diffusion of drugs thus limiting tissue distribution (e.g., central nervous system), reducing absorption (intestine), or increasing excretion (kidney). P-gp present on the luminal surface of enterocytes can regulate the intestinal absorption of some drugs and can therefore promote their excretion through the GI tract. It is also present on the tubular side of the renal epithelium and the biliary side of hepatocytes. Drugs which induce P-gp, such as rifampin, can reduce the bioavailability of drugs by increasing the transport into the intestinal lumen, where it is excreted. Inhibitors of P-gp, such as verapamil or clarithromycin, increase the bioavailability of susceptible drugs by increasing transport into the systemic circulation.

Enterocytes in the stomach and intestine, like hepatocytes, also express the major drug-metabolizing enzyme CYP3A4 [9]. The symbiosis between drug efflux by P-gp and metabolism by CYP3A4 via repeated cycles of absorption and efflux can have a significant effect on drug disposition [15]. As with alterations in metabolism by CYP isoenzymes, drug effects on P-gp might have a greater impact on agents with a narrow therapeutic index.

Beyond drug metabolism, other factors that can affect drug disposition include absorption, distribution, and renal excretion. For inhaled medications, body size may influence systemic exposure, assuming each patient inhales the same amount of drug, a patient with a low body mass index (BMI) can have higher lung and systemic exposure than a larger patient. The typical emphysema patient tends to have a low body mass index. For example, inhaled fluticasone furoate was associated with a higher area under the serum concentration curve (AUC) in Asians compared with White/Caucasians, in part due to differences in body size [16, 17].

Disposition of Drugs Administered by the Inhalational Route

Nearly every COPD patient will be receiving one or more inhaled medications due to the effectiveness and relative safety of therapies administered by this route. Figure 10.1 shows the initial fate of an aerosolized medication after inhalation, where some portion reaches the airways and the remainder is deposited into the oropharynx where it is swallowed [18]. Where the drug is delivered is highly dependent on the inhalational device, drug formulation, and patient factors such as inhalational technique and degree of airflow obstruction. Large aerosol particles tend to deposit by impaction in the oropharynx (>5 um), whereas smaller particles (1–5 um) are deposited by either impaction or gravitational sedimentation in the conducting airways (bronchi, bronchioles) and alveolar regions (terminal bronchioles, alveoli) [7, 19]. Smaller aerosol particles tend to deposit more distally in the lungs and thus can reach the alveoli. The smallest particles (<0.5–1 um) tend to remain suspended via Brownian movement and either rapidly diffuse after impacting onto the epithelium or are exhaled. Drug clearance from the lung occurs through a combination of mucociliary functions, exhalation of aerosol particles, and diffusion into the systemic circulation [7, 19]. Although lipophilicity promotes binding to tissues, it also makes the drug more likely to be removed by mucociliary clearance [19]. Once the drug deposits on the airway surfaces, molecules can diffuse across cell membranes to reach receptor sites. Target receptors of drugs include those in the epithelium, vasculature, airway smooth muscle, inflammatory cells, and mucus-producing glands. Depending on the lipophilicity and other physiochemical characteristics of the drug, molecules reach the receptors and exert pharmacological effects [7, 19].

Typically, inhaled drugs for obstructive lung diseases are lipophilic as to promote activity in the lungs including exerting a prolonged effect, while this characteristic slows the transition of a drug into the systemic circulation [7]. For most inhaled

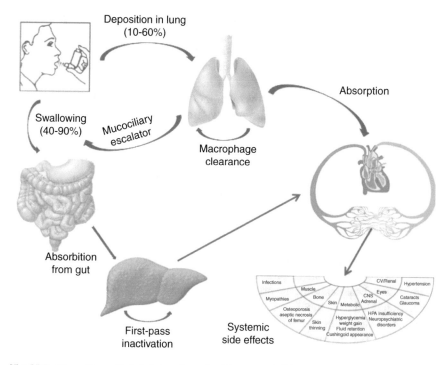

Fig. 10.1 Disposition of inhaled drug therapies Matera et al. [18])

medications, it is the parent drug that exerts the pharmacological effects, whereas for some ICS, the parent drug is inactive and the metabolite exerts the principal pharmacological effects.

The β2- and corticosteroid receptors are distributed throughout the small, medium, and large airways, whereas, although not exclusively, muscarinic receptors are in the medium and large airways [19, 21]. Endogenous substances that interact with these receptors include norepinephrine, epinephrine, acetylcholine, and cortisol among others. Drug therapies for COPD mimic or antagonize the processes affected by these endogenous substances. Not all receptors have to be occupied to exert clinically relevant pharmacological effects nor does a receptor have to remain occupied by the drug for its function to continue to be altered – analogously, there is the pharmacokinetic half-life and there is the pharmacodynamic half-life; the latter is often longer.

Drug metabolism and membrane transporters affect the activity and disposition of drugs in the airways [7, 20]. Excluding what portion is expectorated, drug deposited into the lung may undergo enzyme metabolism in the mucus or lung tissue by CYP450 isoenzymes and be eliminated by active transport or passive diffusion across membranes to reach the pulmonary vascular bed [7, 20]. In the lungs, including in Type I cells, several CYP450 isoforms are expressed as well as other biotransformation enzymes such as esterases, sulfotransferases, and glutathione S-transferases [22]. CYP3A5 and CYP1A1 (the latter inducible by tobacco smoking) appear to be the most common CYP450 enzymes in the lungs. The most abundant liver CYP450 enzyme, CYP3A4, is expressed to a lower degree in pulmonary tissue. CYP3A5 is responsible for most CYP3A-related metabolism in the lungs [7]. There are differences between CYP3A4 and CYP3A5, for example, the latter does not appear to metabolize erythromycin, quinidine, or 17 α-ethinyl estradiol at significant rates [23]. As occurs in other tissues such as the liver, intestines, and kidney, efflux transporters such as P-gp may also affect drug disposition in the lungs. The drug-metabolizing capacity of the lungs is substantially lower than that of the liver. For most inhaled medications in COPD, the lung is usually not the major contributor to systemic drug clearance, except indirectly through diffusion of drug into the blood circulation.

As shown in Fig. 10.2, beclomethasone dipropionate, the first marketed inhaled corticosteroid (ICS) in the United States, is extensively metabolized in the airways [24]. Beclomethasone dipropionate is a prodrug that is converted to the active metabolite, beclomethasone monopropionate, by esterases in the respiratory tract and is further metabolized by CYP3A5 to less active metabolites in the lungs and ultimately the liver. Although esterases are also present in the bloodstream, they contribute little to the overall metabolism of BDP [24]. With the exception of the ICS including ciclesonide, other current inhaled medications do not undergo substantial metabolism in the respiratory tract [25].

For inhaled medications, the principal route where the drug reaches the systemic circulation is from the lungs, rather than absorption from the GI tract [7, 20]. Inhaled drug that reaches the systemic circulation does not undergo initial hepatic first-pass metabolism, but eventually will reach the liver and may undergo metabolism, although some inhaled drugs, like tiotropium [26] and glycopyrrolate [27], rely more on renal clearance. Diffusion of drug from the lungs into the systemic circulation can occur quite rapidly, for many inhaled drugs in a matter of minutes, although for some it takes longer to achieve peak blood levels.

Similar to oral therapies, inhaled drug that is swallowed is exposed to metabolism and transport in enterocytes and subsequently reaches the enterohepatic circulation for further metabolism by the liver microsomes [20]. In some drugs, like albuterol, that have discernible oral absorption, there can be two peak blood levels,

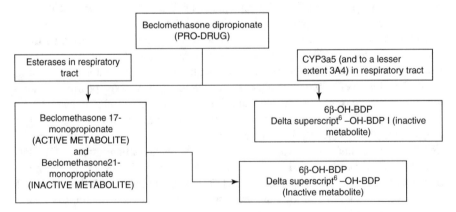

Fig. 10.2 Metabolic pathways of beclomethasone dipropionate (BDP) in the respiratory tract (Roberts [24])

one shortly after inhalation and the second delayed reflecting oral absorption [28]. The extent of absorption of inhaled bronchodilators such as albuterol and salmeterol that reach the GI tract is usually less than 50%, whereas for ICS, systemic bioavailability from the GI tract is quite low because of the significant first-pass effect.

Effect of COPD and Heart Disease on Drug Disposition

In contrast to CHF, there is little evidence that COPD directly alters drug disposition. One study found lower plasma concentrations of fluticasone and budesonide in COPD than in healthy volunteers [29], whereas vilanterol showed essentially no difference [30]. Lower blood levels of nebulized revefenacin were found in COPD than healthy volunteers [31]. Whether this is a function of greater systemic clearance or because of changes in the lungs related to COPD is unknown. Studies have also shown that smoking inhibits tight junctions in the lung resulting in faster drug absorption through the airway epithelia into the systemic circulation; therefore, it is possible that current smokers may have increased systemic exposure to drugs than nonsmokers; however, this has not been well-studied [32], and this was not seen with vilanterol [30]. Smoking can also induce metabolism by CYP1A1 [33], although it is a relatively uncommon source for drug metabolism. There is also some evidence that hypoxia related to pulmonary and/or heart disease may affect drug disposition [34].

It is well documented that CHF can alter the pharmacokinetics of various systemic medications, largely due to decreased blood flow to major organs, thus potentially affecting drug absorption, metabolism, distribution, and excretion [5, 6]. The best example of altered oral absorption related to CHF is that of the loop diuretic, furosemide, where due to poor blood flow to the GI tract and subsequent engorgement, the already poor GI absorption is further impaired [5, 6]. This can be addressed by increasing the oral dose of furosemide, administering intravenously, or switching to a loop diuretic that is less affected such as torsemide.

CHF can affect drug metabolism in the liver by alterations in blood flow [5, 6]. Metabolized drugs can be classified by whether their hepatic clearance is enzyme-limited (extraction ratio <0.3) or blood flow-limited (extraction ratio >0.7). High extraction ratio drugs are dependent on blood flow to the liver, whereas low extraction ratio drugs are primarily dependent on the intrinsic metabolic capability of the liver (affected by cirrhosis or hepatitis) [35]. If the drug is metabolized mainly in the liver, a decrease in metabolic activity as a result of hepatic impairment leads to an increase in the AUC of an orally administered drug. Therefore, CHF is more likely to alter metabolism of a high extraction ratio drug. All ICS including beclomethasone, budesonide, and fluticasone propionate and furoate are high extraction ratio drugs [25], where systemic exposure from oral absorption could be increased in patients with heart failure; however, this has not been studied. Theophylline's metabolism can be substantially affected by heart failure as well as liver impairment [36].

The pharmacokinetics of medications are not always predictable or stable in CHF, particularly as it waxes and wanes; but the net effect of alterations in drug distribution and clearance is that plasma concentrations are usually greater than in healthy persons [5]. If metabolism of a drug is impaired, prolongation of the elimination half-life of that agent leads to higher blood concentrations and delay in reaching steady state; therefore, dosing adjustments and subsequent monitoring of adverse effects should consider this. When possible, pharmacodynamic measures such as blood chemistries used for some anticoagulants or serum drug concentration measurements can be helpful. Theophylline is such an example, but probably should be avoided in heart failure patients.

Pharmacokinetics of Drug Therapies Used to Treat COPD

Corticosteroids

Systemic corticosteroids Systemic corticosteroids are typically reserved for acute worsening of COPD using 5–14-day courses [37], whereas a small portion of patients will be prednisone-dependent. In recent years, doses of prednisone 40 mg for 5 days are being used increasingly for exacerbations in noncritically ill patients [38]; notably doses of methylprednisolone 60 mg IV every 6 hours have been used in the not too distant past. The oral corticosteroids, prednisone, prednisolone, dexamethasone, and methylprednisolone, are well absorbed from the GI tract [39]. Food, nor does the P-gp and CYP3A4 inhibitor grapefruit juice, appear to significantly affect absorption. The serum and biological half-lives of corticosteroids can differ significantly as the on-going effects continue after the drug is no longer present. The typical onset of action of systemic steroids in the lungs occurs in a matter of a few hours, initially upregulating β2-receptors as well as beginning to exert anti-inflammatory effects [39]. The half-life of dexamethasone is significantly greater than others; all are extensively distributed throughout the body and rely upon hepatic clearance for removal. Prednisone is a prodrug where metabolism to the active moiety, prednisolone, is necessary to be pharmacologically active [39]. Even in the presence of hepatic impairment, the conversion of prednisone to prednisolone is still largely complete; however, higher serum levels of prednisolone may occur [40]. Intravenous methylprednisolone sodium succinate and dexamethasone sodium phosphate are also prodrugs that are rapidly converted by hydrolysis to methylprednisolone and dexamethasone in the bloodstream and tissues. Corticosteroids are extensively metabolized by CYP3A4 in the liver microsomes, making them subject to a number of pharmacokinetic drug interactions [39].

ICS ICS are used as a maintenance therapy for COPD in combination with long-acting β2-agonist (LABA). High doses of nebulized budesonide alone can be used in the treatment of exacerbations [37], and although not studied specifically in patients with concurrent COPD and CHF, inhaled budesonide is likely to cause less systemic effects than oral or parenteral corticosteroids [41]. The oral bioavailability of ICS are generally low, ranging from <1% for fluticasone propionate to ~25% for beclomethasone due to a significant hepatic first-pass effect [25]. P-gp may play a greater role in the gut for ICS than systemic corticosteroids [42]. The elimination half-life after inhalation can differ for ICS than when administered systemically. For example, the half-life for fluticasone propionate is ~8 hours after intravenous administration, but increases to ~14 hours after inhalation [25]. The intracellular esterification of budesonide and the ciclesonide active metabolite (and to some extent beclomethasone dipropionate) increases the retention time of these drugs in the airways and thereby prolongs their durations of action [25]. The free parent compound becomes available when these esterified forms are slowly hydrolyzed back to their active form and this mechanism contributes to the prolonged effect duration.

All ICS are substrates to metabolizing enzymes present in the lungs, liver, and intestine [25]. High first-pass metabolism by CYP3A4 occurs in the liver and consequently negligible oral bioavailability occurs with fluticasone furoate, fluticasone propionate, mometasone furoate, and ciclesonide, whereas modestly greater oral bioavailability is found for budesonide (10%) and beclomethasone dipropionate (~25%) [25]. In contrast, inhaled drug that reaches the systemic circulation from the lungs does not undergo first-pass metabolism before it reaches other sites in the body. For BDP, 97% is converted in the lung to the more potent beclomethasone monopropionate (BMP). CYP3A4 and CYP3A5 (predominant in the lungs) metabolize BMP at similar overall rates, although the former is less evident in the lung [24]. For ciclesonide, the conversion rate to its active metabolite in the lung is less complete [25, 43]. Inhaled budesonide is also metabolized by CYP3A5 isoenzymes in the lungs and liver. Figure 10.1 shows multiple potential systemic adverse effects of ICS.

Bronchodilators

Inhaled β2-Agonists In the United States, β2-agonists are primarily given via inhalation, although oral agents are occasionally used, whereas in some other countries [44], the oral route is used more often. The onset and duration of action varies among the inhaled β2-agonists largely due to differences in tissue penetration and interactions with receptors and exo-receptors [21]. Current β2-agonists undergo varying degrees of metabolism in the liver, although dosage adjustments are not normally recommended in the presence of hepatic impairment as the doses are relatively small when administered via the inhalational route [21].

Albuterol, one of the most frequently used inhaled medications used for the treatment of COPD, is a racemic mixture of R- and S-enantiomers. As is the case with epinephrine, the pharmacological effects are due to the R-isomer whose affinity for the β-adrenergic receptor is a hundredfold greater than the S-isomer [45]. In contrast, olodaterol and vilanterol are single enantiomer products that exert full agonist activity [30, 46]. For these enantiomers, the molecule appears as chiral mirror images that are nonsuperimposable (similar to right- and left-hand gloves). These configurations, levo (R) and dextra (S) enantiomers, rotate light in different directions and can be handled differently in the body.

Pharmacokinetic disposition differs between albuterol and levalbuterol [47]. Inhaled albuterol that is swallowed is metabolized through hepatic enzymes and through sulfotransferase enzymes (SULTIA3) present in the GI tract to albuterol 4'-O-sulfate. Metabolic products and unchanged drug are excreted through urine. Stereoselective metabolism of both the R- and S-enantiomers occurs where sulfotransferases work more effectively on the former. The bioavailability of the S-isomer is significantly greater than the R-enantiomer, particularly at high doses, resulting in higher S- than R-salbutamol plasma concentrations. The S-enantiomer is less pharmacologically active, although it has been suggested it is more likely to contribute to adverse effects. However, comparative study has found no difference in CV effects between albuterol and levalbuterol in COPD [48].

Formoterol is moderately lipophilic and hydrophilic, exerting a faster onset of action than the more lipophilic salmeterol – the latter diffuses more slowly to reach β2-receptors [21, 49]. Formoterol is metabolized primarily by direct glucuronide conjugation and O-demethylation (CYP2D6 and CYP2C19) in the liver to metabolites with reduced activity [48]. Some patients may be deficient in CYP2D6 or 2C19 or both; however, the clinical implications are not known [49]. A patient exhibiting intolerance to formoterol (e.g., excessive tachycardia) may be deficient in CYP2D6; thus, changing to a β2-agonist not dependent on metabolism by this CYP450 enzyme such as vilanterol and indacaterol may be helpful. Pharmacokinetic studies of formoterol in hepatic or renal failure have not been conducted [49]. As the main route of clearance is hepatic, patients with significant liver impairment or receiving concomitant drugs altering CYP2D6 metabolism should be monitored more closely.

Salmeterol is extensively metabolized by hydroxylation by CYP3A4 to α-hydroxysalmeterol, and the less active metabolite is eliminated predominantly in the feces [50]. The package insert indicates that because salmeterol is predominantly cleared by hepatic metabolism and that liver dysfunction may lead to accumulation of salmeterol in plasma, such patients should be closely monitored [50]. Because of the reliance upon CYP3A4, a number of potential drug interactions can occur with salmeterol (see section "Drug-Drug Interactions in the COPD Patient with Comorbid Cardiac Disease") [50].

Indacaterol, the first commercially available ultralong-acting LABA, has a rapid onset of action, and depending on the dose, up to a 24-hour duration [51]. Indacaterol undergoes metabolism by CYP3A4 to a hydroxylated metabolite, as well as other minor pathways [52, 53]. Unmetabolized drug accounts for about one-third of total systemic drug exposure [52, 53]. In vitro studies showed that indacaterol is a low-affinity substrate for P-gp. The pharmacokinetics of indacaterol was studied in patients with mild and moderate hepatic impairment, where no relevant changes in peak blood level or AUC of indacaterol occurred [52]. Studies in subjects with severe hepatic impairment were not performed. Due to the very low contribution of the urinary pathway to total body elimination, renal dysfunction is not expected to alter drug clearance.

Vilanterol, which has a relatively quick onset of action and extended duration [54], is also principally metabolized by CYP3A4 (O-dealkylation) to less active metabolites. The package insert recommends caution when considering the coadministration of vilanterol with strong CYP3A4 inhibitors [30] (e.g., itraconazole). Vilanterol is also a substrate of P-gp, where the effect of inhibitors (e.g., verapamil) or inducers of this membrane transporter can affect gastric absorption of a swallowed drug and therefore systemic bioavailability. Closer monitoring is recommended when used in patients with moderate to severe hepatic impairment.

Olodaterol has a fast onset and 24-hour duration of action [46]. It is metabolized by direct glucuronidation and by O-demethylation with the only metabolite, an unconjugated demethylation product, also having activity by binding to β2-receptors. However, according to the package insert, this metabolite was not detectable in plasma after chronic inhalation at the recommended dose [46]. CYP2C9 and CYP2C8 are the principal enzymes responsible for metabolizing in the liver, with minimal contribution of CYP3A4; therefore, poor metabolizers for these isoenzymes may alter the systemic response to olodaterol; however, this has not been studied. The package insert reports that olodaterol blood levels were increased by approximately 40% in subjects with severe renal impairment. Data in patients with less severe renal impairment were not reported [46]. In contrast, patients with mild to moderate liver impairment showed minimal changes in systemic drug exposure [55].

Inhaled Antimuscarinics The onset of effect of ipratropium is evident within 20–30 minutes with a duration of action approaching 6–8 hours [56]. It is a quaternary compound, poorly absorbed in the GI tract with most of the swallowed drug excreted in the feces. Ipratropium is partially metabolized to multiple, largely inactive, metabolites primarily by ester hydrolysis and conjugation [57]. The pharmacokinetics of ipratropium has not been studied in patients with renal or liver impairment, perhaps because of drug regulatory requirements for inhaled medications at the time the drug was marketed in the 1980s. Following intravenous administration, nearly 50% is excreted unchanged in the urine. Although not included in the package insert, a conservative approach would be to monitor adverse effects more closely in patients with severe renal dysfunction.

Tiotropium was developed as a structural analog of glycopyrrolate and was the first long-acting antimuscarinic approved for COPD [58]. It exerts its bronchodilatory effects within 30 minutes and has a duration of action of at least 24 hours [54]. Biotransformation of tiotropium appears to be minimal as nearly three-fourths of the drug is renally excreted unchanged and metabolites do not bind to muscarinic receptors [58]. Although, ex vivo experiments with hepatocytes show CYP2D6 and CYP3A4 are involved in tiotropium metabolism, the relatively small portion of metabolized drug would indicate enzyme inhibitors or inducers or pharmacogenetic differences are unlikely to cause significant changes in drug disposition. A very small fraction (<5%) of the swallowed portion of inhaled tiotropium is absorbed through the GI tract [26]. According to the package insert, patients with moderate to severe renal impairment (ClCr <60 mL/min) receiving tiotropium should be monitored closely for anticholinergic side effects [26]. The effects of hepatic impairment on the pharmacokinetics of tiotropium have not been studied, but would likely be insignificant except perhaps in the most severe cases.

Aclidinium exerts bronchodilatory effects within 30 minutes and has a duration of action of ~12 hours [54]. Clinical pharmacokinetic studies of aclidinium indicate that the major route of metabolism is chemical and enzymatic hydrolysis by esterases in the respiratory tract [59]. Metabolites do not bind to muscarinic receptors and thus are pharmacologically inactive. Blood levels quickly decline after inhalation due to the rapid hydrolysis by esterases [60]. No significant differences in pharmacokinetics of aclidinium were found in patients with varying degrees of renal impairment. The reliance on esterases on metabolism would indicate that hepatic impairment would have minimal effects on aclidinium disposition. This may be the preferred LAMA in patients with severe renal or liver impairment, particularly if the patient is predisposed or is experiencing anticholinergic side effects.

Glycopyrrolate was originally used in the 1980s where the parenteral formulation was nebulized. It is now commercially available in the United States as a twice-daily LAMA for COPD in MDI, DPI, and nebulized formulations [61]. It exerts bronchodilatory effects within 30 minutes and has a duration of action of ~12 hours [54]. The majority of glycopyrrolate that reaches the systemic circulation goes through the lungs as oral absorption is incomplete [54]. Renal elimination of the parent drug accounts for about two-thirds of total clearance of systemically available glycopyrrolate, whereas nonrenal clearance processes including metabolism also occur. According to the package insert, the AUC and elimination half-life of intravenous glycopyrrolate were significantly altered (up to 2.2-fold) in patients with mild to severe renal impairment [27]. In vitro investigations showed that multiple CYP isoenzymes contribute to the oxidative biotransformation, whereas glucuronide and/or sulfate conjugates of glycopyrrolate in the urine account for about 3% of the dose [27].

Umeclidinium exerts its bronchodilatory effects within 1 hour and has a duration of action of at least 24 hours [62]. It is primarily metabolized to metabolites with decreased activity by CYP2D6 followed by conjugation, with little contribution by CYP3A4. As the blood levels of this drug decline very quickly after inhalation, it is uncertain whether esterases may play a role in its metabolism. No clinically significant difference in systemic exposure to umeclidinium was observed following repeat inhaled dosing in CYP2D6 normal, ultrarapid, extensive, and intermediate metabolizers and poor metabolizer subjects [63]. Patients with mild to moderate hepatic impairment showed no decrement in clearance, and severe disease was not studied [64]. There was no evidence of significantly altered pharmacokinetics in severe renal impairment [65]. Although it is a substrate for P-gp, oral bioavailability is poor, where systemic exposure of umeclidinium is mostly through the lung after inhalation [66].

Revefenacin, a nebulized LAMA, exerts bronchodilatory effects in less than an hour, peaks at 1–2 hours, and has a duration of 24 hours [31, 67]. The absolute oral bioavailability of revefenacin is low (<3%). It is primarily metabolized via hydrolysis to an active metabolite, the latter at much higher concentrations than the former. The active metabolite is formed by hepatic metabolism and possesses activity at target muscarinic receptors lower (approximately one-third to one-tenth) than revefenacin, but could potentially contribute to systemic antimuscarinic effects at therapeutic doses. The manufacturer recommends avoiding this drug in hepatic impairment. There are modest changes in excretion of revefenacin in patients with renal impairment [66]. Although revefenacin is a substrate for efflux transporters such as P-gp and uptake transporters such as OATP1B1, its low blood levels and less active metabolite lead to a low probability of significant pharmacokinetic drug interactions. Like aclidinium, revefenacin may be preferred in patients with significant renal disease to decrease the risk of systemic adverse effects.

Theophylline Theophylline, a nonselective phosphodiesterase inhibitor, has been used for over 60 years in obstructive lung diseases and as an oral sustained-release product since the 1980s. Theophylline, including oral sustained-release products, is rapidly and completely absorbed when administered orally under fasting conditions [36]. Aminophylline, 80% theophylline, is also well absorbed when administered orally. It is primarily eliminated by hepatic biotransformation, predominantly CYP1A2 but also CYP3A4 and to a lesser extent by urinary excretion (10–15%) [36]. At higher doses, theophylline can exhibit nonlinear pharmacokinetics, causing blood levels to rise disproportionately with dose increases. Although blood concentrations are determined mainly by hepatic metabolism, they may also be increased in congestive heart failure, where the half-life markedly increases [36]. Targeting lower blood levels (<10 mcg/ml by using "low" doses) is currently recommended to decrease the risk of serum concentration-related adverse effects and these blood levels have been shown to exert anti-inflammatory effects [68].

Roflumilast Roflumilast, a selective phosphodiesterase inhibitor indicated for the COPD phenotype with severe disease and frequent exacerbations, is currently available as an oral formulation [69]. The oral bioavailability of roflumilast is ~80%, and although food delays absorption, it does not decrease the extent of absorption [70, 71]. Therefore, if given with food, it may improve GI tolerability. Roflumilast is eliminated through hepatic metabolism by CYP1A2 and CYP3A4, primarily to the active metabolite roflumilast N-oxide [72]. The metabolite roflumilast N-oxide is substantially more active than the parent compound and is responsible for much of its effects. In contrast to theophylline, tobacco smoking has little effect on the clearance of roflumilast or its active metabolite [72]. With regards to liver disease, roflumilast was studied in subjects with mild to moderate hepatic impairment (Child-Pugh A and B) where the serum AUC for roflumilast and roflumilast N-oxide were increased by 51–92% and 24–41%, respectively. Renal clearance is minimal for roflumilast; thus, dosing adjustments are not necessary, although use in end-stage renal disease may warrant closer monitoring for adverse effects.

Drug-Drug Interactions in the COPD Patient with Comorbid Cardiac Disease

Drug-drug interactions (DDIs) are a common cause of medication adverse effects, particularly in the elderly due to susceptibility, polypharmacy, and multi-morbidities [9, 73]. In the era of electronic records and order entry, the prescriber is confronted with drug therapy alerts in nearly every patient and sorting through this myriad of drug information can be difficult, particularly in these complex patients with multiple drug interactions or alerts. DDIs can be classified into two main types: (1) pharmacokinetic alterations in absorption, distribution, metabolism, and excretion of one drug by another and (2) pharmacodynamic that can be divided into three subtypes, (a) interference with a physiological or biological control process, (b) direct effect on receptor function, and (c) additive or opposed pharmacological effect(s). Little has been published regarding drug interactions specifically in the COPD patient with CVD. One study reported the type and frequency of drug interactions that occur in hospitalized patients with COPD and CHF [74]. The median number of drugs patients were receiving upon admission was six and there was a median of six drug interactions in each patient encountered. The use of concomitant β-blockers and β2-agonist, a pharmacodynamic drug interaction, was found in two-thirds of patients, although, as will be discussed later in this chapter, this is generally not a clinically relevant interaction when using a cardioselective β1-blocker. Other interactions included angiotensin-converting enzyme inhibitors with medications that can increase serum potassium.

The principal source of pharmacokinetic DDIs of medications used for COPD is through alterations of drug metabolism. ICS, systemic corticosteroids, roflumilast, theophylline, and most β2-agonists are primarily dependent on drug metabolism to facilitate removal from the body, whereas most inhaled antimuscarinics rely more on excretion through the kidney and/or biliary tract. For azithromycin, little metabolism occurs, and most of the drug is excreted through the biliary and GI tract [75]. For drugs used in the treatment of CVD, agents subject to DDIs include amiodarone and dronedarone (strong metabolizing enzyme inhibitors), verapamil (moderate potency P-gp inhibitor), warfarin (substrate), statins (substrate), and digoxin (substrate) [9]. Pharmacodynamic drug interactions with CVD medications are numerous including ACEI, loop diuretics, β-blockers, and potassium-sparing diuretics among others. It should be noted that not every patient will exhibit a clinically significant drug interaction when two interacting medications are combined, or there may be no significant interaction at all.

There are other comorbid pulmonary conditions in the COPD patient where drug interactions are relatively common including lung transplantation and pulmonary hypertension [76, 77]. In lung transplantation, numerous agents are subject to drug interactions including immunosuppressives (e.g., cyclosporine, mycophenolate, azathioprine, corticosteroids, sirolimus) and antibiotics (e.g., quinolones, azoles, and caspofungin) [76]. Drug interactions that may be seen in the patient with pulmonary hypertension include the concurrent use of bosentan and warfarin [78] or the use of rifampin and treprostinil [79]. The focus of this section will be on the interactions of drugs typically used in the management of the COPD patient with comorbid CVD and will not cover DDIs in the lung transplant or pulmonary hypertension patient populations.

Systemic and Inhaled Corticosteroids

The potential for DDIs is significant with corticosteroids, largely because of the dependence on metabolism by CYP3A4 and the implications of systemic effects [39]. All currently available systemic and inhaled corticosteroids are subject to CYP enzyme inhibition or induction, principally through altering the function of CYP3A4 and CYP3A5 [80]. Examples of clinical scenarios of such drug interactions include the development of an adrenal crisis when a prednisone-dependent patient receives rifampin (strong enzyme inducer) [81] or the development of Cushingoid side effects when itraconazole is coadministered in the long term with inhaled fluticasone propionate [82]. Whereas drug interactions with systemic steroids may be evident soon after the interacting drugs are coadministered, systemic effects that can occur as a consequence of interactions with ICS would likely take much longer to manifest.

Table 10.1 shows the pharmacokinetic interactions that may occur with corticosteroids. Drug classes prone to impair the metabolism of corticosteroids include macrolides, azoles, and HIV medications [80]. Cobicistat and ritonavir are some of the HIV medications documented to interact with corticosteroids. Grapefruit juice can increase methylprednisolone systemic exposure by altering P-gp and CYP3A4 activity [83]. It should be noted that not all triazoles or macrolides will impair CYP3A metabolism [84] where fluconazole and voriconazole have less effect on CYP3A4; in contrast, itraconazole and posaconazole are strong inhibitors of CYP3A4 [85]. Notably, voriconazole is less likely to interact with corticosteroids than itraconazole [85] or posaconazole [86–88]. For macrolides, erythromycin and clarithromycin are much more likely to impair CYP3A4 than azithromycin [89].

For systemic steroids, metabolizing enzyme inducers include rifampin, phenobarbital, phenytoin, and carbamazepine [90]. Phenobarbital increased the total body clearance of methylprednisolone twofold, phenytoin fivefold, and carbamazepine threefold. Rifampin is a very strong inducer of drug metabolism; even a few days of treatment can alter metabolism. Erythromycin for 1 week decreased the clearance of methylprednisolone by nearly one-half [91]. In addition, ketoconazole increased the methylprednisolone and prednisone AUC by more than twofold [92].

There are also a number of pharmacodynamic interactions of drugs with systemic corticosteroids as shown in Table 10.2 [39]. Corticosteroids, like prednisone, commonly increase blood sugar by decreasing insulin receptor sensitivity and

Table 10.1 Pharmacokinetic drug interactions with corticosteroids

Substrate drug	Principal pathways of metabolism	Inhibitors	Inducers
Beclomethasone dipropionate	Esterases in respiratory tract convert prodrug beclomethasone dipropionate to active metabolite beclomethasone 17-monopropionate, further metabolized by CYP3A4 and CYP3A5	Azoles (ketoconazole, itraconazole, posaconazole) Macrolides (clarithromycin, erythromycin) Antiretrovirals (cobicistat and ritonavir)	Rifampin, St. John's wort, phenytoin
Ciclesonide	Esterases in respiratory tract convert prodrug ciclesonide to active metabolite des-ciclesonide, which is further metabolized by CYP3A4 and CYP3A5	Azoles (ketoconazole, itraconazole, posaconazole) Macrolides (clarithromycin, erythromycin) Antiretrovirals (cobicistat and ritonavir)	Rifampin, St. John's wort, phenytoin
Budesonide, fluticasone propionate, fluticasone furoate, mometasone	Metabolized by CYP3A4	Azoles (ketoconazole, itraconazole, posaconazole) Macrolides (clarithromycin, erythromycin) Antiretrovirals (cobicistat and ritonavir)	Rifampin, St. John's wort, phenytoin
Prednisone, prednisolone, methylprednisolone, dexamethasone	Prodrug prednisone converted by liver CYP3A4 to prednisolone	Azoles (ketoconazole, itraconazole, posaconazole, voriconazole) Macrolides (clarithromycin, erythromycin) Antiretrovirals (cobicistat and ritonavir)	Rifampin, St. John's wort, phenytoin

increasing gluconeogenesis [93]. This typically occurs within 1–2 days after initiation in susceptible patients and is dose-dependent. Systemic corticosteroids may also increase blood pressure by sodium retention and thus decrease the effectiveness of antihypertensives [94]. Systemic corticosteroids can also increase potassium excretion through the kidneys and promote hypokalemia.

Table 10.2 Pharmacodynamic drug interactions with systemic corticosteroid therapy

Antidiabetic agents	Antagonism of blood glucose lowering; hyperglycemia; effects of corticosteroids on blood glucose are dose-dependent and occur quickly
NSAIDs and salicylates	Increased risk for gastrointestinal bleeding (consider using concurrent acid blockers)
Antihypertensives	Antagonism of hypotensive effects
Inhaled β2-agonist	Increased risk of hypokalemia, tachycardia, and tremors
Warfarin	Increased or decreased effect of warfarin, increased risk of GI bleeding
Vaccines	Reduced effectiveness of vaccines

Inhaled β2-Agonists

Pharmacokinetic and pharmacodynamic drug interactions are reported with inhaled β2-agonists and may have particular implications in the CVD patient. Potential cardiac effects include tachycardia, hypokalemia, and ECG changes; noncardiac effects include tremors and nausea [95]. Each of the LABAs undergo extensive metabolism; therefore, pharmacokinetic drug interactions can occur. As the net effect of these drug interactions is increased systemic exposure of the LABA, the patient with underlying heart disease may be more susceptible to these side effects.

Table 10.3 shows DDIs for the LABAs. For indacaterol, reported drug interaction studies include verapamil (P-gp inhibitor), erythromycin (CYP3A4 and P-gp inhibitor), ketoconazole, and ritonavir – leading to increases in systemic exposure (AUC) ranging from 1.4- to 2-fold [52]. Compared to doses approved in the United States, these interactions may be more relevant with the higher doses approved in Europe. As inhibition of metabolism by drugs may be slow, multiple days of concomitant therapy may be necessary to assess the potential for increased β-agonist side effects such as tachycardia. For olodaterol, studies in healthy subjects showed no interaction with fluconazole, whereas ketoconazole (potent CYP3A4 and P-gp inhibitor) increased olodaterol AUC by 68% [46]. The drug interaction between salmeterol and ketoconazole was quite profound where the AUC increased 16-fold – considered due to increased systemic bioavailability [50]. Although not studied, one would expect a similar interaction with itraconazole and salmeterol. Erythromycin was reported to increase the salmeterol peak blood level by 40% [50]. For formoterol and arformoterol, metabolism is primarily through CYP2D6 and CYP2C19 [96, 97]. Although DDIs are not documented, inhibitors of CYP2D6 such as amiodarone, bupropion, fluoxetine, and propafenone could theoretically increase systemic exposure to these drugs.

Pharmacodynamic interactions with β2-agonists include diuretics, corticosteroids, β-blockers, and drugs that prolong the QT interval [21]. In a dose-dependent manner, β2-agonists can augment hypokalemia and associated ECG changes via the shift of potassium from the extracellular fluid to intracellular fluid compartment, thus augmenting the effects of diuretics [21]. Systemic corticosteroids can also contribute to hypokalemia through their mineralocorticoid and glucocorticoid effects causing increased excretion of potassium [39]. The COPD patient with concomitant CHF would be at

Table 10.3 Pharmacokinetic drug interactions with long-acting β2-agonists

LABA	Mechanism of DDI	Inhibitors	Inducers
Arformoterol, formoterol	CYP2D6, CYP2C19	NR	Rifampin St. John's wort
Indacaterol	CYP3A4, P-gp	Erythromycin ketoconazole ritonavir, verapamil	NR
Olodaterol	CYP2C8, CYP2C9, CYP3A4, P-gp	Ketoconazole	NR
Salmeterol	CYP3A4, P-gp	Erythromycin ketoconazole	NR
Vilanterol	CYP3A4, P-gp	Ketoconazole verapamil	NR

particular risk of hypokalemia when aggressive diuretic dosing is combined with inhaled β2-agonists. Additional cardiac effects of corticosteroids when combined with β2-agonists include tachycardia that may occur due to augmenting the effect of adrenergic bronchodilators on the myocardium [98]. Inhaled β2-agonist can prolong QT interval modestly, usually <5 milliseconds (ms) at normal doses; however, it may be additive to other agents that increase the QT [21] including some tricyclic antidepressants, fluoroquinolones, macrolides, amiodarone, and antiarrhythmics among others.

A pharmacodynamic drug interaction occurs between β-blockers and β2-agonists where the effects of each may be opposed on the β2-adrenoreceptor [99]. However, if using cardioselective β1-blockers, there is a small probability of worsening respiratory status in the COPD as the predominant β-adrenoreceptors in the lungs are β2 [99, 100]. The effects of β-blockers on pulmonary function and clinical outcomes will be further discussed under Pulmonary Effects of Drug Therapies for CVD.

Inhaled Antimuscarinics

As most inhaled antimuscarinics primarily depend on renal excretion, drug interactions are most often pharmacodynamic in nature, potentially leading to anticholinergic effects such as urinary retention, blurred vision, constipation, and dry mouth – albeit much less frequently than seen with systemic agents [101, 102]. These effects are largely due to inhaled drug reaching the systemic circulation, whereas dry mouth may occur as a local as well as a systemic side effect. Infrequently, tachycardia attributable to these agents may be encountered in susceptible patients receiving higher doses.

Additive effects due to concurrent inhaled and systemic anticholinergics are most likely to occur in the elderly patient with polypharmacy. Examples include concomitant amitriptyline or nortriptyline used as a hypnotic or a medication used for urinary retention such as oxybutynin. Whereas combining short-acting and long-acting β2-agonists is considered acceptable, it is not recommended to combine ipratropium with a LAMA. Little additional bronchodilation and added side effects occur when ipratropium is added to tiotropium – likely the same holds true for other LAMAs [101]; thus, the risk/benefit does not favor combining these two therapies. There may be differences in propensities for anticholinergic topical adverse effects among the different inhalers – e.g., tiotropium Respimat® [26] has a lower reported frequency of dry mouth than the tiotropium Handihaler® [102], possibly related to differences in aerosol particle size and oropharyngeal deposition.

Pharmacokinetic interactions can occur with umeclidinium and glycopyrrolate as alterations in membrane transporter function have been reported one study found coadministration of verapamil, a moderate P-gp inhibitor, with umeclidinium led to ~1.4-fold increase in AUC in healthy volunteers [103]. In another study involving healthy subjects, cimetidine, an inhibitor of organic cation transport (contributes to the renal excretion of glycopyrrolate) increased the systemic exposure (AUC) of glycopyrrolate by 22% and decreased overall renal clearance by 23% [104]. In these studies of umeclidinium and glycopyrrolate in healthy volunteers, the minimal adverse effects observed from increased drug exposure are not necessarily indicative of what may occur in an elderly patient with impaired drug clearance because of organ dysfunction and/or greater susceptibility because of underlying CVD. Therefore, monitoring is warranted for anticholinergic adverse effects, especially when initiating these therapies in the presence of interacting drugs.

Theophylline

Theophylline is subject to both pharmacokinetic and pharmacodynamic drug interactions [68] (Table 10.4). Because of its narrow therapeutic index, drug interactions should always be considered [105]. However, lower target blood levels used today significantly decrease the likelihood of clinically significant drug interactions. By the nature of one of its pharmacological mechanisms, theophylline can antagonize adenosine [106]; thus, when a patient is receiving parenteral adenosine in the treatment of atrial arrhythmias, an inadequate clinical response may result in the presence of theophylline.

There are numerous pharmacokinetic drug interactions with theophylline, largely due to alterations in hepatic metabolism, primarily with CYP1A1 and CYP1A2 and less so with CYP3A4 [105] (Table 10.4). Interacting drugs prescribed in the COPD patient include the inhibitors cimetidine, ciprofloxacin, erythromycin, and clarithromycin as well as the inducers phenytoin and rifampin. Ciprofloxacin is well-known to increase blood levels of theophylline by inhibiting CYP1A2 isoenzyme, typically within a few days after coadministration. Inhalation of hydrocarbons such as tobacco smoking can induce metabolism of theophylline by CYP1A1 quite substantially [36, 105, 107]. If a patient is receiving theophylline and quits smoking, it should be expected that blood levels will increase, typically within a week. Inhalation or ingestion of nicotine alone would not be expected to alter theophylline metabolism.

Table 10.4 Pharmacokinetic drug interactions with theophylline and roflumilast

Theophylline	Metabolized by CYP1A2 and CYP 3A4	Ciprofloxacin, cimetidine, itraconazole, posaconazole, clarithromycin, erythromycin	Rifampin, St. John's wort, phenytoin
Roflumilast	Metabolized by CYP1A2 and CYP3A4	Itraconazole, posaconazole, clarithromycin, erythromycin	Rifampin, St. John's wort

Roflumilast

Due to the dependence of roflumilast on metabolism by CYP3A4, it is subject to drug interactions [72]. Gastrointestinal side effects of roflumilast tend to be dose-dependent, and like theophylline, GI side effects are usually worse when initiating therapy and lessen with continuation. It was found that initiating roflumilast at 250-mcg doses for 4 weeks led to better tolerance than initiating at 500 mcg daily [108]. Among the different drug interaction studies in healthy volunteers of roflumilast, erythromycin and ketoconazole, both CYP 3A4 inhibitors, were shown to increase the AUC of roflumilast by 70% and 99%, respectively [72] (Table 10.4). It is recommended that the following drugs be given cautiously in persons receiving roflumilast (cimetidine, erythromycin [109], ketoconazole [110], fluvoaxamine [111], enoxacin, and gestodene and ethinylestradiol [72]. There is no data evaluating the potential interaction between roflumilast and grapefruit juice (flavonoids) or itraconazole; however, these could be a clinically relevant interaction through CYP3A4 inhibition. It is also recommend that the strong enzyme inducer, rifampin, not be given with roflumilast [112]. Although not recommended by the manufacturer, because of the 99% binding of roflumilast to albumin, it is reasonable to monitor warfarin effects more closely for a short time period after starting roflumilast.

Antibiotics

Some macrolides, fluoroquinolones, and triazoles are well documented to cause drug interactions by impairing metabolism of other drugs [9, 84, 85, 87]. In general, β-lactams do not effect CYP metabolism to a significant extent; however, nafcillin can impair CYP3A4 activity [89]. Long courses of antimicrobials, such as an itraconazole for Aspergillus infection in a COPD patient, may increase the risks associated with these drug interactions. In addition to drug interactions involving drug metabolism, anti-infectives can be associated with prolongation of the QT interval and will be further discussed in the section "Cardiac Effects of Medications Used in the Treatment of COPD".

Antimicrobials differ in their ability to bind and inhibit metabolizing isoenzymes such as CYP3A4 [9, 11]; thus, generalizations of pharmacokinetic drug interactions are not valid on the basis of drug class, as often occurs in drug information databases. In contrast to erythromycin and clarithromycin, azithromycin has been shown to interfere poorly with the cytochrome P450 system in vitro, where numerous drug interaction studies have shown a very low risk of altered drug clearance associated with azithromycin [84]. For the macrolides like erythromycin and clarithromycin, it typically takes at least several days to a week of administration before the pharmacokinetic interaction is maximal.

All azoles inhibit the metabolism of CYP3A4, therefore having the potential to interact with drugs used in the treatment of COPD, although some have been determined to be nonsignificant interactions [85]. Among the commonly used triazoles, itraconazole is the azole most likely to be an inhibitor of membrane transporters including P-gp [85]. Voriconazole can be a strong inhibitor of several other CYP isoenzymes including CYP2C19 and CYP2C9. Posaconazole has little effect on CYP2C9 and CYP2D6. The newest triazole, isavuconazonium sulfate (prodrug for isavuconazole), appears to affect CYP metabolism coenzymes similar to voriconazole, with some differences [113]. The voriconazole package insert has a number of drugs that are either contraindicated or strong warnings about monitoring with coadministration of sirolimus, warfarin, and benzodiazepines, among others [86].

Among the azoles, itraconazole is most likely to decrease metabolism of systemic and inhaled corticosteroids [85]. Both voriconazole and isavuconazole have been shown to have a minimal effect on the metabolism of methylprednisolone in healthy volunteers [85, 114]. Ketoconazole is typically used for superficial fungal infections and thus is used infrequently in the COPD patient; however, it is used for drug interaction studies during Phase 2 development as it is a prototype CYP3A4 enzyme and P-gp inhibitor. Based on pharmacokinetic studies for indacaterol, olodaterol, vilanterol, and salmeterol demonstrating an interaction with ketoconazole, it is anticipated that itraconazole would interact with these drugs to increase systemic exposure and potential adverse effects.

Among the fluoroquinolones, ciprofloxacin has the greatest potential to impair hepatic metabolism of substrate drugs, although levofloxacin and moxifloxacin can also alter drug metabolism [89]. In contrast to macrolides, the effects of fluoroquinolones on metabolism of the substrate drug occurs more rapidly, such as seen with ciprofloxacin and theophylline. Fluoroquinolones have less effect on CYP3A4 than azoles and macrolides and greater effects on isoenzymes such as CYP1A2, particularly ciprofloxacin. In the COPD patient, an important drug interaction with fluoroquinolones is reduced oral bioavailability by caused by coadministration of cations [89] such as calcium for osteoporosis prevention or enteral feeds for cachexia in the COPD patient. In serious respiratory tract infections, parenteral quinolones may be preferred.

Cardiac Effects of Medications Used in the Treatment of COPD

Effect of Heart Disease on Myocardial Adrenergic and Muscarinic Receptors

Changes in β-receptors and muscarinic receptors can occur in heart disease. CHF is characterized by adaptive responses that lead to abnormal neurohormonal activation to compensate for left ventricular function decline [115], and increased activity of the sympathetic nervous system is well-known [116]. As a result of excessive and persistent sympathetic overstimulation, the β1-receptors downregulate substantially and β2-receptors become more prominent [116, 117]. A study in heart failure patients showed that β1 receptors are less evident, whereas β2-receptors increase such that the β2:β1 ratio is ~1:2, which essentially reverses to ~2:1 in the failing myocardium [118]. This may partially explain why the patient with heart failure may be more susceptible to inhaled β2-agonists. Also, changes in the muscarinic system occur in heart failure where the interaction between muscarinic and adrenoceptors changes such that the sympathetic ganglia convert more to a cholinergic phenotype [115]. However, differences in the number and function of muscarinic receptors in the failing human heart are not substantially changed [119].

Corticosteroids

Systemic corticosteroids are used widely in COPD largely because of effectiveness, low costs, and wide availability, although side effects are quite common even with low-dose, short courses [38]. Corticosteroid effects are mediated by the intracellular glucocorticoid receptors and the mineralocorticoid receptors; both are expressed in the myocardium and blood vessels. Both glucocorticoid and mineralocorticoid effects of corticosteroids could lead to CV effects via upregulated β-receptor sensitivity as well as other effects on the myocardium and sodium/fluid retention [39]. In the REDUCE trial evaluating systemic corticosteroids for COPD exacerbations, prednisone 40 mg daily for 5 days caused worsening heart failure in some patients [38]. However, it has also been reported that low doses of prednisone (10 mg/day) may promote the activity of diuretics in patients with CHF [94]. As shown in Table 10.5, differences exist among the synthetic glucocorticoids with regards to anti-inflammatory and sodium-retaining potencies [39].

Methylprednisolone has modestly lesser mineralocorticoid effects than prednisolone; however, when given IV and higher doses are used, this would likely negate that advantage. Dexamethasone has little mineralocorticoid effect compared to other corticosteroids, a potential advantage in the CHF patient, although it is

Table 10.5 Relative anti-inflammatory and mineralocorticoid potencies of systemic glucocorticoids

Compound	Equivalent potency (mg)	Relative anti-inflammatory potency	Relative sodium-retaining potency	Biological half-life
Cortisone	20	1	1	8–12
Hydrocortisone	20	1	0.8	8–12
Prednisone	5	4	0.8	18–36
Prednisolone	5	5	0.8	18–36
Methylprednisolone	4	5	0.5	18–36
Dexamethasone	0.75	25	0 or slight	36–54

Modified from Becker [39]

generally not used in COPD because of its long half-life and potential for adrenal suppression. However, if using dexamethasone instead of prednisone for the treatment of a COPD exacerbation in a prednisone-dependent patient, the lack of mineralocorticoid effects may lead to a decrease in blood pressure.

Both short-term and long-term administration of corticosteroids have been reported to be associated with an increased risk of ischemic heart disease, hypertension, atrial arrhythmias, and CHF. In a population-based study (non-COPD), the risk for CHF, myocardial infarction, stroke, and transient ischemic attacks combined was 3.7, 3.3, 1.7, and 7.4 (risk ratio), respectively [120]. However, another study in patients exposed and unexposed to glucocorticoids found no difference in CV events [121]. Risk of atrial fibrillation and flutter have been reported to be increased in those on high doses of glucocorticoids [122, 123]. However, low dose was reported to decrease the risk of arrhythmias in patients who had undergone coronary artery bypass surgery [124].

Glucocorticoids are associated with weight gain, likely related to increased appetite and fluid retention [125]. Some studies suggest that moderate or higher doses of prednisone promote fluid retention [120], whereas other studies have not supported this association [126]. In some patients, systemic corticosteroids have been shown to worsen heart failure, largely through mineralocorticoid effects leading to fluid retention [127].

ICS have thus far not been associated with worse CV outcomes and may even have positive cardiac effects. In the TORCH study, the fluticasone propionate arm did not show worsened CV outcomes compared to placebo or in combination with salmeterol [128]. The SUMMIT trial (Study to Understand Mortality and MorbidITy) trial was an international, multicenter trial of patients with COPD and either a history of CVD or heightened risk for CVD in 16,485 patients [129, 130]. When comparing ICS/LABA, ICS, LABA, and placebo over 1 year in COPD patients at high risk of CVD, there was a nonsignificant trend towards improved CV survival (adjudicated) with ICS compared to placebo (hazard ratio = 0.90, p = 0.12) [130]. Additional research is warranted with ICS in COPD patients with heart disease, particularly over extended time periods.

β2-Agonists and Antimuscarinics

The principal mechanisms that inhaled bronchodilators cause CV side effects are through alterations to the sympathetic and parasympathetic nerve pathways in the heart and vasculature [131] (Figs. 10.3 and 10.4). For the muscarinic system, M_2 is the predominant muscarinic isoform present in the heart, while in the coronary circulation subtype, M_3 is present [132]. Muscarinic receptors are coupled to the Gi-protein, where vagal activation decreases cAMP. Gi-protein activation also leads to the activation of K_{ACh} channels that increase potassium efflux and hyperpolarizes the cells to regulate the heart rate by altering the electrical activity of the sinoatrial node. By inhibiting the regulatory actions of acetylcholine, muscarinic receptor antagonists block the effects of vagal innervation on the heart, principally to the SA and AV node, thus increasing heart rate and conduction velocity. In ventricular preparations, anticholinergics decrease the force of contraction previously activated by cAMP-elevating agents such isoproterenol [117].

Activation of the β1- and β2-adrenoceptors in the human heart leads in coupling G-proteins to activate adenylyl cyclase, increasing the intracellular level of cAMP, promoting calcium influx and thus enhancing myocardial function [117]. The density of β2-adrenoreceptors on the heart and skeletal muscle is much lower than

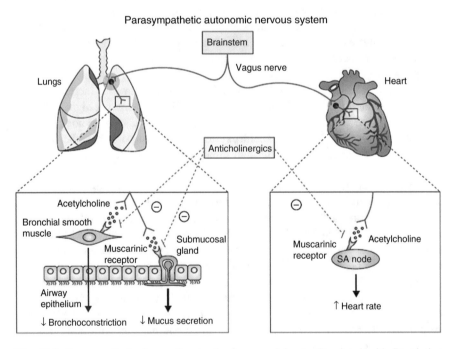

Fig. 10.3 Parasympathetic innervation to the lungs and heart. (Reprinted with Permission from 131)

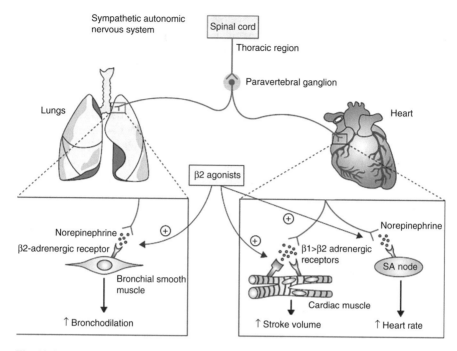

Fig. 10.4 Sympathetic innervation to the lungs and heart. (Reprinted with Permission from 131)

airway smooth muscle cells. β2-agonists bind principally to the β2-adrenoreceptors located in the nodal tissue, conducting system, and contracting myocytes. β2-agonists can be arrhythmogenic because of chronotropic and inotropic effects, depolarization, repolarization, and cellular potassium shifts [21]. These β2-cardioselecetive inhaled agents exhibit minimal agonist effects on the β1-receptor, and β2-agonist-induced tachycardia results from the direct stimulation of cardiac β_2-adrenoceptors in the SA node as well as indirect activation of peripheral receptors leading to vasodilatation and reflex vagal withdrawal. If tachycardia is significant enough, this may increase myocardial oxygen consumption and electrical instability – possibly detrimental in the failing heart.

β2-agonists induce cardiac-related side effects in a dose-dependent manner and include an increase in myocardial oxygen consumption, changes in blood pressure, tachycardia, arrhythmias, and hypokalemia [21]. β2-agonist-related ECG changes include flattening of the T wave, prolongation of the QT interval, and ST segment depression. One study showed that COPD patients with preexisting cardiac arrhythmias and hypoxcmia exhibited dose-dependent effects of formoterol on the myocardium [133].

Other relevant effects of β2-agonists on the CV system are shifting of potassium intracellularly into skeletal muscle, liver-induced glycogenolysis thus increasing blood glucose, and increased renin from the kidney [21]. Both tremors and hypokalemia are due to direct stimulation of β_2-receptors in skeletal muscle and occur in a dose-dependent manner. Long-term use of β2-agonists can lead to receptor desensitization through dampening of the signaling or downregulation of β2-receptor numbers (e.g., tachyphylaxis), which may lessen reported side effects such as tachycardia and tremor over time [21]. Ventilation/perfusion mismatches can occur when first administering inhaled β2-agonists; however, this may not be clinically significant in the COPD patient [21].

In general, the effects of inhaled β2-agonists on the QT interval are modest – however, such effects may be additive and therefore relevant – whereas inhaled antimuscarinics have minimal, if any, effects on QT. A double-blind, placebo, and active-control (moxifloxacin) study in healthy volunteers showed dose-dependent changes with indacaterol in QTc of 2.7, 3.0, and 3.3 ms following doses of 150, 300, and 600 mcg, respectively [134]. Olodaterol was also shown to have minor effects on QTc where supratherapeutic doses led to an increase in QTc of ~6 ms, and near-normal doses only increased the QTc by ~2 ms [135]. At 8 times the recommended dose for 10 days, umeclidinium did not prolong the QTc to any clinically relevant extent in more than 80 subjects [66]. In a study of aclidinium 200 mcg and 800 mcg administered to healthy volunteers for 3 days, no effects on prolongation of the QT interval were observed [58].

It has also been reported that inhaled β2-agonists may improve cardiac performance by enhancing cardiac and stroke volume and reducing peripheral vascular resistance, although the clinical significance is unknown [136, 18]. In addition, recent studies have evaluated the effects of LABA, LAMA, and ICS on arterial stiffness in COPD [137–139]. In a non-placebo-controlled study, arterial stiffness, measured by aortic pulse wave velocity, was lower with both ICS/LABA and LAMA in COPD [139]. Another study comparing ICS/LABA and placebo did not show a significant effect of arterial stiffness; however, a post hoc analysis did show a subgroup who benefited from ICS/LABA treatment [137]. In a more recent placebo-controlled study by Bhatt et al., LABA or ICS/LABA over 24 weeks did not alter arterial stiffness [138].

Theophylline

It is well documented that at "toxic" blood concentrations of theophylline, cardiac side effects like supraventricular and ventricular arrhythmias can occur and at very high levels, e.g., >40 mcg/ml can cause cardiac-related death [68, 140–142]. At blood concentrations more than 20 mcg/ml, sinus tachycardia, supraventricular ectopic beats, and ventricular premature beats are common. More evidence has substantiated this finding but has also added to the evidence that this effect can also happen during so-called nontoxic therapeutic doses. One study found that patients with toxic levels associated with the chronic use of theophylline were more likely to experience arrhythmias and death than acute overdoses [141].

Theophylline can induce alterations in ECGs including significant reductions in the atrioventricular and His-Purkinje conduction intervals and SA node conduction time [142].

Antimicrobials

Antibiotics are used commonly in COPD, fluoroquinolones for exacerbations and macrolides for the treatment as well as prevention of exacerbations. Azoles used for the short-term and long-term treatment of fungal infections in the COPD patient are reported to cause adverse CV effects, albeit infrequently. A number of warnings regarding antibiotics have come from the US FDA over the last 2 decades regarding cardiac toxicities. In 2001, a warning was issued regarding the increased risk of worsened CHF with itraconazole; the mechanism is unknown [143].

The potential adverse cardiac effects of azithromycin came under scrutiny in 2012 by the FDA and then in 2013 when the warning in the package insert was updated [143]. The change in the package insert was largely in response to a retrospective study in one US state's Medicaid population [144] and by FDA review indicating there is a risk of cardiac events associated with azithromycin.

In 2016, a warning concerning the multiple and potentially serious side effects of fluoroquinolones was issued by the FDA. The FDA discourages the use of this drug class unless other antibiotics are not a good option [145]. In 2018, the US FDA issued a warning about the cardiotoxicity of clarithromycin [146] in patients with stable coronary artery disease based on a 10-year follow-up study [147]. Notably the risk was evident beginning about 1 year after receiving 2-week courses of clarithromycin. The hazard ratio was 1.1 (95% CI 1.0–1.21), which was significant over the 10-year period, and a greater risk was evident in the first 4 years after therapy and was most evident in persons not taking statins [8]. It is unclear how a 2-week course of clarithromycin would affect CV outcomes over a multiyear period.

Effects of these anti-infectives may be due to direct actions on the myocardium leading to arrhythmias or heart failure as well as indirectly through drug interactions by increasing systemic exposure of other medications that can affect the heart. One of the leading proposed mechanisms that these agents adversely affect cardiac function is through prolongation of the QT interval increasing the risk of developing the ventricular arrhythmia torsades de pointes (TdP). Drugs have been associated with this arrhythmia for many years but regulatory awareness was heightened when terfenadine, an oral antihistamine, was reported to cause cardiac deaths in the early 2000s. It was determined that slowed CYP3A4 metabolism of the parent drug was associated with the arrhythmia [148]. Since then, an emphasis has been placed on the proarrhythmic risk of drug therapies, principally based on the likelihood of prolonging the QT interval. Although QT interval prolongation is considered the major proarrhythmic mechanism, it is perhaps better considered a surrogate for TdP [148,

149]. Drugs that prolong the QT interval range from having potent torsadogenic activity to no proarrhythmic action and even antiarrhythmic effects [148]. Blockade of hERG channels is the primary cause of TdP, but blockade/activation of other channels can also be torsadogenic. While it appears that the standard assays (hERG channel activity, action potential duration, and QT/QTc interval) are very good at predicting the risk of QT interval prolongation, they are less useful in determining the proarrhythmic effects of agents [148]. Thus, drug-induced QT prolongation is considered by some to be a suboptimal surrogate for TdP and other ventricular arrhythmias.

TdP from antimicrobials is a low-frequency event, but can be life-threatening, particularly in susceptible persons [148, 150, 151]. Risk factors for developing TdP include older age, electrolyte disturbances, baseline prolonged QTc, increases in QT interval >60 ms, and administration of multiple drugs that prolong the QT interval [148, 150] (Table 10.6). Typically, for a patient to develop TdP, multiple risk factors must be present. The obtainment of an EKG with interpretation is recommended in some instances. CredibleMeds, a program of the Arizona Center for Education and Research on Therapeutics, maintains an evidence-based list of potential QT-prolonging medications stratified by their risk of TdP (risk, possible, conditional, and avoided) [152].

The US FDA provides guidance on determining risks of TdP [153] including a recommendation to have a positive control group – moxifloxacin can be used (as noted in the indacaterol study previously described [134]). After initial studies looking at the potential for drugs to affect the mechanisms associated with QTc prolongation, such as I_{kr} channels, it is required to conduct such studies using therapeutic doses of the investigational drugs with metabolic inhibitors. These investigations tend to be done late in drug development.

Table 10.6 Risk factors for drug-induced torsades de pointes

Prolonged QTc >500 ms or increase in QTc >60 ms from offending agent
Concomitant use of other QTc-prolonging agents
Excessive doses of an agent that can induce TdP
Elderly
Female gender
Underlying CV disease including history of MI and CHF
Electrolyte abnormalities (hypokalemia, hypomagnesemia, hypocalcemia)

Clinical Studies Evaluating CV Safety of COPD Medications

Inhaled Bronchodilators

Studies evaluating the cardiac safety of inhaled antimuscarinics and β2-agonists in COPD have reported mixed findings. Since the mid-1990s, there have been more than 25 observational studies and 60 clinical trials reporting on CV effects of inhaled β2-agonists and antimuscarinics, with or without ICS [131]. There have also been a number of pooled and meta-analysis. The vast majority of the prospective clinical trials excluded patients with significant CV disease and thus may not be indicative of the efficacy and safety of these agents in a COPD patient with comorbid CVD, although heart disease is present in some patients without being properly diagnosed. Only recently have prospective studies of inhaled therapies been conducted in patients with significant CV risks where the primary outcome was cardiac events [130, 154, 155]. Regulatory agencies such as the FDA-mandated post-marketing safety studies and EMA post-authorization safety studies (PASS) will continue to assess CV safety of these agents.

Among retrospective observational studies reported in the review by Lahousse, approximately one-half showed significantly higher CV risks in COPD patients who received inhaled bronchodilator therapy [131]. In retrospective, observational studies, numerous variables come into play; perhaps the most important is that these patients are very complex and proper diagnosis and assignment of outcomes to any particular factor is very difficult retrospectively. Further, there are inaccuracies in documentation in medical records and lack of control on medication compliance – thus should be considered hypothesis-generating awaiting prospective trials. A study in more than 200 hospitalized COPD patients showed ~20% of the patients never used their ICS/LABA inhaler after discharge, and in those that did, the majority used it incorrectly [156]. In a post hoc analysis, medication nonadherence in COPD was found to be a risk factor for mortality among subjects in the TORCH study [157]. Nonadherence to COPD and other medications may pose a greater risk of CV events and is unaccounted for in retrospective database studies.

COPD patients appear to be most susceptible to CVD events during or shortly after hospitalization for a COPD exacerbation. Using an administrative database in the UK, a study evaluating COPD exacerbations and CVD relationships, among COPD patients, prescriptions for oral antibiotics and corticosteroids were associated with a higher risk for myocardial infarction and stroke [158]. Similarly, in the recent SUMMIT study, where overall, there were no increased CV risks with fluticasone furoate or vilanterol, there was an increased risk of CVD events in the post-hospitalization period [159]. A retrospective analysis of patients in Taiwan health system by Wang attributed worse CV outcomes in the 30-day period posthospitalization with the use of long-acting bronchodilators [44].

β2-Agonists Both short-acting and long-acting β2-agonists can be associated with adverse cardiac effects. Regarding the short-term use of short-acting β2-agonists like albuterol, a Cochrane analysis reported no serious adverse effects [160]. In the extensive review by Lahousse of cardiac toxicity of pulmonary medications in COPD [131], among 39 prospective studies of LABA alone or in combination with other inhaled therapies such as ICS, only one study reported statistically significant worse CV outcomes – specifically in a placebo-controlled study of arformoterol by nebulization [161]. In the largest of these prospective studies, the Towards a Revolution in COPD Health (TORCH) over 3 years, COPD patients were randomized to placebo, fluticasone propionate alone, salmeterol alone, or their combination in greater than 6000 COPD patients [162]. All-cause mortality was the primary outcome and deaths were adjudicated during the study. Patients at high risk of dying within 3 years were excluded. ICS/LABA combination product had the lowest proportion of patients who withdrew from the study (34% vs 44% in the placebo group) and had a nonsignificant decrease in all-cause mortality compared with placebo ($p = 0.052$). A post hoc analysis of the TORCH trial addressed CV-related secondary outcomes where it was found that one in five subjects reported a CV event during the 3-year study and there were no increased risks for either salmeterol monotherapy or the fixed-combination treatment [128]. There appeared to be some cardioprotective effects of the ICS/LABA combination in this post hoc analysis.

Based on this finding in TORCH as well as other evidence, a large prospective study (SUMMIT) of a newer ICS/LABA combination of vilanterol and fluticasone furoate was conducted [130]. The study was conducted for at least 1 year in more than 16,000 moderate COPD patients with or at high risk of CV disease. The primary endpoint (all-cause mortality) was not significantly affected by combination therapy (HR 0.88, $p = 0.14$). It is possible that longer-term studies of ICS/LABA may show benefits as these drugs are administered for years, especially in light of the trend for better CV outcomes in the SUMMIT study. However, as shown in other studies, all treatments did reduce the rate of moderate and severe exacerbations. In a secondary analysis of CV events, individual or combination inhaled therapies were not associated with CV outcomes different than that of placebo [163]. In a post hoc analysis of SUMMIT, using the sensitive troponin I as a marker of cardiac risk, neither inhaled B2 or combination ICS/LABA resulted in higher blood levels [164].

Some clinical trials have employed Holter monitoring in a subset or all study subjects receiving LABA therapy. In a study in COPD patients, using Holter monitors, dose-dependent effects of formoterol on supraventricular tachycardia and plasma potassium were observed [133]. Among more than 700 patients with Holter monitoring comparing nebulized arformoterol, salmeterol, and placebo, it was found that in nearly 42%, atrial arrhythmias were evident at baseline and this increased by 2–5% over placebo after randomization to inhaled bronchodilator [165]. Rates of serious arrhythmias did not increase over the 12-week study period.

One important consideration of the safety of inhaled bronchodilators is that nearly all studies have evaluated therapies administered by multi-dose inhalers and not by nebulization where doses are typically much higher (ipratropium, formoterol, and arformoterol). It has been shown that the type of device and particle size affect systemic drug concentrations [19]. It was found in a 1-year study that measuring serial electrocardiograms while receiving arformoterol by nebulization resulted in an approximately 3.0-ms higher QTc compared to salmeterol inhaler [96].

Antimuscarinics One of the first prospective clinical studies to suggest CV safety issues existed with an inhaled antimuscarinic was the Lung Health Study [166]. This randomized controlled trial assessed the effects of different interventions on long-term outcomes including the cardiovascular risk of inhaled ipratropium. This study observed a relationship between ipratropium and a higher risk of death and hospitalization secondary to CV disease. Notably, there was a failure to adjust p-values for multiple statistical comparisons, and a reanalysis of the data showed that the increased risk of CV morbidity and mortality was largely among patients who were randomized to the ipratropium group but who did not take ipratropium and thus would be defined as nonadherent [167].

Among the 20 prospective clinical studies of inhaled antimuscarinics reported in the review by Lahousse, none showed significantly worse CV outcomes [131]. As with studies of inhaled LABAs, a weakness of these studies is the exclusion of patients with substantial cardiac risks. In the largest prospective study evaluating the efficacy and safety of tiotropium (UPLIFT) [168], the relative risks of CHF, angina, myocardial infarction (MI), and cardiac failure were significantly lower with tiotropium than placebo [169]. Around that time, a meta-analysis by Singh indicated a higher risk of CV events with tiotropium, but did not include the UPLIFT study in that meta-analysis [170]. In 2010, the Food and Drug Administration (FDA) concluded that because of the limitations of that meta-analysis and the strengths of the UPLIFT trial, there was no increased risk of MI or death was associated with tiotropium DPI [171]. In a combined analysis of multiple clinical trials in 727 patients using Holter monitoring, tiotropium DPI or SMI was not associated with changes in heart rate, supraventricular premature beats, or ventricular premature beats and pauses compared with placebo or the pretreatment baseline period [172]. In 2013, a pooled safety analysis by Halpin showed either no difference or lower rates of serious adverse events or fatal CV events to tiotropium SMI or Handihaler® compared to placebo [173]. A meta-analysis in 2013 by Dong also showed an association with tiotropium SMI and ICS/LABA with CV deaths in severe COPD, but not tiotropium DPI [174].

Because of the concerns of potentially greater CV events with the tiotropium SMI, the manufacturer undertook a large prospective study comparing two doses of tiotropium SMI with tiotropium dry powder inhaler (DPI) in patients with CV risks – TIOSPIR [155]. Patients with COPD and concomitant cardiac disease were included unless they had unstable CVD (MI in the last 6 months, admission to hospital admission for New York Heart Association Functional class III or IV, or unstable or life-threatening arrhythmia in the previous 12 months), as well as moderate to severe renal impairment. Among nearly 17,000 patients, tiotropium SMI was found to be noninferior to tiotropium DPI with respect to the risk of death (hazard ratio 0.96). The incidence of major cardiovascular adverse events (MACE) was also similar between the two tiotropium groups, although a trend towards an increased incidence of myocardial infarction was reported in the SMI group as compared with the DPI group (hazard ratio 1.4, $p = 0.06$).

The most recent prospective studies to evaluate the CV safety of a LAMA were the 3-year ASCENT study for aclidinium in subjects with CV disease or risk factors [154] and a report on the effect of revefenacin on MACE in Phase III studies [175]. The primary objectives of the long-term Aclidinium Bromide on Long-Term Cardiovascular Safety and COPD Exacerbations in PatieNTs with Moderate to Very Severe COPD were to evaluate the long-term effects of twice-daily aclidinium on MACE, overall safety, and COPD exacerbations in patients with moderate to very severe disease with a history or significant risk factors for CV comorbidities and renal insufficiency (ClCr <60 ml/min) [154]. Aclidinium met its primary safety endpoint, demonstrating a favorable CV safety profile, with the time to patients experiencing a first MACE similar to placebo.

LAMA/LABA Dual Bronchodilators Several new LAMA/LABA combination products are available including umeclidinium/vilanterol, glycopyrronium/formoterol, and tiotropium/olodaterol. A LAMA with a LABA dual bronchodilator product provides greater bronchodilation than that achieved with an ICS/LABA combination and may have similar or greater effects on COPD exacerbations [176].

Among 3 clinical trials for indacaterol and glycopyrronium in more than 3000 subjects, there were no safety signals for CV events. A pooled safety analysis in 11,404 patients also reported that there were no greater risks on death, MACE, and atrial arrhythmias of the combination vs placebo or tiotropium [177]. MACE tended to occur in patients with a body mass index >30 kg/m^2 given glycopyrronium vs placebo.

The clinical studies of tiotropium/olodaterol, aclidinium/formoterol, and umeclidinium/vilanterol did not show a safety signal regarding CV events; however, as other key clinical trials for individual long-acting bronchodilators, subjects with significant CV were excluded [131]. A 52-week study of glycopyrrolate/formoterol MDI in 3274 moderate to very severe COPD patients also did not show an increased risk of CV events including in comparison to tiotropium [178].

It appears that in certain COPD patients, bronchodilation can produce favorable effects on the myocardium [179, 180]. A 2015 study in COPD patients with hyperinflation and heart disease showed cardiac benefits of indacaterol [179]. A crossover study of indacaterol/glycopyrronium for 14 days vs placebo was undertaken to assess effects on cardiac function. Treatment with indacaterol and glycopyrronium increased left ventricular end-diastolic volume by ~6 ml/m^2 as well as improvements in right ventricular end-diastolic volume and cardiac output [180].

Anti-infectives

Fluoroquinolones Fluoroquinolones are widely used for COPD exacerbations due to their spectrum of activity, availability of oral and IV formulations, modest cost, and clinical trials supporting efficacy in COPD exacerbations. Fluoroquinolones are associated with rare CV adverse effects, most often reported to be related to QTc prolongation [181, 182]. Fluoroquinolones exhibit the potential, as do most other agents that can cause QT prolongation, to block the cardiac voltage-gated potassium channels, particularly the rapid component (I_{Kr}) of the delayed rectifier potassium current (IK) [148, 181, 182]. Prolongation of the QT interval does not solely have adverse cardiac effects, but, by causing early after depolarizations, may induce TdP. Fluoroquinolones downregulate a gene involved in cardiac repolarization, which can cause prolongation of the QT interval [148]. Grepafloxacin was withdrawn from the market because of cardiac toxicity, whereas the cardiac risks of those currently in clinical use are less clear. Data concerning CV risks of fluoroquinolones are based on animal studies, drug development clinical studies, case reports, and retrospective studies using large healthcare databases. Early clinical trials are apt to not show this side effect as it tends to be rare and typically high-risk patients are excluded from the Phase 2 and 3 studies.

In one study, 2 European healthcare databases were used to estimate the risk of arrhythmias among adults treated with fluoroquinolones in Denmark (1997–2001) and Sweden (2006–2013). Sixty-six cases of arrhythmia were identified among more than 900,000 fluoroquinolone courses [183]. The low rate was nearly identical to the rate of arrhythmia in an equally large control group that received penicillin V. The most commonly prescribed fluoroquinolones were ciprofloxacin (83%) and norfloxacin (12%); both of these fluoroquinolones have a relatively low arrhythmic potential. A 2017 meta-analysis by Liu found that levofloxacin and moxifloxacin were associated with an increased risk of TdP, whereas ciprofloxacin was not [184]; this is consistent with the potential for QTc prolongation of these fluoroquinolones. It has been shown that the higher the fluoroquinolone dose and serum AUCs, the higher the QT prolongation risk and subsequently the risk of TdP [181].

Macrolides Of the three principal macrolides on the US market, azithromycin is the most commonly used for COPD exacerbations and as a maintenance therapy to decrease exacerbation risks [185]. Like fluoroquinolones, the mechanism that macrolides can cause a prolongation of the QT interval is blockade of the rapid delayed rectifier potassium current (I_{Kr}) conducted by the human ether-a-go-go-related gene (hERG)-encoded potassium channel [186]. In a study reported in the package insert, azithromycin doses of 500 mg, 1000 mg, and 1500 mg were administered to 113 heathy subjects [75]. There was a dose-dependent effect of azithromycin on the QTc interval of 5 ms, 7, ms, and 9 ms, respectively. A 2012 FDA guidance on drugs that can be proarrhythmic reports that an increase in the QTc of 5 milliseconds (ms) should lead to additional studies evaluating potential cardiac effects [153]. Thus, the effect of a azithromycin 500 mg dose based on a 5-ms increase in QT would indicate that there is a low risk of CV adverse effects.

Oral azithromycin has low oral bioavailability of ~30% [75]; thus, intravenous azithromycin would yield much higher concentrations and may have a greater risk of cardiac events in the hospitalized setting where this route of administration might be employed. The difference in potential cardiac effects of azithromycin between oral and intravenous has not been elucidated. Intravenous erythromycin has been shown to have a higher risk of QT interval prolongation than oral administration [187].

Published data concerning the potential cardiac effects associated with azithromycin include animal studies, published case reports, prospective clinical trials of macrolides for acute infections and anti-atherogenesis effects in coronary artery disease, retrospective studies using healthcare databases, FDA spontaneous adverse event reporting system [188], and studies of chronic azithromycin for COPD. Animal studies indicate azithromycin has a lower potential for prolonging the QT interval than erythromycin and clarithromycin. At much higher concentrations than achieved clinically in humans, animal studies showed that azithromycin exhibited either a very low [189–191] or no [192] potential for QT interval prolongation. One study indicated even though azithromycin prolonged QT interval at very high concentrations, ventricular arrhythmias did not occur because of the manner of the drug affecting cardiac conduction [190]. Bradycardia was reported with very elevated concentrations of azithromycin [190]. Macrolides, like clarithromycin and erythromycin, are considered to have an increased risk of causing TdP because of "metabolic liability," that is, some macrolides are strong inhibitors of CYP3A4. Azithromycin therefore has low metabolic potential [182].

Case reports have been sporadic [193] – this is notable considering the more than 40 million prescriptions for azithromycin during 1 year [145]. Data from FDA Adverse Event Reporting System showed that between 2004 and 2011, there were a total of 203 reports of azithromycin-associated QT prolongation, torsades de pointes, ventricular arrhythmia, and/or sudden cardiac death resulting in a total of 65 fatalities [194]. Clarithromycin was associated with a similar number of reports. The time frame that included the US and European databases likely reflects several hundred million patients who received azithromycin, manyfold greater than for clarithromycin.

Several retrospective studies using healthcare databases have been published regarding potential azithromycin-associated cardiac effects [144, 195–198]. Studies in the Tennessee Medicaid population [144] and the Veterans Administration health system [196] reported an increased risk of cardiac events with azithromycin compared to amoxicillin; the latter study also showed that levofloxacin was associated CV greater risks. In the Medicaid study [144], although the authors attempted to adjust for cardiac risk factors, among 20+ measures that may have affected outcomes in these patients, 21 were worse in those persons receiving azithromycin. In both of these studies, the increased cardiac events were more likely to occur in the first 5 days. One might expect that if it was a function of tissue concentrations in cardiac tissues, the effects would be more likely to occur a week or longer into therapy as the drug accumulated due to its 70-hour half-life [75]. Notably, in a retrospective study in patients hospitalized for community-acquired pneumonia, the overall 90-day mortality was lower in those who received azithromycin [198]. In that study, there was either no difference in overall cardiac events and a slight increase of myocardial infarction with azithromycin. Two large European retrospective studies – one in Denmark and another using various databases throughout Europe – found no difference in cardiac events between azithromycin and amoxicillin [195, 197]. Both studies also found the risk was greater for azithromycin and amoxicillin than no antibiotic therapy. Although these studies tried to account for other cardiac risk factors, the reality is that quinolones and macrolides are more likely to be used in sicker patients than amoxicillin as well as in patients not receiving antibiotics.

A meta-analysis was published that included 12 prospective placebo-controlled clinical trials ($n = 15,558$). Four of the studies were of azithromycin for acute infections and five studies assess potential benefits of macrolides against Chlamydiae-related atherogenesis in patients with coronary heart disease [199]. The latter represents a population at high risk for CV events. No increased risks for total mortality or CV events were found with azithromycin compared with placebo. These prospective studies may represent the strongest evidence for the lack of significant cardiac risks associated with azithromycin among the general adult population.

Several prospective studies have been conducted of chronic azithromycin to prevent COPD exacerbations, where each of these studies excluded patients with known prolonged QT intervals and significant cardiac risk factors [200, 201]. Neither study found an increased risk of cardiac events, although they excluded high-risk patients. In all likelihood, the intense scrutiny of CV events and related costs related to the use of azithromycin in COPD is disproportionate to the actual risk associated with the drug.

Azoles Some azoles have rarely been associated with the development of TdP and worsening of heart failure [182, 202]. Effects on the QT interval are slight and the principal mechanism for these drugs is through inhibition of metabolism of other agents. Itraconazole appears to be unique among the azoles as it has been reported to worsen heart failure. The FDA recommends avoiding itraconazole in patients with ventricular dysfunction or a history of heart failure for onychomycosis and only to consider itraconazole in case of life-threatening fungal infections [203]. In the COPD patient population, with the typical long courses of itraconazole for aspergillus lung infections in COPD patients, the development or worsening of cardiotoxicity should be monitored. The mechanisms of this adverse effect are unknown; however, potential etiologies include inhibition of metabolism of endogenous hormones and negative inotropic effects.

Adverse Effects of Cardiovascular Medications on the Respiratory Tract

A number of cardiovascular drug therapies can cause adverse effects to the respiratory system. Adverse effects include bronchoconstriction, upper airway angioedema, cough, interstitial pneumonitis, organizing pneumonia, and eosinophilic pneumonia. However, these adverse effects are uncommon, although they can be associated with significant morbidity in some patients, rarely leading to death. Considering the number of patients affected, perhaps the most important among these is the concern that β-blockers can cause bronchoconstriction and thus worsening respiratory status in the COPD patient, leading to underutilization of a drug class that is well established to decrease CV-related mortality.

Angiotensin-Converting Enzyme Inhibitors

All of the angiotensin-converting enzyme (ACE) inhibitors can induce a dry, persistent, and sometimes nocturnal cough (in 5–20% of patients); yet these agents are unlikely to worsen COPD or asthma [204]. It is more common in women, nonsmokers, and African Americans [205]. The mechanism of the cough is due to mast cell degranulation. The cough may develop within hours of the first dose to months later, but usually occur within 1–2 weeks after initiation. The cough typically resolves 1–4 weeks after discontinuation of the ACE inhibitor, but in a subgroup, resolution may take longer. An increased incidence of cough does not appear to occur with the angiotensin II receptor antagonists and switching from an ACEI to one of these agents usually leads to resolution of the cough. ACEI can also be associated with angioedema and in its most severe form can cause airway obstruction [206].

Antiarrhythmics

Amiodarone and dronedarone (an analogue of amiodarone), used for atrial as well as ventricular arrhythmias, are the principal antiarrhythmics reported to cause acute interstitial pneumonitis [207, 208], typically reversible if identified early and effectively managed effectively including discontinuing the drug. Initially, it was thought that dronedarone did not cause pulmonary toxicity; however, in 2012 the FDA issued a warning after reports of toxicity occurred [209]. Amiodarone and dronedarone pneumonitis have been reported to occur in as many as 5% of patients [210]. It can present in an insidious or rapidly progressive manner, as soon as within days after initiation of the drug or as long as years later [210].

Amiodarone and its metabolites as well as dronedarone produce lung damage directly by a cytotoxic effect and indirectly by an immunological reaction [211, 212]. It appears to occur in a dose-dependent manner, and when amiodarone was first marketed, doses of 400 mg daily were widely used, but today lower doses are typically used and are less likely to cause pneumonitis. It has also been reported that total cumulative dose may also be predictive of the risk of pneumonitis [211]. Although toxicity can occur at any time after treatment is initiated, those considered at greatest risk are individuals who have received a daily dose of 400 mg or more for more than 2 months, or lower doses, commonly 200 mg daily, for more than 2 years [213]. It occurs more frequently in men and increases with age [214]. Individuals with preexisting lung disease and males appear to be more susceptible [213, 214]. Systemic corticosteroids may provide benefit and drug discontinuation is necessary in many patients, depending on the type of lung damage [210].

β-Blockers

β-Blockers decrease mortality and improve cardiac-related symptoms in patients with CHF and ischemic heart disease; however, they are underutilized in patients with concurrent COPD [215]. Reasons for underuse include the concern for worsening respiratory status in obstructive lung disease in part due to the exclusion of COPD patients from key clinical trials of β-blockers in heart failure and ischemic heart disease. In a retrospective international study of patients admitted for acute heart failure, it was found that COPD patients were underprescribed β-blockers both upon admission and at discharge compared to those without COPD [216]. Another study found that non-cardioselective β-blockers were used in 3% of the patients with atrial fibrillation and 26% of those with CHF – principally carvedilol [217].

The mechanisms that β-blockers can improve outcomes in COPD patients include benefits associated with the treatment of concurrent CHF and ischemic heart disease, improved bronchodilator responsiveness by upregulation of β-receptors within the lung, and decreased deleterious effects of β2-agonists on the myocardium. β2-Agonists are unlikely to antagonize the effects of cardioselective β1-blockers on adrenergic receptors in the heart; however, β2-agonist do stimulate β2-receptors in the heart, which are known to be increased in the presence of CHF [218]. Studies evaluating the effects of cardioselective β-blockers have found no consistently deleterious effects on exacerbation risks [219–223], on pulmonary function [219–222], or on exercise capacity [220] as well as showing mortality benefits [222, 223].

Although decreases in FEV_1 can be significant in some patients with nonselective β-blockers like propranolol and carvedilol, cardioselective β1-blockers (atenolol, metoprolol, and bisoprolol) do not reduce FEV_1 either acutely or with long-term use. In a study of 12 COPD patients, it was found that metoprolol did not impede the bronchodilator effects of isoprenaline, whereas propranolol did – two subjects needed treatment of acute dyspnea when given propranolol during the investigation [224]. In a study by Agostini in patients with CHF, changes in pre- and post-bronchodilator (albuterol) FEV_1 were greater with bisoprolol than carvedilol and DLCO changes also favored the cardioselective β-blocker [225]. In another study comparing bisoprolol and carvedilol in patients with COPD and CHF, FEV_1 increased to a greater extent with the cardioselective agent [226]. One study did find at high doses that cardioselective β-blockers may adversely affect the bronchodilator response to albuterol, which was not observed with lower doses [227]. A Cochrane review of 20 randomized trials of cardioselective β1-blockers in COPD found no significant effect on FEV_1 or bronchodilator response after a single dose or up to 12 weeks of treatment [100].

Mortality benefits of β-blockers appear to be maintained in COPD patients in the acute care and long-term settings. Two studies were performed in acute settings [219, 223]. A single-center analysis found that β-blocker use in COPD was an independent predictor of survival to hospital discharge, with no evidence that these agents reduce the beneficial effects of short-acting β2-agonist use [228]. In a cohort of patients with cardiovascular disease admitted due to acute COPD exacerbation to 404 acute care hospitals, there was no association between β-blocker therapy and in-hospital mortality, 30-day readmission, or late mechanical ventilation [219]. Of note, receipt of nonselective β-blockers was associated with an increased risk of 30-day readmission compared with β1-selective blockers. In a meta-analysis of 15 retrospective studies of 21,596 patients with COPD, the pooled estimate for reduction in overall mortality attributed to the use of β-blockers was 28% and for exacerbations was 38%. The reduction in mortality was 26% (95% CI, 7–42%) in the subgroup with known HF [222]. A 2019 study, (BLOCKCOPD), [229] investigated the role of cardioselective metoprolol to decrease exacerbations in COPD patients in whom β-blockers were not otherwise clinically indicated such as in CHD. This placebo-controlled study was terminated early because of increased severe COPD exacerbations and a trend towards mortality in the treatment arm, although the time to first exacerbation was shorter with metoprolol. This suggests that primary benefits of cardioselective β-blockers in COPD occur at least in part due to cardiac effects.

Adverse Effects of Drugs Used for the Treatment of Pulmonary Hypertension in the COPD Patient

Pulmonary arterial hypertension (PAH) occurs in a minority of COPD patients, typically occurring late in the disease in those with chronic hypoxemia or those with combined pulmonary fibrosis and emphysema. As COPD progresses, hypoxia may activate vasoconstriction meant to increase the amount of oxygen transferred to the blood, where chronic hypoxic vasoconstriction leads to PAH. PAH in the COPD patient is classified as World Health Organization Group III [230]. Numerous drugs are now available for the treatment of PAH including phosphodiesterase inhibitors such as sildenafil and tadalafil, endothelin receptor blockers such as bosentan and macitentan, and prostacyclins such as IV epoprostenol and oral, IV, and inhaled trepostinil [231, 232]. Newer agents include selexipag and riociguat that work through somewhat different mechanisms, affecting the same pathways on vascular smooth muscle. Selexipag is a highly selective, high-affinity agonist of the prostacyclin receptor. Riociguat acts on the nitric oxide pathway by promoting the production of cyclic guanosine monophosphate through sensitizing to endogenous nitric oxide and directly stimulating soluble guanylate cyclase independent of its effects on nitric oxide. These medications can exhibit both vasodilatory and antiproliferative effects that help to decrease the load on the right ventricle.

Side effects of these medications are widely varied depending on the mechanisms and individual agent within classes including hypotension, liver dysfunction, headaches, blood disorders, GI intolerance, and dermatological disorders, among others [231, 232]. The primary pulmonary-related concern is worsened respiratory status. Deterioration of oxygenation due to ventilation/perfusion mismatching is the primary reason for deterioration of respiratory status. However, these agents can improve respiratory status including exercise capacity among other benefits in COPD patients.

Use of drug therapies for PAH in patients with COPD remains poorly defined, largely owing to sparse evidence. A survey of US pulmonary hypertension treatment centers reported various approaches to treating the COPD/pulmonary hypertension patient including using FEV$_1$ and right heart catheterization data. The minority indicated they do not use drug therapies to treat these patients [233]. Studies are conflicting regarding risk of worsened hypoxia when initiating these agents in COPD patients. In a placebo-controlled pilot study in severe PAH in 28 GOLD stage II and III COPD patients, with modest oxygen requirements and not in decompensated heart failure, it was found that sildenafil had a favorable hemodynamic effect, with no significant effect on gas exchange and a good safety profile [234]. They also observed a statistically significant increase in the DLCO% in the treated group (32.8–35.0%). Another study evaluated 20 COPD patients with PAH before and after a randomized single dose of sildenafil (20 or 40 mg), where both doses improved pulmonary hemodynamics at rest and during exercise, but worsened arterial oxygenation at rest [235]. A 2017 meta-analysis of five randomized clinical trials of sildenafil and tadalafil among 257 COPD patients showed that symptoms were not reduced, nor reduced pulmonary artery pressure and pulmonary vascular resistance; however, hypoxia was not worsened [236].

In a randomized study of bosentan in 30 patients with severe COPD, 20% with pulmonary hypertension at rest showed no significant functional benefit, and it was found that arterial oxygenation and quality of life declined in patients taking bosentan compared with placebo [237]. A placebo-controlled trial of 16 COPD patients in severe acute respiratory failure and mild PH showed that intravenous epoprostenol treatment was associated with a transient improvement in pulmonary pressures, but also with a significant decrease in oxygenation, rendering intravenous prostacyclins as nonselective vasodilators [238]. Inhaled prostacyclins may work preferentially in ventilated regions of the lung due to deposition to unobstructed areas of the lung, avoiding nonselective vasodilation and worsening ventilation/perfusion mismatch. Inhaled treprostinil in nine COPD patients with PAH showed that most patients tolerated the drug, although the minority had moderate to severe adverse reactions including worsening shortness of breath and exacerbation. FEV$_1$, FVC, and DLCO declined, whereas measures like 6MWT and ABG overall did not change [239]. In an acute vasodilator study in ten COPD patients with PAH (based on echocardiography), inhaled iloprost was associated with improvement in ventilation/perfusion matching [240]. Another study in COPD/PAH patients showed that inhaled prostanoids can acutely reduce mean pulmonary artery pressures while largely maintaining gas exchange [241].

Based on current evidence, treatment of PAH due to chronic respiratory conditions centers on the optimization of the management of the underlying lung disease. One group of authors suggested that drug therapy for pulmonary hypertension should be considered (1) when pulmonary hypertension persists despite the normal care being optimal such as using nonpharmacological interventions like supplemental oxygen and COPD medications and (2) when pulmonary hypertension is considered to be disproportionate to the degree of airflow limitation. Data is sparse, and based on the list from clintrials.gov in early 2018, the newer agents do not have any ongoing studies for COPD patients with PAH.

Conclusion

In the spirit of the first rule of Hippocrates – first do no harm – minimizing adverse effects of drug therapies used for COPD patients with cardiac disease is important when prescribing and monitoring medications. This is challenging if the mechanism that the drug benefits one condition can also worsen the other. Compared to oral or parenteral medications, inhaled therapies are relatively safe; however, it can cause extrapulmonary side effects as most of each inhaled dose is eventually absorbed into the bloodstream.

By the inherent mechanisms of action of the principal COPD drugs – β2-agonists, antimuscarinics, and corticosteroids – all have the potential to adversely affect the CV system. In the case of inhaled bronchodilators, reported side effects include tachycardia, arrhythmias, hypertension, myocardial infarction, and stroke. Some retrospective studies and meta-analysis have indicated that inhaled bronchodilators are associated with increased cardiac events. These studies are limited by the ability to control for the numerous factors that can influence outcomes – yet may provide some indication that LABA and LAMA may affect CV outcomes in the "real world." However, there are now several large prospective studies in COPD patients with heart disease that show these inhaled bronchodilators exhibit an acceptable risk/benefit – and may even have positive effects in heart disease under certain circumstances.

Whereas inhaled steroids are not associated with adverse cardiac effects, systemic steroids can worsen heart failure and contribute to tachycardia. In contrast, there is some evidence that inhaled steroids either do not affect or possibly could benefit heart disease. Systemic steroids have also been associated with a decreased risk of arrhythmias.

Medications to treat heart disease can have significant adverse effects on the respiratory system including β-blockers, some antiarrhythmics, and ACEI. As long as β2-cardioselective β-blockers are utilized in the COPD patient, there is minimal negative effects on respiratory function and may improve cardiac and pulmonary outcomes including exacerbations and mortality. Likewise, drugs for the treatment of pulmonary hypertension can provide cardiopulmonary benefits, yet they may also worsen respiratory status in the COPD patient.

Anti-infectives, used in the short term for exacerbations or in the long term for prevention, may also be associated with adverse cardiac effects by directly affecting the heart or indirectly through drug interactions. Differences in the potential for drug interactions and cardiac effects among the anti-infectives should be considered when using these agents. Assigning a potential drug interaction to a class of anti-infectives is incorrect as there can be substantive differences among the similar agents within that class.

There is a significant amount of pharmacokinetic and pharmacodynamic data of inhaled and oral therapies, although not always specifically studied, considering disease-related disposition and relevant drug interactions could lessen adverse effects. Thus, the information presented in the chapter could be used to guide selection and monitoring of drug therapies. Notably, considering many of the inhaled drugs are heavily dependent on liver metabolism, the effect of CHF on hepatic drug clearance is largely unstudied. It is not possible to avoid these inhaled or systemic drugs in the COPD patient with heart disease; otherwise, the consequences would be quite profound considering limitations from debilitating shortness of breath and health impairment. Therefore, we must continue to strive to best understand how to optimize these therapies at the population level and in individual patients.

References

1. https://www.cdc.gov/nchs/products/databriefs/db267.htm.
2. http://www.who.int/mediacentre/factsheets/fs310/en/.
3. Pleasants R, Herrick H, Liao W. Chronic obstructive lung disease in North Carolina: prevalence, characteristics and impact. N C Med J. 2013;74:376–83.
4. Institute of Medicine (US) Committee on Quality of Health Care in America. In: Kohn LT, Corrigan JM, Donaldson MS, editors. To err is human: building a safer health system. Washington, DC: National Academies Press; 2000.
5. Ogawa R, Stachnik JM, Echizen H. Clinical pharmacokinetics of drugs in patients with heart failure: an update (Part 2, drugs administered orally). Clin Pharmacokinet. 2014;53:1083–114.
6. Lainscak M, Vitale C, Seferovic P, Spoletini L, Cavn K, Guuseppe T, Rosano MC. Pharmacokinetics and pharmacodynamics of cardiovascular drugs in chronic heart failure. Intl J Cardiol. 2016;224:191–8.
7. Olsson B, Bondesson E, Bongstrom L, Edsbäcker S, Eirefelt S, Ekelund K, Gustavsson L, Hegelund-Myrbäck T. Pulmonary drug metabolism, clearance, and absorption. In: Smyth HDC, Hickey AJ, editors. Controlled pulmonary drug delivery. New York: Springer; 2011. p. 21–50.
8. Kararli TT. Gastrointestinal absorption of drugs. Crit Rev Ther Drug Carrier Syst. 1989;6(1):39–86.
9. Lynch T, Price A. The effect of cytochrome P450 metabolism on drug response, interactions, and adverse effects. Am Fam Physician. 2007;76:391–6.
10. Nelson DR, Koymans L, Kamataki T, Stegeman JJ, Feyereisen R, Waxman DJ, Waterman MR, Gotoh O, Coon MJ, Estabrook RW, Gunsalus IC, Nebert DW. P450 superfamily: update on new sequences, gene mapping, accession numbers and nomenclature. Pharmacogenetics. 1996;6(1):1–42.
11. Meyer UA. Overview of enzymes of drug metabolism. J Pharmacokinet Biopharm. 1996;24(5):449–59.
12. Foti RS, Dalvie DK. Cytochrome P450 and non–cytochrome P450 oxidative metabolism: contributions to the pharmacokinetics, safety, and efficacy of xenobiotics. Drug Metab Dispos. 2016;44:1229–45.

13. Zanger UM, Schwab M. Cytochrome P450 enzymes in drug metabolism: regulation of gene expression, enzyme activities, and impact of genetic variation. Pharmacol Ther. 2013;138(1):103–41.
14. Klein K, Zanger UM. Pharmacogenomics of cytochrome P450 3A4: recent progress toward the "missing heritability" problem. Front Genet. 2013;4:12.
15. Srivalli KMR, Lakshmi PK. Overview of P-glycoprotein inhibitors: a rational outlook. Braz J Pharm Sci. 2012;48(3):353–67.
16. Siederer S, Allen A, Yang S. Population pharmacokinetics of inhaled fluticasone furoate and vilanterol in subjects with chronic obstructive pulmonary disease. Eur J Drug Metab Pharmacokinet. 2016;41(6):743–58.
17. Allen A, Siederer S, Yang S. Population pharmacokinetics of inhaled fluticasone furoate and vilanterol in adult and adolescent patients with asthma. Int J Clin Pharmacol Ther. 2016;54(4):269–81.
18. Matera MG, Martuscelli E, Cazzola M. Pharmacological modulation of adrenoceptor function in patients with coexisting chronic obstructive pulmonary disease and chronic heart failure. Pulm Pharmacol Ther. 2010;23:1–8.
19. Laube BL, Janssens HM, de Jong FHC, Devadason FG, Dhand R, et al. ERS/ISAM task force report. What the pulmonologist should know about new inhalational therapies. Eur Respir J. 2011;37:1308–31.
20. Winkler J, Hochhaus G, Derendorf H. How the lung handles drugs: pharmacokinetics and pharmacodynamics of inhaled corticosteroids. Proc Am Thorac Soc. 2004;1: 356–63.
21. Cazzola M, Page CP, Calzetta L, Matera MG. Pharmacology and therapeutics of bronchodilators. Pharmacol Rev. 2012;64:450–504.
22. Hukkanen J, Pelkonen O, Hakkola J, Raunio H. Expression and regulation of xenobiotic- metabolizing cytochrome P450 (CYP) enzymes in human lung. Crit Rev Toxicol. 2002;32:391–411.
23. Wrighton SA, Brian WR, Sari MA, Iwasaki M, Guengerich FP, Raucy JL, Molowa DT, Vandenbranden M. Studies on the expression and metabolic capabilities of human liver cytochrome P450IIIA5 (HLp3). Mol Pharmacol. 1990;38:207–13.
24. Roberts JK, Moore CD, Ward RM, Yost GM, Reilly CA. Metabolism of beclomethasone dipropionate by cytochrome P450 3A enzymes. J Pharmacol Exp Ther. 2013;345(2):308–16.
25. Daley-Yates P. Inhaled corticosteroids: potency, dose equivalence and therapeutic index. Br J Pharmacol. 2015;80(3):372–80.
26. Spiriva Respimat® PI. Boehringer Ingelheim Pharmaceuticals, Inc. Ridgefield, CT 06877 USA. February 2017. Accessed 15 Feb 2018.
27. Seebri® PI. Sunovion Pharmaceuticals Inc. Marlborough, MA. July 2017. Accessed 15 Feb 2018.
28. Seheult JN, O'Connell P, Tee KC, Bhola TH, Bannai HA, Sulaiman I, et al. The acoustic features of inhalation can be used to quantify aerosol delivery from a Diskus® dry powder inhaler. Pharm Res. 2014;31:2735–47.
29. Dalby C, Polanowski T, Larsson T, Borgström L, Edsbäcker S, Harrison TW. The bioavailability and airway clearance of the steroid component of budesonide/formoterol and salmeterol/fluticasone after inhaled administration in patients with COPD and healthy subjects: a randomized controlled trial. Respir Res. 2009;10:104.
30. Anoro® PI. GlaxoSmithKline. Research Triangle Park, NC. October 2017. Accessed 15 Feb 2018.
31. Quinn D, Barnes CN, Yates W, Bourdet L, Moran EJ, et al. Safety of revefenacin (TD-4208), a long-acting muscarinic antagonist, in patients with chronic obstructive pulmonary disease (COPD): results of two randomized, double-blind, phase 2 studies. Pulm Pharmacol Ther. 2018;48:71–9.
32. Schamberger AC, Mise N, Jia J, Genoyer E, Yildirim AÖ, Meiners S, Eickelberg O. Cigarette smoke-induced disruption of bronchial epithelial tight junctions is prevented by transforming growth factor-β. Am J Respir Cell Mol Biol. 2014;50(6):1040–52.

33. Zevin S, Benowitz NL. Drug interactions with tobacco smoking. An update. Clin Pharmacokinet. 1999;36(6):425–38.
34. Donovan L, Welford SM, Haaga J, Lamanna J, Strohl KP. Hypoxia—implications for pharmaceutical developments. Sleep Breath. 2010;14(4):291–8.
35. Brunton L, Knollman B, Hilal-Dandan R. Goodman and Gilman's the pharmacological basis of therapeutics. 13th ed. New York: McGraw Hill Professional; 2017.
36. Hendeles L, Massanari M, Weinberger M. Update on the pharmacodynamics and pharmacokinetics of theophylline. Chest. 1985;88(Supp 2):103S–11S.
37. Global Initiative for Chronic Obstructive Lung Disease. 2018th ed. Global Initiative for Chronic Obstructive Lung Disease, Inc; 2018. Available at: http://goldcopd.org/vg. Accessed 15 Feb 2018.
38. Leuppi JD, Schuetz P, Bingisser R, et al. Short-term vs conventional glucocorticoid therapy in acute exacerbations of chronic obstructive pulmonary disease: the REDUCE randomized clinical trial. JAMA. 2013;309(21):2223–31.
39. Becker DE. Basic and clinical pharmacology of glucocorticosteroids. Anesth Prog. 2013;60(1):25–31.
40. Renner E, Horber FF, Jost G, Frey BM, Frey FJ. Effect of liver function on the metabolism of prednisone and prednisolone in humans. Gastroenterology. 1986;90:819–28.
41. Maltais F, Ostinelli J, Bourbeau J, Tonnel AB, Jacquemet N, Haddon J, Rouleau M, Boukhana M, Martinot JB, Duroux P. Comparison of nebulized budesonide and oral prednisolone with placebo in the treatment of acute exacerbations of chronic obstructive pulmonary disease: a randomized controlled trial. Am J Respir Crit Care Med. 2002;165:698–703.
42. Crow A, Tan AM. Oral and inhaled corticosteroids: differences in P-glycoprotein (ABCB1) mediated efflux. Toxicol Appl Pharmacol. 2012;260(3):294–302.
43. Van der Molen T, Kocks JWH. The efficacy and safety of inhaled corticosteroids: are we ignoring the potential advantages of ciclesonide? NPJ Prim Care Respir Med. 2014;24:14013.
44. Wang MT, Liou J, Lin CW, Tsai CL, Wang UH, Hsu YJ, et al. Association of cardiovascular risk with inhaled long-acting bronchodilators in patients with chronic obstructive pulmonary disease: a nested case-control study. JAMA Intern Med. 2018; [Epub ahead of print]. https://jamanetwork.com/journals/jamainternalmedicine/article-abstract/2666790?redirect=true.
45. Boulton DW, Fawcett JP. The pharmacokinetics of levosalbutamol: what are the clinical implications? Clin Pharmacokinet. 2001;40(1):23–40.
46. Striverdi® PI. Boehringer Ingelheim, Inc. Ridgefield, CT. July 2014. Accessed 15 Feb 2018.
47. Lötvall J. Pharmacological similarities and differences between beta2-agonists. Respir Med. 2001;95(Suppl B):S7–11.
48. Donohue JF, Hanania NA, Ciubotaru RL, et al. Comparison of levalbuterol and racemic albuterol in hospitalized patients with acute asthma or COPD: a 2-week, multicenter, randomized, open-label study. Clin Ther. 2008;30(6):989–1002.
49. Foradil® PI. Merck and Company. Whitehouse Station, NJ. November 2012. Accessed 15 Feb 2018.
50. Serevent® PI. GlaxoSmithKline. Research Triangle Park, NC. September 2017. Accessed 15 Feb 2018.
51. Dente FL, Bacci E, Vagaggini B, Paggiaro P. Role of indacaterol in the management of asthma and chronic obstructive pulmonary disease. Clin Investig. 2011;1(4):473–84.
52. Arcapta® PI. Sunovion Pharmaceuticals. Marlborough, MA. Rcah 2017. Accessed 15 Feb 2018.
53. Kagan M, Dain J, Peng L, Reynolds C. Metabolism and pharmacokinetics of indacaterol in humans. Drug Metab Dispos. 2012;40(9):1712–22.
54. Cazzola M, Beeh KM, Price D, Roche N. Assessing the clinical value of fast onset and sustained duration of action of long-acting bronchodilators for COPD. Pulm Pharmacol Ther. 2015;31:68–78.
55. Kunz C, Luedtke D, Unseld A, Hamilton A, Halabi A, Wein M, Formella S. Pharmacokinetics and safety of olodaterol administered with the Respimat Soft Mist inhaler in subjects with impaired hepatic or renal function. Int J Chron Obstruct Pulmon Dis. 2016;11:585–95.

56. Pakes GE, Brogden RN, Heel RC, Speight TM, Avery GS. Ipratropium bromide: a review of its pharmacological properties and therapeutic efficacy in asthma and chronic bronchitis. Drugs. 1980;20(4):237–66.
57. Atrovent® HFA PI. Boehringer Ingelheim Pharmaceuticals, Inc. Ridgefield, CT. April 2012. Accessed 15 Feb 2018.
58. Barnes PJ. The pharmacological properties of tiotropium. Chest. 2000;117(2 Suppl):63S–6S.
59. Turdoza® PI. AstraZeneca Pharmaceuticals LP. Wilmington, DE. June 2017. Accessed 15 Feb 2018.
60. Gavald A, Ramos I, Carcasona C, Calama E, Otal R, et al. The in vitro and in vivo profile of aclidinium bromide in comparison with glycopyrronium bromide. Pulm Pharmacol Ther. 2014;28:114e121.
61. Santus P, Radovanovic D, Cristiano A, Valenti V, Rizzi M. Role of nebulized glycopyrrolate in the treatment of chronic obstructive pulmonary disease. Drug Des Devel Ther. 2017;11:3257–71.
62. Tal-Singer R, Cahn A, Mehta R, Preece A, Crater G, Kelleher D, Pouliquen I. Initial assessment of single and repeat doses of inhaled umeclidinium in patients with chronic obstructive pulmonary disease: two randomised studies. Eur J Pharmacol. 2013;701:40–8.
63. Cahn A, Mehta R, Preece A, Blowers J, Dona A. Safety, tolerability and pharmacokinetics and pharmacodynamics of inhaled once-daily umeclidinium in healthy adults deficient in CYP2D6 activity: a double-blind, randomized clinical trial. Clin Drug Investig. 2013;33:653–64.
64. Mehta R, Hardes D, Kelleher D, Preece A, Tombs L, Brealey N. Clinical effects of moderate hepatic impairment on the pharmacokinetic properties and tolerability of umeclidinium and vilanterol in inhalational umeclidinium monotherapy and umeclidinium/vilanterol combination therapy: an open-label, nonrandomized study. Clin Ther. 2014;36:1016–27.e.2.
65. Mehta R, Hardes K, Brealey N, Tombs L, Preece A, Kelleher D. Effect of severe renal impairment on umeclidinium and umeclidinium/vilanterol pharmacokinetics and safety: a single-blind, nonrandomized study. Int J COPD. 2015;10:15–23.
66. Incruse® PI. GlaxoSmithKline. Research Triangle Park, NC. October 2017. Accessed 1 June 2019.
67. Yupleri®. Mylan. Morgantown, WV. 2019. Accessed 1 June 2019.
68. Barnes PJ. Theophylline. Pharmaceuticals. 2010;3(3):725–47.
69. Rabe KF. Roflumilast for the treatment of chronic obstructive pulmonary disease. Expert Rev Respir Med. 2010;4(5):543–55.
70. Bethke TD, Lahu G. High absolute bioavailability of the new oral phosphodiesterase-4 inhibitor roflumilast. Int J Clin Pharmacol Ther. 2011;49:51–7.
71. Hauns B, Hermann R, Hunnemeyer A, Herzog R, Hauschke D, Zech K, Bethke TD, et al. Investigation of a potential food effect on the pharmacokinetics of roflumilast, an oral, once-daily phosphodiesterase 4 inhibitor, in healthy subjects. J Clin Pharmacol. 2006;46(10):1146–53.
72. Daliresp® (Roflumilast) package insert. AstraZeneca Pharmaceuticals LP. Wilmington, DE 19850. August 2017. Accessed 15 Feb 2018.
73. Palleria C, Di Piallo A, Galleli L. Pharmacokinetic drug-drug interaction and their implication in clinical management. J Res Med Sci. 2013;18(7):601–10.
74. Roblek T, Trobec K, Mrhar A, Lainscak M. Potential drug-drug interactions in hospitalized patients with chronic heart failure and chronic obstructive pulmonary disease. Arch Med Sci. 2014;5(10):920–32.
75. Zithromax® package insert. Pfizer Labs. New York, NY. February 2017. Accessed 15 Feb 2018.
76. Adegunsoye A, Strek ME, Garrity E, Guzy R, Bag R. Comprehensive care of the lung transplant patient. Chest. 2017;152(1):150–64.
77. Ciracì R, Tirone G, Scaglione F. The impact of drug-drug interactions on pulmonary arterial hypertension therapy. Pulm Pharmacol Ther. 2014;28(1):1–8.

78. Tracleer® PI. Actelion Pharmaceuticals US, Inc. South San Francisco, CA. Accessed 15 Feb 2018.
79. Remodulin® PI. United Therapeutics Corp. Research Triangle Park, NC. 2014. Accessed 15 Feb 2018.
80. Daveluy A, Raignoux C, Miremont-Salamé G, et al. Drug interactions between inhaled corticosteroids and enzymatic inhibitors. Eur J Clin Pharmacol. 2009;65(7):743–5.
81. McAllister WA, Al-Habet SM, Rogers HJ. Rifampicin reduces effectiveness and bioavailability of prednisolone. Br Med J (Clin Res Ed). 1983;286(6369):923–5.
82. Parmar JS, Howell T, Kelly J, Bilton D. Profound adrenal suppression secondary to treatment with low dose inhaled steroids and itraconazole in allergic bronchopulmonary aspergillosis in cystic fibrosis. Thorax. 2002;57:749–50.
83. Varis T, Backman JT, Kivistö KT, Neuvonen PJ. Grapefruit juice can increase the plasma concentrations of oral methylprednisolone. Eur J Clin Pharmacol. 2000;56:489–93.
84. Westphal JF. Macrolide -induced clinically relevant drug interactions with cytochrome P-450A (CYP) 3A4: an update focused on clarithromycin, azithromycin and dirithromycin. Br J Clin Pharmacol. 2000;50(4):285–95.
85. Gubbins PO, Heldenbrad S. Clinically relevant drug interactions of current antifungals. Mycoses. 2010;53:95–113.
86. Vfend® PI. Pfizer, Roerig. New York, NY. January 2019. Accessed 1 June 2019.
87. Bruggemann RJM, Alffenaar JC, Blijlevens NMA, Eliane M, Billaud EM, Kosterink JGW, Verweij PE, Burger DM. Clinical relevance of the pharmacokinetic interactions of azole antifungal drugs with other coadministered agents. Clin Infect Dis. 2009;48:1441–58.
88. Noxafil®. Merck and Co. Whitehouse Station, NJ. March 2019. Accessed 1 June 2019.
89. Bolhuis MS, Panday PN, Pranger AD, Kosterink JG, Alffenaar JW. Pharmacokinetic drug interactions of antimicrobial drugs: a systematic review on oxazolidinones, rifamycines, macrolides, fluoroquinolones, and beta-lactams. Pharmaceutics. 2011;3(4):865–913.
90. Czock D, Keller F, Rasche FM, Haussler U. Pharmacokinetics and pharmacodynamics of systemically administered glucocorticoids. Clin Pharmacokinet. 2005;44:61–98.
91. Laforce CF, Szefler SJ, Miller MF, Ebling W, Brenner M. Inhibition of methylprednisolone elimination in the presence of erythromycin therapy. J Allergy Clin Immunol. 1983;72(1):34–9.
92. Glynn AM, Slaughter RL, Brass C, D'Ambrosio R, Jusko WJ. Effects of ketoconazole on methylprednisolone pharmacokinetics and cortisol secretion. Clin Pharmacol Ther. 1986;39(6):654–9.93.
93. Liu D, Ahmet A, Ward L, Krishnamoorthy P, Mandelcorn ED, Leigh R, et al. A practical guide to the monitoring and management of the complications of systemic corticosteroid therapy. Allergy Asthma Clin Immunol. 2013;9:30.
94. Liu C, Zhao Q, Zhen Y, Zhai J, Liu G, Zheng M, et al. Effect of corticosteroid on renal water and sodium excretion in symptomatic heart failure: prednisone for renal function improvement evaluation study. J Cardiovasc Pharmacol. 2015;66(3):316–22.
95. Cazzola M, Page CP, Rogliani P, Matera MG. β2-agonist therapy in lung disease. Am J Respir Crit Care Med. 2013;187:690–6.
96. Brovana® PI. Sunovion Pharmaceuticals Inc. Marlborough, MA 01752 USA. February 2014. Accessed 1 June 2019.
97. Performist® PI. Mylan Specialties. Morgantown, WV. March 2013. Access 1 June 2019.
98. Guideri G, Barletta MA, Lehr D. Extraordinary potentiation of isoproterenol cardiotoxicity by corticoid pretreatment. Cardiovasc Res. 1974;8(6):775–86.
99. Hawkins NM, Petrie MC, MacDonald MR, Jhund PS, Fabbri LM, Wikstrand J, et al. Heart failure and chronic obstructive pulmonary disease: the quandry of beta-blockers and beta-agonists. J Am Coll Cardiol. 2011;57:2127–38.
100. Salpeter S, Omiston T, Salpeter E. Cardioselective betablockers for chronic obstructive pulmonary disease. Cochrane Database Syst Rev. 2005;(4):CD003566.
101. Cole JM, Sheehan AH, Jordan JK. Concomitant use of ipratropium and tiotropium in chronic obstructive pulmonary disease. Ann Pharmacother. 2012;46(12):1717–21.

102. Spiriva Handihaler®. Boehringer Ingelheim Pharmaceuticals, Inc. Ridgefield, CT 06877 USA. February 2018. Accessed 15 Feb 2018.
103. Mehta R, Kelleher D, Preece A, Hughes S, Crater G. Effect of verapamil on systemic exposure and safety of umeclidinium and vilanterol: a randomized and open-label study. Int J Chron Obstruct Pulmon Dis. 2013;8:159–67.
104. Dumitras S, Sechaud R, Drollmann A, Pal P, Vaidyanathan S, Camenisch G, Kaiser G. Effect of cimetidine, a model drug for inhibition of the organic cation transport (OCT2/MATE1) in the kidney, on the pharmacokinetics of glycopyrronium. Int J Clin Pharmacol Ther. 2013;51(10):771–9.
105. Jonkman JH. Therapeutic consequences of drug interactions with theophylline pharmacokinetics. J Allergy Clin Immunol. 1986;78(4 part 2):736–42.
106. Bertolet BD, Luiz B, Avasarala K, Calhoun WB, Franco EA, Nichols WM, Kerensky RA, Hill JA. Differential antagonism of cardiac actions of adenosine by theophylline. Cardiovasc Res. 1996;32:839–45.
107. Kroon LA. Drug interactions with smoking. Am J Health Sys Pharm. 2007;64(18):1917–21.
108. Facius A, Bagul N, Gardiner P, Watz H. Pharmacokinetics of a 4 week up-titration of roflumilast in the OPTIMIZE study. Am J Respir Crit Care. 2017;195:A1337.
109. Lahu G, Hünnemeyer A, Herzog R, et al. Effect of repeated doses of erythromycin on the pharmacokinetics of roflumilast and roflumilast N-oxide. Int J Clin Pharmacol Ther. 2009;47(4):236–45.
110. Lahu G, Hünnemeyer A, von Richter O, et al. Effect of single and repeated doses of ketoconazole on the pharmacokinetics of roflumilast and roflumilast N-oxide. J Clin Pharmacol. 2008;48(11):1339–49.
111. von Richter O, Lahu G, Hünnemeyer A, et al. Effect of fluvoxamine on the pharmacokinetics of roflumilast and roflumilast N-oxide. Clin Pharmacokinet. 2007;46(7):613–22.
112. Nassr N, Hünnemeyer A, Herzog R, et al. Effects of rifampicin on the pharmacokinetics of roflumilast and roflumilast N-oxide in healthy subjects. Br J Clin Pharmacol. 2009;68(4):580–7.
113. Groll AH, Desai A, Han D, Howieson C, Kato K, et al. Pharmacokinetic assessment of drug-drug interactions of isavuconazole with the immunosuppressants cyclosporine, mycophenolic acid, prednisolone, sirolimus, and tacrolimus in healthy adults. Clin Pharmacol Drug Dev. 2017;6(1):76–85.
114. Varis T, Kaukonen KM, Kivistö KT, Neuvonen PJ. Plasma concentrations and effects of oral methylprednisolone are considerably increased by FDA. Clin Pharmacol Ther. 1998;64(4):363–8.
115. Fernandez SF, Canty JM. Adrenergic and cholinergic plasticity in heart failure. Circ Res. 2015;116(10):1639–42.
116. Packer M. The neurohormonal hypothesis: a theory to explain the mechanism of disease progression in heart failure. J Am Coll Cardiol. 1992;20(1):248–54.
117. Brodde O, Michel MC. Adrenergic and muscarinic receptors in the human heart. Pharmacol Rev. 1999;51(4):651–89.
118. Bristow MR, Ginsburg R, Umans V, Fowler M, Minobe W, Rasmussen R, Zera P, et al. B1- and B2-adrenergic-receptor subpopulations in nonfailing and failing human ventricular myocardium: coupling of both receptor subtypes to muscle contraction and selective B1-receptor down-regulation in heart failure. Circ Res. 1986;59:297–309.
119. Brodde O, Konschak U, Becker K, Rüter F, Poller U, Jakubetz J, Radke J, Zerkowski H. Cardiac muscarinic receptors decrease with age in vitro and in vivo studies. J Clin Invest. 1998;101:471–8.
120. Wei L, MacDonald TM, Walker BR. Taking glucocorticoids by prescription is associated with subsequent cardiovascular disease. Ann Intern Med. 2004;141:764.
121. Kremers H, Reinaldi MS, Crowson CS, Davis JM, Hunder GG, Gabriel SE. Glucocorticoids and cardiovascular and cerebrovascular events in polymyalgia rheumatica. Arthritis Rheum. 2007;57(2):279–86.

122. van der Hooft CS, Heeringa J, Brusselle GG, et al. Corticosteroids and the risk of atrial fibrillation. Arch Intern Med. 2006;166:1016.
123. Huerta C, Lanes SF, García Rodríguez LA. Respiratory medications and the risk of cardiac arrhythmias. Epidemiology. 2005;16:360.
124. Halonen J, Halonen P, Järvinen O, et al. Corticosteroids for the prevention of atrial fibrillation after cardiac surgery: a randomized controlled trial. JAMA. 2007;297(14):1562–7.
125. Curtis JR, Westfall AO, Allison J, et al. Population-based assessment of adverse events associated with long-term glucocorticoid use. Arthritis Rheum. 2006;55(3):420–6.
126. Whitworth JA, Gordon D, Andrews J, Scoggins BA. The hypertensive effect of synthetic glucocorticoids in man: role of sodium and volume. J Hypertens. 1989;7(7):537–49.
127. Greene MA, Gordon A, Boltax AJ. Clinical and cardiodynamic effects of adrenocortical steroids in congestive heart failure. Circulation. 1960;21:661–71.
128. Calverley PMA, Anderson JM, Celli B, Ferguson GT, Jenkins C, et al. Cardiovascular events in patients with COPD: TORCH study results. Thorax. 2010;65:719e725.
129. Celli B, Anderson JA, Brook R, Calverley P, Crim C, Andrew AP, et al. LABA/ICS in COPD patients with CV disease or risk: a factorial analysis of the SUMMIT trial. Am J Respir Crit Care Med. 2018;197(12):1641–4. https://doi.org/10.1164/rccm.201710-2052LE.
130. Vestbo J, Anderson JA, Brook RD, et al. Fluticasone furoate and vilanterol and survival in chronic obstructive pulmonary disease with heightened cardiovascular risk (SUMMIT): a double-blind randomized controlled trial. Lancet. 2016;387:1817–26.
131. Lahousse L, Verhamme KM, Stricker BH, Brusselle GG. Cardiac effects of current treatments of chronic obstructive pulmonary disease. Lancet Respir Med. 2016;4:149–64.
132. Dhein S, VanKoppen CJ, Brodde E. Muscarinic receptors in the mammalian heart. Pharmacol Res. 2001;44(3):161–82.
133. Cazzola M, Imperatore F, Salzillo A, Di Perna F, Calderaro F, Imperatore A, Matera M. Cardiac effects of formoterol and salmeterol in patients suffering from COPD with preexisting cardiac arrhythmias and hypoxemia. Chest. 1998;114:411–5.
134. Khindri S, Ronald Sabo R, Harris S, Woessner R, Jennings S, Drollmann AF. Cardiac safety of indacaterol in healthy subjects: a randomized, multidose, placebo- and positive controlled, parallel-group thorough QT study. BMC Pulm Med. 2011;11:31.
135. Troost J, Pivovarova A, Kunz C, Hamilton A. Evaluation of the effects of the long-acting B2-agonist olodaterol on the QT and QTc interval in healthy subjects. Am J Respir Crit Care Med. 2013;187:A2603.
136. Maak CA, Tabas JA, McClintock DE. Should acute treatment with inhaled beta agonists be withheld from patients with dyspnea who may have heart failure? J Emerg Med. 2011;40(2):135–45.
137. Dransfield MT, Cockcroft JR, Townsend RR, et al. Effect of fluticasone propionate/salmeterol on arterial stiffness in patients with COPD. Respir Med. 2011;105(9):1322–30.
138. Bhatt SP, Dransfield MT, Cockcroft JR, Wang-Jairaj J, Midwinter DA, et al. A randomized trial of once-daily fluticasone furoate/vilanterol or vilanterol versus placebo to determine effects on arterial stiffness in COPD. Int J Chron Obstruct Pulmon Dis. 2017;12:351–65.
139. Pepin JL, Cockcroft JR, Midwinter D, Sharma S, Rubin DB, Andreas S. Long-acting bronchodilators and arterial stiffness in patients with COPD: a comparison of fluticasone furoate/vilanterol with tiotropium. Chest. 2014;146:1521–30.
140. Patel AK, Skatrud JB, Thomson JH. Cardiac arrhythmias due to oral aminophylline in patients with chronic obstructive pulmonary disease. Chest. 1981;80:661–5.
141. Shannon M. Life-threatening events after theophylline overdose: a 10-year prospective analysis. Arch Intern Med. 1999;159(9):989–94.
142. Sessler CN, Cohen MD. Cardiac arrhythmias during theophylline toxicity. A prospective continuous electrocardiographic study. Chest. 1990;98:672–8.

143. U.S. Food and Drug Administration Drug Information. FDA drug safety communication: azithromycin (Zithromax or Zmax) and the risk of potentially fatal heart rhythms. Available at: http://www.fda.gov/Drugs/DrugSafety/ucm341822.htm. Accessed 1 Feb 2018.

144. Ray WA, Murray KT, Hall K, Arbogast PG, Stein CM. Azithromycin and the risk of cardiovascular death. N Engl J Med. 2012;366(20):1881–90.

145. https://www.fda.gov/Safety/MedWatch/SafetyInformation/SafetyAlertsforHumanMedical Products/ucm597862.htm. Accessed 1 June 2019.

146. https://www.fda.gov/drugs/drug-safety-and-availability/fda-drug-safety-communication-fda-review-finds-additional-data-supports-potential-increased-long.

147. Winkel P, Hilden J, Fischer Hansen J, Gluud C, et al. Clarithromycin for stable coronary heart disease increases all-cause and cardiovascular mortality and cerebrovascular morbidity over 10 years in the CLARICOR randomised, blinded clinical trial. Int J Cardiol. 2015;182:459–65.

148. Roden DM. Predicting drug-induced QT prolongation and torsades de pointes. J Physiol. 2016;594:2459–68.

149. Lawrence CL, Pollard CE, Hammind TG, Valentin JP. In vitro models of proarrhythmia. Br J Pharmacol. 2008;154:1516–22.

150. Li M, Ramos LG. Drug-induced QT prolongation and torsades de pointes. Pharm Ther. 2017;42:473–7.

151. Albert RK, Schulleri JL. Macrolide antibiotics and the risk of cardiac arrhythmias. Am J Respir Crit Care Med. 2014;189(10):1173–80.

152. https://crediblemeds.org.

153. Guidance for industry E14, clinical evaluation of QT/QTc interval prolongation and proarrhythmic potential for non-antiarrhythmic drugs. U.S. Department of Health and Human Services, Food and Drug Administration, Center for Drug Evaluation and Research, Center for Biologics Evaluation and Research. Oct 2012. https://www.fda.gov/downloads/Drugs/GuidanceComplianceRegulatoryInformation/Guidances/UCM073153.pdf.

154. Wise RA, Chapman KR, Scirica BM, et al. Effect of aclidinium bromide on major cardiovascular events and exacerbations in high-risk patients with chronic obstructive pulmonary disease: the ASCENT-COPD randomized clinical trial. JAMA. 2019;321(17):1693–701.

155. Wise RA, Anzueto A, Cotton D, Doll R, Devins T, Disse B, et al., and the TIOSPIR Investigators. Tiotropium Respimat inhaler and the risk of death in COPD. N Engl J Med. 2013;369:1491–501.

156. Sulaiman I, Cushan B, Greeen G, et al. Objective assessment of adherence to inhalers by patients with chronic obstructive pulmonary disease. Am J Respir Crit Care Med. 2017;195:1333–43.

157. Vestbo J, Anderson JA, Calverley PM, Celli B, Ferguson GT, Jenkins C, Knobil K, Willits LR, Yates JC, Jones PW. Adherence to inhaled therapy, mortality and hospital admission in COPD. Thorax. 2009;64(11):939–43.

158. Donaldson GC, Hurst JR, Smith CJ, Hubbard RB, Wedzicha JA. Increased risk of myocardial infarction and stroke following exacerbation of COPD. Chest. 2010;137:1091–7.

159. Kunisaki KM, Dransfield MT, Anderson JA, Brook RD, Calverley PMA, et al. Exacerbations of chronic obstructive pulmonary disease and cardiac events: a cohort analysis. Am J Respir Crit Care Med. 2018;198(1):51–7. https://doi.org/10.1164/rccm.201711-2239OC.

160. Sestini P, Renzoni E, Robinson S, Poole P, Ram FS. Short-acting B2-agonists for stable chronic obstructive pulmonary disease. Cochrane Database Syst Rev. 2002;4: CD001495.

161. Donohue JF, Hanania NA, Make B, et al. One-year safety and efficacy study of arformoterol tartrate in patients with moderate to severe COPD. Chest. 2014;146:1531–42.

162. Calverley PMA, Anderson JA, Celli B, et al., and the TORCH investigators. Salmeterol and fluticasone propionate and survival in chronic obstructive pulmonary disease. N Engl J Med. 2007;356:775–89.

163. Brook RD, Anderson JA, Calverley PMA, Celli B, Crim C, et al. Cardiovascular outcomes with an inhaled beta2-agonist/corticosteroid in patients with COPD at high cardiovascular risk. Heart. 2017;103:1536–42.

164. Adamson PD, Anderson JA, Brook RD, et al. Cardiac troponin I and cardiovascular risk in patients with chronic obstructive pulmonary disease. J Am Coll Cardiol. 2018;72(10):1126–37.
165. Baumgartner RA, Hanania NA, Calhoun WJ, Sahn SA, Sciarappa K, Hanrahan JP. Nebulized arformoterol in patients with COPD: a 12-week, multicenter, randomized, double-blind, double-dummy, placebo- and active-controlled trial. Clin Ther. 2007;29(2):261–78.
166. Anthonisen NR, Connett JE, Enright PL, Manfreda J, and the Lung Health Study Research Group. Hospitalizations and mortality in the Lung Health Study. Am J Respir Crit Care Med. 2002;166:333–9.
167. Lanes S, Golish W, Mikl J. Ipratropium and lung health study [letter]. Am J Respir Crit Care Med. 2003;167(7):801.
168. Tashkin DP, Celli B, Senn S, Burkhart D, Kesten S, Menjoge S, et al., and the UPLIFT Study Investigators. A 4-year trial of tiotropium in chronic obstructive pulmonary disease. N Engl J Med. 2008;359:1543–54.
169. Celli B, Decramer M, Leimer I, Vogel U, Kesten S, Tashkin DP. Cardiovascular safety of tiotropium in patients with COPD. Chest. 2010;137(1):20–30.
170. Singh S, Loke YK, Enright PL, Furberg CD. Mortality associated with tiotropium mist inhaler in patients with chronic obstructive pulmonary disease: systematic review and meta-analysis of randomised controlled trials. BMJ. 2011;342:d3215.11.
171. Michele TM, Pinheiro S, Iyasu S. The safety of tiotropium—the FDA's conclusions. N Engl J Med. 2010;363:1097–9.
172. Hohlfeld JM, Furtwaengler AM, Könen-Bergmann K. Cardiac safety of tiotropium in patients with COPD: a combined analysis of Holter-ECG data from four randomised clinical trials. Int J Clin Pract. 2015;69(1):72–80.
173. Halpin DMG, Dahl R, Hallmann C, Mueller A, Tashkin D. Tiotropium Handihaler and Respimat in COPD: a pooled safety analysis. Int J Chron Obstruct Pulmon Dis. 2015;10:239–59.
174. Dong Y, Lin H, Shau W, Wu Y, Chang C, Lai M. Comparative safety of inhaled medications in patients with chronic obstructive pulmonary disease: systematic review and mixed treatment comparison meta-analysis of randomised controlled trials. Thorax. 2013;68:48–56.
175. Donohue JF, Feldman G, Sethi S, Barnes CN, Pendyala S, et al. Cardiovascular safety of revefenacin, a once-daily, lung-selective, long-acting muscarinic antagonist for nebulized therapy of chronic obstructive pulmonary disease: evaluation in phase 3 clinical trials. Pulm Pharmacol Ther. 2019;57:101808.
176. Cazzola M, Ora J, Puxeddu E, Rogliani P. Indacaterol/glycopyrronium combination for COPD. Pulm Ther. 2017;3:45–57.
177. Wedzicha JA, Dahl R, Buhl R, et al. Pooled safety analysis of the fixed-dose combination of indacaterol and glycopyrronium (QVA149), its monocomponents, and tiotropium versus placebo in COPD patients. Respir Med. 2014;108:1498–507.
178. Hannania N, Tashkin DP, Kerwin EM, Denebberg M, O'Donnlee DE, et al. Long-term safety and efficacy of glycopyrrolate/formoterol metered dose inhaler using novel Co-Suspension™ delivery technology in patients with chronic obstructive pulmonary disease. Respir Med. 2017;126:105–15.
179. Santus P, Radovanovic D, DiMarco S, et al. Effect of indacaterol on lung deflation improves cardiac performance in hyperinflated COPD patients: an interventional, randomized cross-over trial. Int J Chron Obstr Pulmon Dis. 2015;10:1917–23.
180. Hohlfeld JM, Vogel-Claussen J, Biller H, Berliner D, Berschneider K, Tillman HC, et al. Effect of lung deflation with indacaterol plus glycopyrronium on ventricular filling in patients with hyperinflation and COPD (CLAIM): a double-blind, randomised, crossover, placebo-controlled, single-centre trial. Lancet Respir Med. 2018;6(5):368–78.
181. Rubenstein E, Camm J. Cardiotoxicity of fluoroquinolones. J Antimicrob Chemother. 2002;49:593–6.
182. Owens RC, Nolin TD. Antimicrobial-associated QT interval prolongation: pointes of interest. Clin Infect Dis. 2006;43:1603–11.

183. Inghammar M, Svanström H, Melbye M, et al. Oral fluoroquinolone use and serious arrhythmia: bi-national cohort study. BMJ. 2016;352:i843.
184. Liu X, Ma J, Huang L, Zhu W, Yuan P, Wan R, Hong K. Fluoroquinolones increase the risk of serious arrhythmias: a systematic review and meta-analysis. Medicine. 2017;96(44):e8273.
185. Wedzicha J, Calverley PMA, Albert RK, Anzueto A, Criner GJ, Hurst JR, et al. Prevention of COPD exacerbations: a European Respiratory Society/American Thoracic Society guideline. Eur Respir J. 2017;50(3):1602265.
186. Havercamp W, Eckhardt L, Monnig G, Schulae-Bahr E, Wedekind H, Kirchhof P, Havercamp F, Breithardt G. Clinical aspects of ventricular arrhythmias associated with QT prolongation. Eur Heart J. 2001;3(Suppl K):K81–8.
187. Ohtani H, Taninaka C, Hanada E, Kotaki H, Sato H, Sawada Y, Iga T. Comparative pharmacodynamic analysis of Q-T interval prolongation induced by the macrolides clarithromycin, roxithromycin, and azithromycin in rats. Antimicrob Agents Chemother. 2000;44(10):2630–7.
188. Mosholder AD, Mathew J, Alexander JJ, Smith H, Nambiar S. Cardiovascular risks with azithromycin and other antibacterial drugs. N Engl J Med. 2013;368(18):1665–8.
189. Atli O, Ilgin S, Altuntas H, Burukoglu D. Evaluation of azithromycin induced cardiotoxicity in rats. Int J Clin Exp Med. 2015;8(3):3681–90.
190. Zhang M, Xie M, Li S, et al. Electrophysiologic studies on the risks and potential mechanism underlying the proarrhythmic nature of azithromycin. Cardiovasc Toxicol. 2017;17(3):434–40.
191. Ohara H, Nakamura Y, Watanabe Y, Cao X, Yamazaki Y, Izumi-Nakaseko H, et al. Azithromycin can prolong QT interval and suppress ventricular contraction, but will not induce torsade de pointes. Cardiovasc Toxicol. 2015;15(3):232–40.
192. Milberg P, Eckardt L, Bruns HR, Biertz J, Ramtin S, Reinsch N, et al. Divergent proarrhythmic potential of macrolide antibiotics despite similar QT prolongation: fast phase 3 repolarization prevents early after depolarizations and Torsade de Pointes. J Pharmacol Exp Ther. 2002;303(1):218–25.
193. Hancox JC, Masnain M, Vieweg WVR, Breden EL. Azithromycin, cardiovascular risks, QTc interval prolongation, torsade de pointes, and regulatory issues: a narrative review based on the study of case reports. Ther Adv Infect Dis. 2013;1(5):155–65.
194. Raschi EPE, Koci A, Moretti U, Sturkenboom M, De Ponti F, Moretti U, Spina E, Behr ER, et al. Macrolides and torsadogenic risk: emerging issues from the FDA pharmacovigilance database. J Pharmacovigilance. 2013;1(6):467–79.
195. Svanstrom H, Pasternak B, Hviid A. Use of azithromycin and death from cardiovascular causes. N Engl J Med. 2013;368(18):1704–12.
196. Rao GA, Mann JR, Shoaibi A, Bennett CL, Nahhas G, Sutton SS, et al. Azithromycin and levofloxacin use and increased risk of cardiac arrhythmia and death. Ann Fam Med. 2014;12(2):121–7.
197. Trifirò G, de Ridder M, Sultana J, Oteri A, Rijnbeek P, Pecchioloi S, et al. Use of azithromycin and risk of ventricular arrhythmia. CMAJ. 2017;189(15):E560–8.
198. Mortensen EM, Halm EA, Pugh MJ, Copeland LA, Metersky M, Fine MJ, et al. Association of azithromycin with mortality and cardiovascular events among older patients hospitalized with pneumonia. JAMA. 2014;311(21):2199–208.
199. Almalki ZS, Guo JJ. Cardiovascular events and safety outcomes associated with azithromycin therapy: a meta-analysis of randomized controlled trials. Am Health Drug Benefits. 2014;7(6):318–28.
200. Albert RK, Connett J, Bailey WC, Casaburi R, Cooper JAD Jr, Criner GJ, Curtis JL, Dransfield MT, Han MK, Lazarus SC, et al. COPD Clinical Research Network. Azithromycin for prevention of exacerbations of COPD. N Engl J Med. 2011;365:689–98.
201. Uzun S, Djamin RS, Kluytmans JA, Mulder PG, van't Veer NE, Ermens AA. Azithromycin maintenance treatment in patients with frequent exacerbations of chronic obstructive pulmonary disease (COLUMBUS): a randomised, double-blind, placebo-controlled trial. Lancet Respir Med. 2014;2(5):361–8.
202. Bril F, Gonzalez CD, Di Girolamo G. Antimicrobial agents-associated with QT interval prolongation. Curr Drug Saf. 2010;5(1):85–92.

203. Advisory for fungal drugs. FDA Consum. 2001;35(4):4.
204. Dicpinigaitis PV. Angiotensin-converting enzyme inhibitor-induced cough: ACCP evidence-based clinical practice guidelines. Chest. 2006;129:169S–73S.
205. Sica DA. Angiotensin-converting enzyme inhibitors side effects—physiologic and non-physiologic considerations. J Clin Hypertension. 2004;6(7):410–6.
206. Bezalel S, Mahlab-Guri K, Asher I, Werner B, Sthoeger ZM. Angiotensin-converting enzyme inhibitor-induced angioedema. Am J Med. 2015;128:120–5.
207. Cordarone® (amiodarone) package insert. Wyeth Pharmaceuticals Inc. Philadelphia, PA. 2017.
208. Multaq® package insert. Sanofi-Aventis U.S., LLC. Bridgewater, NJ. 2017.
209. Droneradone FDA Warning Letter. 9 Sept 2012. https://www.accessdata.fda.gov/drugsatfda_docs/appletter/2012/022425Orig1s016,s017,s018ltr.pdf.
210. Papiris SA, et al. Amiodarone: review of pulmonary effects and toxicity. Drug Saf. 2010;33:539–58.
211. Wolkove N, Baltzan M. Amiodarone pulmonary toxicity. Can Respir J. 2009;16(2):43–8.
212. Lee YR, Wilson EJ, Pate PL. Dronedarone-induced pulmonary toxicity – a case report and literature review. J Hosp Clin Pharm. 2016;2(2):70–5.
213. Jessurum GA, Crijns HJG. Amiodarone pulmonary toxicity. BMJ. 1997;314:619–20.
214. Camus P, Martin WJ II, Rosenow EC III. Amiodarone pulmonary toxicity. Clin Chest Med. 2004;25:65–75.
215. Onishi K. Total management of chronic obstructive pulmonary disease (COPD) as an independent risk factor for cardiovascular disease. J Cardiol. 2017;70:128–34.
216. Parissis JT, Andreoli C, Kadoglou N, et al. Differences in clinical characteristics, management and short-term outcome between acute heart failure patients chronic obstructive pulmonary disease and those without this co-morbidity. Clin Res Cardiol. 2014;103:733–41.
217. Lorgunpai SJ, Grammas M, Lee DS, McAvay G, Charpentier P, Tinetti ME. Potential therapeutic competition in community-living older adults in the U.S.: use of medications that may adversely affect a coexisting condition. PLoS One. 2014;9(2):e89447.
218. Hawkins NM, MacDonald MR, Petrie MC, Chalmer MC, Carter GW, et al. Bisoprolol in patients with heart failure and moderate to severe chronic obstructive pulmonary disease: a randomized controlled trial. Eur J Heart Fail. 2009;11:684–90.
219. Stefan MS, Rothberg MB, Priya A, Pekow PS, Au DH, Lindenhauer PK. Association between β-blocker therapy and outcomes in patients hospitalized with acute exacerbations of chronic obstructive lung disease with underlying ischaemic heart disease, heart failure or hypertension. Thorax. 2012;67:977–84. https://doi.org/10.1136/thoraxjnl-2012-201945.
220. Bhatt SP, Wells JM, Kinney GL, Washko GR, Budoff M, Kim Y, et al. Beta-blockers are associated with a reduction in COPD exacerbations. Thorax. 2016;71:8–14.
221. Duffy S, Marron R, Voelker H, Albert R, Connett J, Bailey W, et al. Effect of beta-blockers on exacerbation rate and lung function in chronic obstructive pulmonary disease (COPD). Respir Res. 2017;18:124.
222. Du Q, Sun Y, Ding N, Yu L, Chin YI. Beta-blockers reduced the risk of mortality and exacerbation in patients with COPD: a meta-analysis of observational studies. PLoS One. 2014;9:e113048.
223. Dransfield MT, McAllister DA, Anderson JA, Brook RD, Calverley PMA, et al. Beta-blocker therapy and clinical outcomes in patients with moderate COPD and heightened cardiovascular risk: an observational sub-study of SUMMIT. Ann Am Thorac Soc. 2018;15:608–14.
224. Tivenius L. Effects of multiple doses of metoprolol and propranolol on ventilatory function in patients with chronic obstructive lung disease. Scand J Respir Dis. 1976;57:190–6.
225. Agostini P, Contini M, Cattadori G, Apostolo A, Sciomer S, Bussotti M, et al. Lung function with carvedilol and bisoprolol in chronic heart failure: is β selectivity relevant? Eur J Heart Fail. 2007;9:827–33.
226. Lainscak M, Podbregar M, Kovacic D, Rozman J, von Haehling S. Differences between bisoprolol and carvedilol in patients with chronic heart failure and chronic obstructive pulmonary disease: a randomized trial. Respir Med. 2011;105(Suppl 1):S44–9.

227. Chang CL, Mills GD, McLachlan JD, Karalus NC, Hancox RJ. Cardio-selective and non-selective beta-blockers in chronic obstructive pulmonary disease: effects on bronchodilator response and exercise. Intern Med J. 2010;40(3):193–200.

228. Dransfield MT, Rowe SM, Johnson JE, Bailey WC, Gerald LB. Use of b blockers and the risk of death in hospitalised patients with acute exacerbations of COPD. Thorax. 2008;63:301–5.

229. Bhatt SP, Connett JE, Voecker H, et al. B-blockers for the prevention of acute exacerbations of chronic obstructive pulmonary disease (BLOCK COPD): a randomized controlled study protocol. BMJ Open. 2016;6:e102292.

230. COPD with PAH Group WHO Classification. Proceedings of the 4th world symposium on pulmonary hypertension, February 2008, Dana Point, CA. J Am Coll Cardiol. 2009;54(1 Suppl):S1–S117.

231. Minai OA, Chaouat A, Adnot A. Pulmonary hypertension in COPD: epidemiology, significance, and management pulmonary vascular disease: the global perspective. Chest. 2010;137(6 Suppl):39S–51.

232. Tsai H, Sung YK, Perez VJ. Recent advances in the management of pulmonary arterial hypertension. F1000Res. 2016;5:2755.

233. Trammell AW, Pugh ME, Newman JH, Hemnes AR, Robbin IM. Use of pulmonary arterial hypertension–approved therapy in the treatment of non–group 1 pulmonary hypertension at US referral centers. Pulm Circ. 2015;5(2):356–63.

234. Vitulo P, Stanziola A, Confalonieri M, et al. Sildenafil in severe pulmonary hypertension associated with chronic obstructive pulmonary disease: a randomized controlled multicenter clinical trial. J Heart Lung Transplant. 2017;36:166–74.

235. Blanco I, Gimeno E, Munoz PA, Pizarro S, Gistau C, Rodriguez-Roisin R, et al. Hemodynamic and gas exchange effects of sildenafil in patients with chronic obstructive pulmonary disease and pulmonary hypertension. Am J Respir Crit Care Med. 2010;181:270–8.

236. Prins KW, Duval S, Markowitz J, Pritzker M, Thenappan T. Chronic use of PAH-specific therapy in World Health Organization Group III pulmonary hypertension: a systematic review and meta-analysis. Pulm Circ. 2017;7:145–55.

237. Stolz D, Rasch H, Linka A, Di Valentino M, Meyer A, Brutsche M, Tamm M. A randomised, controlled trial of bosentan in severe COPD. Eur Respir J. 2008;32:619–28.

238. Archer SL, Mike D, Crow J, Long W, Weir EK. A placebo-controlled trial of prostacyclin in acute respiratory failure in COPD. Chest. 1996;109(3):750–5.

239. Bajwa AA, Shujaat A, Patel M, Thomas C, Rahaghi F, Burger CD. The safety and tolerability of inhaled treprostinil in patients with pulmonary hypertension and chronic obstructive pulmonary disease. Pulm Circ. 2017;7(1):82–8.

240. Dernaika TA, Beavin M, Kinasewitz GT. Iloprost improves gas exchange and exercise tolerance in patients with pulmonary hypertension and chronic obstructive pulmonary disease. Respiration. 2010;79(5):377–82.

241. Boeck L, Tamm M, Grendelmeier P, Stolz D. Acute effects of aerosolized iloprost in COPD related pulmonary hypertension—a randomized controlled crossover trial. PLoS One. 2012;7:e52248.

Chapter 11
Cardiovascular Co-Morbidity in Chronic Lung Disease: Exercise Training

Rachael A. Evans

Clinical Pearls

- Unstable cardiac disease must be optimally managed prior to participation in an exercise program, but patients with co-morbid cardiac disease should not be routinely excluded from participation.
- Recommended components of an exercise training program such as combined aerobic and resistance training are strikingly similar for both cardiac and pulmonary conditions.
- The pulmonary rehabilitation team should receive adequate training on different cardiac conditions and symptoms of decompensation akin to understanding chronic lung diseases and exacerbations.

Introduction

Although the services of cardiac rehabilitation (CR) and pulmonary rehabilitation (PR) are organised according to specialty, this is a slight misnomer as the main benefits of both services occur via the systemic features of the conditions. Many patients do not fit neatly into one disease or specialty category. The prevalence of cardiovascular disease in patients with COPD referred for PR is estimated to be between 20% and 50% [1, 2]. In a CR population, only 6% had underlying respiratory conditions but this is likely to be an underestimate either due to under-diagnosis

R. A. Evans (✉)
National Institute of Health Research Biomedical Research Centre, Respiratory Sciences, University of Leicester, Leicester, UK

Department of Respiratory Medicine, Thoracic Surgery and Allergy, Glenfield Hospital, University Hospitals of Leicester NHS Trust, Leicester, UK
e-mail: re66@leicester.ac.uk

© Springer Nature Switzerland AG 2020
S. P. Bhatt (ed.), *Cardiac Considerations in Chronic Lung Disease*,
Respiratory Medicine, https://doi.org/10.1007/978-3-030-43435-9_11

or referral bias [3]. The prevalence of COPD when systematically assessed in patients undergoing percutaneous coronary intervention was nearly 25%. There is therefore a need to consider how services are organised for patients to maximise benefit both in terms of access and in receiving a tailored program which best serves their individual needs.

This chapter provides an overview of the existing CR and PR models, but will focus on how all elements of the PR model can be best tailored for the patient with chronic lung disease and a cardiovascular co-morbidity.

Breathlessness and the Role of Pulmonary Rehabilitation for Chronic Lung Disease

Despite differing underlying pathology among chronic lung diseases, the consequent symptomatology is extremely similar. Exertional breathlessness is one of the most commonly experienced symptoms and results in a variety of clinical problems. Early on, sufferers reduce either the distance walked or the walking speed to reduce breathlessness. Although almost undetectable initially, partly due to assumptions that 'slowing down' is a natural part of aging, over time activity reduces to the point where it is unacceptable to the person and typically triggers a visit to a healthcare professional for assessment. Physical inactivity and deconditioning are associated with the well-described skeletal muscle impairment in chronic lung disease which increases the load on an already burdened ventilatory system, thus worsening breathlessness. Further negative consequences impair almost all aspects of life including work, social activities, hobbies, and family life. The feeling of breathlessness is very frightening and evokes anxiousness, and coupled with the social impacts above, depressive symptoms become very common.

PR targets all the described extra-pulmonary manifestations of chronic lung diseases such as skeletal muscle impairment, mood disturbances, and bone and cardiovascular diseases causing improvements in dyspnea, walking distance, and health-related quality of life [4]. There are no improvements in lung function and hence this is not the mechanism of benefit. The recommended components of PR are individually prescribed exercise training, multidisciplinary education, self-management, and psychosocial support. It developed through the 1970s with the first randomised controlled trial of PR versus usual care published in the 1980s. Subsequently, a body of work evolved and a recent meta-analysis confirmed PR as one of the, if not the most, effective treatments for patients with chronic lung disease [5]. PR results in reduction in dyspnea, improvements in health-related quality of life, and increased walking distance. Although much of the original research involved predominantly patients with COPD, PR is beneficial for many patients with chronic lung disease such as interstitial lung diseases and bronchiectasis, and inclusion in PR programs is recommended [4]. Patients with severe disease should not be excluded including those with respiratory failure and cor pulmonale [4]. Benefits of PR extend to a reduction in hospital bed-days in the year post-PR with improvements in known prognostic factors such as exercise capacity. To date, there are no trials with an adequate sample size to definitively report the effects upon survival and it may be unethical to conduct such trials contemporarily.

Secondary Prevention in Cardiovascular Disease and the Role of Cardiac Rehabilitation

The traditional population for CR includes patients who are post-myocardial infarction, coronary artery bypass grafting, percutaneous coronary intervention, and non-coronary heart surgery. The process of CR has three phases and is initiated at the point of the 'event':

- Phase 1 – Initiated while the patient is still in the hospital
- Phase 2 – A supervised ambulatory outpatient program typically lasting 8 to 12 weeks
- Phase 3 – A lifetime maintenance phase in which physical fitness and additional risk factor reduction are emphasised

The typical components of phase 2 include the management of nutrition, weight, blood pressure, lipids, diabetes, tobacco cessation, psychosocial issues, physical activity counselling, and exercise training. A recent meta-analysis of exercise-based CR versus usual care showed the intervention to be associated with an improvement in health-related quality of life and a reduction in admissions. However, despite a reduction in cardiovascular mortality, but not overall mortality, the risk of myocardial infarction is unchanged [6].

Data from the UK National Audit of Cardiac Rehabilitation (NACR) showed that only 27% patients received a measure of exercise performance perhaps inferring that aerobic training prescription is not routinely individually prescribed in practice [7]. The American Heart Association guidelines recommend 30 minutes of at least moderate-intensity physical activity a minimum of five times a week [8]. However, importantly a physical activity history is provided as an alternative to an exercise test to guide prescription. This is particularly relevant to patients with heart failure as individually prescribed moderate- to high-intensity aerobic exercise training was an essential part of the Heart Failure: A Controlled Trial Investigating Outcomes of Exercise Training (HF-ACTION) trial [9]. The positive results of the latter trial contributed a large part to Medicare supporting reimbursement for CR in patients with heart failure in 2014. A question therefore remains as to which model of rehabilitation (cardiac or pulmonary) is most relevant to the breathless patient with heart failure [10].

Cardiovascular Risk in Chronic Lung Disease and Breathlessness in Heart Failure

As described in Chap. 5, cardiovascular disease is a common co-morbidity of many chronic lung diseases by shared risk factors of smoking and physical inactivity and potentially underlying systemic inflammatory pathways. In a cohort of patients with COPD attending PR, arterial stiffness was increased in comparison to healthy controls [11] and similar data has recently been reported in bronchiectasis [12]. The PR population typically has multiple co-morbidities including cardiovascular disease and they do as well from PR [13]. Other data suggests a prognostic role of cardiovascular disease as patients with mild to moderate COPD more commonly die from cardiovascular disease than respiratory failure. Although improving exercise capacity may improve cardiovascular risk, currently cardiovascular risk reduction is not part of the assessment, process, or outcome of PR.

Abdominal aortic aneurysms (AAA) are common in patients with COPD due to shared risk factors and there is often concern about the safety of exercise, particularly of high-intensity exercise. Expert opinion suggests participation in PR for AAA <5.5 cm; for aneurysms >5.5 cm, surgery is indicated depending on fitness. In cases where surgery is contraindicated, mild to moderate exercise, with the avoidance of exercise that precipitates transient increases in blood pressure such a high load resistance training, is recommended [14].

Exercise training is recommended for patients with heart failure and a meta-analysis of exercise rehabilitation versus usual care reported improvements in the intervention group in health status with a reduction in healthcare utilisation but no difference at 1 year in mortality [15]. Exercise training may also improve left ventricular function through remodelling. Patients with heart failure (particularly those with reduced ejection fraction where the literature is greatest) are currently referred to CR but their symptoms and disability have more in common with patients with chronic lung disease than the traditional CR population. Currently, only a small proportion of patients with heart failure who might benefit receive CR in the UK which is likely to be mirrored in other countries. In the USA, less than 30% of the traditional patients post-MI and CABG are referred for CR [16]; it is therefore reasonable to assume an even lower proportion for patients with heart failure since reimbursement via Medicare only became available within the last 5 years.

Patients with pulmonary hypertension are another potential outlier to the current exercise rehabilitation service structure. Exercise training improves exercise performance and health-related quality of life and appears to be safe for patients with pulmonary hypertension but which service should they be referred to? They are similarly breathless on exertion to patients with chronic lung disease and therefore would benefit from the symptom-based approach of PR, but their demographics and potential need for cardiac monitoring would be more similar to a patient with cardiac disease.

There is a growing rationale to combine the approaches of CR and PR. However, as the focus of this book is to understand cardiovascular disease in chronic lung disease, the following section will focus on any adaptations necessary to the process of PR for a patient with conditions across both cardiac and pulmonary specialities.

The Process of Pulmonary Rehabilitation and Modifications Needed for Cardiovascular Disease

Assessment

The assessment is the time to further inform patients about the aims and the process of pulmonary rehabilitation. There should be a systematic assessment of the inclusion and exclusion criteria. The main inclusion criterion is breathlessness limiting exertion commonly assessed by the Medical Research Council (MRC) dyspnea scale of ≥2. Guidelines recommend MRC grades 3–5 but patients with milder breathlessness (MRC 2) also benefit and are often included [17]. Exclusion criteria include major neurological or musculoskeletal deficit preventing ability to exercise or safety concerns such as unstable cardiac disease, for example, a myocardial infarction within 4 weeks, unstable arrhythmias, unstable angina, and unstable heart failure or severe aortic stenosis. Patients with pulmonary hypertension, right heart failure, heart failure with reduced or preserved ejection fraction, angina, atrial arrhythmias, or other cardiovascular disease should not be routinely excluded from participation in a PR program, but should be optimally managed by an appropriately skilled healthcare professional prior to referral. As described in Chap. 8, patients with chronic lung disease and co-existent cardiac disease have more symptoms, worse exercise performance and health-related quality of life, and so it is important that they are not excluded from a therapy with known benefit.

An assessment of dyspnea, exercise performance, and health status before and after the program is standard and can inform both individual progress and program quality. An exercise assessment is performed to inform the exercise prescription, requirements for safety, and as a baseline for the exercise outcome. It is increasingly performed using simple, inexpensive field tests rather than expensive laboratory-based exercise equipment. Blood pressure (BP) monitoring should be performed before and after exercise. Symptoms of chest tightness causing exercise cessation, symptomatic reduction of 10 mmHg in systolic BP, and either pre-syncope or syncope on the exercise test should all precipitate a medical review prior to participation. The need for electrocardiography throughout an exercise test for cardiovascular disease is debated (but mostly employed), whereas this is rarely performed for a PR assessment.

Patients with resting hypoxia should exercise with supplemental oxygen. The criterion for ambulatory oxygen varies among jurisdictions. Those who desaturate markedly on exercise to oxygen saturation <85% are often offered supplementary oxygen during training but to date there is no evidence of superior efficacy. There is often concern around patients who desaturate but this is frequently an everyday occurrence for the individual. The American College of Sports Medicine advises to only terminate exercise tests if the desaturation is accompanied by a complication such as arrhythmia, pre-syncope, or chest pain.

Outcome Measures

Cardiopulmonary exercise test is described in detail in Chap. 10.

The following field tests have been validated in both pulmonary and cardiac conditions and would therefore be appropriate for patients with both chronic lung and cardiovascular disease.

Six-Minute Walk Test

The most commonly used field test is the six-minute walk test (6MWT) which is completed over a 30-meter flat course. It is self-paced, and standardised instructions are given as the distance walked can be influenced by encouragement. Patients are asked to walk as far as they can for 6 minutes and the result is usually presented as the distance walked, although the speed can be calculated. The test is reproducible after two practice tests and is responsive in both chronic lung and cardiovascular diseases. Normal reference values for many different populations are available. It is often referred to as a measure of functional capacity but in more severe disease it can reflect maximal exercise capacity. The 6MWT distance is highly correlated with other outcomes such as mortality for both chronic lung and cardiovascular diseases and is featured in a multidimensional severity index, the BODE index, for COPD. It is used to set exercise prescription for PR (usually as a percentage of the overall speed), but the intensity will vary between individuals, will often reflect only mild to moderate intensity training, and therefore may not be the best test available for this purpose.

Incremental Shuttle Walk Test

The incremental shuttle walk test (ISWT) is a symptom-limited, externally paced test, conducted along a 10-meter course, and reflects maximal exercise capacity. The walking speed increases every minute until the patient is too breathless or fatigued to continue or can no longer maintain the required speed. The result is presented as the total distance achieved. It is reproducible after a single practice test. In contrast to the 6MWT, the ISWT has a graded physiological response. However, normal reference values are not currently available. The test is also reliable, valid, and interpretable, making it an excellent evaluative test.

Endurance Shuttle Walk Test

The endurance shuttle walk test (ESWT) was developed as a test of submaximal exercise capacity. It is similarly symptom-limited and externally paced and uses the same 10-meter course as the ISWT. After a two-minute warm-up, the patients walk at the set speed until they can no longer maintain the required speed or are too breathless or fatigued to continue. The result is presented as the time walked after the warm-up and is reproducible after a familiarisation test. The advantage of the ISWT and ESWT is the ability to develop individualised exercise prescriptions for pulmonary rehabilitation. The speed of the walk can be set at a high intensity (85% of the predicted peak oxygen consumption) derived from the ISWT distance. The duration of the walk can then be progressed throughout the program. Both the ISWT and ESWT are responsive outcome measures.

Peripheral Muscle Strength

Increasingly, measures of strength are included in a PR assessment most commonly either finger grip strength or quadriceps strength. Isometric strength can be measured using a handheld dynamometer or a strain gauge. A one-repetition maximum (1-RM), the maximum weight a person can lift in one manoeuver, can be used with knee extensor gym equipment. Isokinetic dynamometry is less frequently used for clinical purposes.

Health-Related Quality of Life

Health-related quality of life is commonly assessed by questionnaires for clinical and research purposes. Generic questionnaires such as the short-form 36 (SF-36) and the EuroQol (EQ-5D) have been validated in both cardiac and respiratory populations and tend to be discriminative but less responsive. The EQ-5D has the added value of enabling cost-effectiveness to be calculated. They are also helpful in assessing the multi-morbid patient. However, disease-specific questionnaires have been developed in order to be more specific and are often more responsive to interventions. The Chronic Heart Questionnaire (CHQ) and the Chronic Respiratory Questionnaire (CRQ) are almost identical except for one question despite being developed in different populations by the same research team. They are valid and responsive, and pragmatically either would be a good option to use for patients with combined chronic respiratory and cardiovascular disease.

Anxiety and Depression

The Hospital Anxiety and Depression scale has been extensively used in a variety of chronic cardiac and pulmonary diseases separately (and in many other long-term conditions) and therefore pragmatically would be reasonable to use this for the patient with combined cardiopulmonary disease.

Dyspnea

The Medical Research Council dyspnea scale assesses the degree of activity limitation caused by breathlessness and is valid and reproducible. It is most commonly used as an inclusion criterion for referral to PR rather than as an outcome measure.

The Borg breathless scale is commonly used to assess the degree of breathlessness experienced at the end of an exercise test and is not disease-specific. However, it is important to understand the impact of breathlessness on quality of life for which there is the dyspnea domain of either the CHQ or the CRQ. However, scientifically it is not recommended to report sections of questionnaires that have been validated as a whole. Two questionnaires have been validated in both cardiac and pulmonary conditions: the Multidimensional Dyspnea Profile questionnaire (MDP) [18] and the Dyspnea-12 Questionnaire in patients with COPD, interstitial lung disease, and chronic heart failure [19], and therefore either would be suitable for use for the patient with both a pulmonary and cardiac condition.

Frailty Measures

Fried and colleagues defined frailty as a clinical syndrome in which three or more of the following criteria are present: unintentional weight loss (10 lbs in the past year), self-reported exhaustion, weakness (grip strength), slow walking speed, and low physical activity. Measures associated with frailty such as the Short Physical Performance Battery (SPPB) and Timed Up and Go (TUG) have recently been extensively evaluated in patients with chronic lung disease, and PR can modify frailty [20]. The results may indicate a need for a targeted intervention such as balance training or strength training.

Exercise Prescription

The Effects of Physiological Aerobic Training

In health, the physiological effects of aerobic training occur predominantly within the cardiovascular system and the skeletal muscle of the lower limbs. The cardiovascular effects are both central and peripheral. The central effects result in a lower resting heart rate by improving the efficiency of each heartbeat, i.e. increase in stroke volume. With regular training, the oxidative capacity of the skeletal muscle is increased by increasing peripheral vasculature particularly capillarisation and thereby increasing blood flow, increasing the proportion of type 1 (slow-twitch non-fatigable muscle fibre type), increasing the oxidative enzymes, and increasing mitochondrial number. All these effects result in more efficient energy production and utilisation, and therefore increase performance. There are also psychological effects of training such as increasing tolerance of physical discomfort.

In chronic lung diseases, the effects of high-intensity aerobic training are largely secondary to skeletal muscle adaptations. Central cardiovascular effects are rarely achieved probably due to the low absolute training intensities achieved. The results after training for the individual are either performing the same task with less dyspnea or improving physical performance for the same degree of dyspnea. There may also be improved tolerance of dyspnea. Overall exercise training as part of PR programs results in increased health-related quality of life. The same benefits are not seen if the training component is removed.

Patients with heart failure can also improve their exercise performance with high-intensity aerobic training. The lower limb skeletal muscle improvements are similar to that seen in patients with COPD. However, left ventricular remodelling may also occur for patients with heart failure, whereas underlying pulmonary function is not altered by exercise training for patients with chronic lung diseases. The mechanisms of benefit of aerobic training in patients with coronary heart disease are predominantly similar to those in health.

Fundamental Principles Behind the Aerobic Exercise Prescription:

- The 'currency' for exercise is energy and in mammals 'dollars' are molecules called 'adenine trinucleotide phosphates' or ATP.
- Different foods have a different energy equivalent per gram, for example, fat approximately equates to 8 kcal and carbohydrate to 4 kcal and are utilised differently by different organs.
- Skeletal muscle uses fatty acids (fats), glucose (carbohydrate), and amino acids (protein) to generate energy.
- This energy needs replenishing in order to sustain exercise and different substrates are used depending on the duration and intensity of exercise.
- In its simplest definition, anaerobic metabolism describes a pathway to make energy without using oxygen and produces lactate as a by-product.
- Aerobic metabolism uses oxygen for glycolysis and energy is made in the mitochondria via the Krebs cycle producing two ATP molecules and the electron transport chain producing 36–38 ATP molecules.
- The anaerobic threshold can be identified by the inflection point when the volume of oxygen utilised (VO_2) is plotted versus volume of carbon dioxide eliminated (VCO_2) or by measuring serial blood lactate levels (see Chap. 10).
- The heart rate and/or oxygen uptake at the anaerobic threshold can be estimated via a maximal incremental exercise test typically on a cycle ergometer.
- Critical power (or speed for walking) is the power below which exercise theoretically can be sustained indefinitely. Critical power would typically fall below the anaerobic threshold. The relationship between power (or speed) and duration is not linear (which is particularly relevant if an endurance test is being used as an outcome measure for an intervention such as pulmonary rehabilitation).
- Usually a maximal exercise test, designed to reach the maximal oxygen uptake (VO_2 max) of the individual, would be used to 'set' the exercise prescription for an endurance exercise session.
- High-intensity training prescribed between 60% and 80% of VO_2 max or heart rate is more effective in improving exercise capacity than low-intensity training for chronic lung and heart diseases.
- For a high-intensity exercise session, the prescription would be set above the anaerobic threshold, but ideally would be sustained for 20–30 minutes before symptom limitation. Even in healthy adults, this is difficult to estimate accurately and some adjustment is often needed.

- During high-intensity training, ideally a plateau of heart rate and peak oxygen consumption will occur at the estimated peak heart rate or peak VO_2 prescribed, but commonly they will continue to increase and exercise will terminate due to symptom limitation before the ideal 20–30 minutes.

Exercise Prescription for Individuals with Chronic Lung Disease or Cardiovascular Disease

To achieve beneficial exercise training, it needs to be prescribed akin to any medication. 'FITT' is a useful acronym which describes the components of the prescription (Table 11.1).

Frequency

A minimum recommendation of three sessions (at least two supervised sessions) per week is recommended for both chronic lung and cardiac conditions.

Intensity

High-intensity lower limb training is recommended for both chronic lung disease and heart failure [4]. The recommendations for desired intensity for patients with coronary artery disease varies across countries; North American, and European guidelines suggest moderate to high-intensity training, whereas UK, Australia, and New Zealand recommend lower-intensity training.

A maximal exercise test is often used to prescribe exercise: a laboratory cardiopulmonary exercise test on either a cycle ergometer or treadmill, or a field test such as the incremental shuttle walk test (ISWT). Individuals with chronic lung disease are commonly not able to achieve the necessary plateau to represent VO_2 max on an exercise test and therefore the term VO_2 peak is used. A 60–80% peak VO_2, peak power, or peak heart rate is typically used for the exercise prescription.

The formula below is used to estimate the peak VO_2 for the ISWT distance achieved.

$$\text{Predicted VO}_2 \text{ peak}\left[\text{ml}/\text{min}/\text{kg}\right] = 4.19 + \left(0.025 \times \text{ISWT distance}\left[\text{m}\right]\right)$$

Table 11.1 The 'FITT' method of exercise prescription

Frequency	Number of exercise sessions per week
Intensity	Intensity of training typically prescribed from a maximal exercise test
Time	Duration of training session and length of exercise program
Type	Mode of exercise

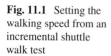

Fig. 11.1 Setting the walking speed from an incremental shuttle walk test

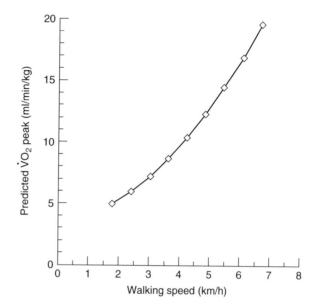

A training intensity of 85% VO_2 peak is frequently used for chronic lung disease when using the ISWT. The walking speed necessary to achieve this VO_2 can be estimated from Fig. 11.1 below and the endurance shuttle walk test (EWST) can be used to externally pace the speed of the walk.

The ESWT can be used both for the exercise prescription and as an outcome of pulmonary rehabilitation. There are 16 levels at different speeds. The same 10-m course for the ISWT is used. The end point of the test is how long the patient walks at the constant endurance speed. The test is stopped by the operator if 20 minutes are achieved.

For example, if the ISWT distance was 400 m, the approximate peak VO_2 is 14.19 ml/min/kg; 85% of peak VO_2 is 12.09, and the walking speed is 4.6 km/h. There are 16 walking speeds for the ESWT so the nearest walking speed should be selected. For this example, the walking speed would be level 11, 4.65 km/h.

Time

The duration of the endurance exercise should be between 20 and 30 minutes.

Type

Walking and cycling are the common training modalities used but other modalities have been used in both chronic lung and cardiac conditions such as water-based training and resistance training.

Exercise Training Prescription Variation Due to a Central Limitation to Exercise

In practice, individuals with COPD rarely achieve 20–30 minutes of continuous high-intensity training at 80% peak VO_2. This is largely due to a ventilatory limitation to exercise caused by a combination of airflow limitation, air trapping and dynamic hyperinflation, and hypoxemia. To respond to the increasing demands during exercise, ventilation (L/min) needs to increase. In people with normal lungs, this is usually achieved without difficulty and the achievement of maximal heart rate typically terminates exercise. In individuals with fixed airflow obstruction, there is a point when ventilation is unable to be increased further as maximum voluntary ventilation ($MVV = FEV_1 \times 37.5$) has been achieved. The only way of matching the demands is to increase the respiratory rate which quickly becomes intolerable.

Alternative exercise strategies have been designed to either increase peak ventilation such as the use of non-invasive ventilation during exercise, long-acting bronchodilators, supplemental oxygen, and breathing helium-hyperoxia. Other strategies have focused on delivering increased stimulus to the skeletal muscle without increasing ventilation demands such as neuromuscular stimulation or reducing the exercising muscle mass by exercising one leg at a time (either cycling one leg at a time or knee extensor training). The latter techniques have also yielded positive results in heart failure. Interval training has also been used by alternating high-intensity training for short periods with either rest or low-intensity training. Overall, the results of interval training are similar to continuous training for chronic lung disease [21] but may be superior in heart failure [22].

Strength Training

Strength training has received much attention over the last two decades and is recommended by international guidelines for both patients with chronic lung disease and cardiovascular disease. Although muscle strength is improved with resistance training compared to endurance training alone, this has not translated to additional improvements in exercise tolerance or health status in either chronic heart or lung conditions. It has been shown to be safe in both conditions. Ideally, resistance training should be individually prescribed, for example, at 40–60% of the one repetition maximum, and progressed through the program. The studies advocating strength training were performed on gym equipment but lower limb exercise in practice often consists of sit to stand, step ups, and leg raises, progressing throughout the program, but these exercises have not been thoroughly evaluated. Ankle weights can also be employed to add resistance.

Other Training Components

There are other components of training such as inspiratory muscle training which may reduce dyspnea in patients with chronic lung disease or heart failure, but similar to strength training, these effects do not translate to additional improvements in walking performance or health status when added to aerobic training.

The Rehabilitation Team

An educated confident multidisciplinary team is key to the success of a PR program. However, identifying the key education needs for a PR team and any additional training to manage cardiovascular disease has not received the same research rigor as the other aspects of a program. Training in cardiovascular diseases similar to recommendations for chronic lung disease would seem necessary. Understanding hypoxemia, arrhythmias, decompensation of heart failure, or cor pulmonale should be included.

Setting

Until the last decade, the most common setting for PR was hospital outpatients mostly due to safety with a hospital acute response or arrest team on standby and medical opinions equally readily available. However, due to the unacceptability of travel to the hospital or group-based therapy, home-based rehabilitation has been evaluated. A recent study comparing home-based PR versus centre-based PR was reported with the former being non-inferior [23] but the results from the centre-based supervised program were lower than typically seen. Recent trials have not reported severe adverse events without routine exclusion of cardiovascular disease. Specific studies are probably warranted before this is widely implemented. Currently, there is no accepted/validated risk stratification for choice of setting which is largely payer or commissioner defined and then patient preference by availability.

Conclusion

Unstable cardiac disease must be optimally managed prior to participation in an exercise program, but patients with co-morbid cardiac disease should not be routinely excluded from participation. The recommended components of an exercise training program such as combined aerobic and resistance training are strikingly similar for both cardiac and pulmonary conditions. The PR team should receive adequate training on different cardiac conditions and symptoms of decompensation akin to understanding chronic lung diseases and exacerbations. In the future, combining the approach of cardiac and pulmonary rehabilitation may be clinically cost-effective.

References

1. Vanfleteren LE, Franssen FM, Uszko-Lencer NH, Spruit MA, Celis M, Gorgels AP, et al. Frequency and relevance of ischemic electrocardiographic findings in patients with chronic obstructive pulmonary disease. Am J Cardiol. 2011;108(11):1669–74.
2. Crisafulli E, Gorgone P, Vagaggini B, Pagani M, Rossi G, Costa F, et al. Efficacy of standard rehabilitation in COPD outpatients with comorbidities. Eur Respir J. 2010;36(5):1042–8.
3. Nonoyama ML, Kin SM, Brooks D, Oh P. Comparison of cardiac rehabilitation outcomes in individuals with respiratory, cardiac or no comorbidities: a retrospective review. Can J Respir Ther. 2016;52(2):43–9.
4. Spruit MA, Singh SJ, Garvey C, Zuwallack R, Nici L, Rochester C, et al. An official American Thoracic Society/European Respiratory Society statement: key concepts and advances in pulmonary rehabilitation. Am J Respir Crit Care Med. 2013;188(8):e13–64.
5. McCarthy B, Casey D, Devane D, Murphy K, Murphy E, Lacasse Y. Pulmonary rehabilitation for chronic obstructive pulmonary disease. Cochrane Database Syst Rev. 2015;(2):CD003793.
6. Anderson L, Oldridge N, Thompson DR, Zwisler AD, Rees K, Martin N, et al. Exercise-based cardiac rehabilitation for coronary heart disease: cochrane systematic review and meta-analysis. J Am Coll Cardiol. 2016;67(1):1–12.
7. National Audit of Cardiac Rehabilitation. British Heart Foundation 2016 [cited 2017 Dec 20]. Available from: www.bhf.org.uk/publications/statistics/national-audit-of-cardiac-rehabilitation-annual-statistical-report-2016.
8. Smith SC Jr, Benjamin EJ, Bonow RO, Braun LT, Creager MA, Franklin BA, et al. AHA/ACCF secondary prevention and risk reduction therapy for patients with coronary and other atherosclerotic vascular disease: 2011 update: a guideline from the American Heart Association and American College of Cardiology Foundation endorsed by the World Heart Federation and the Preventive Cardiovascular Nurses Association. J Am Coll Cardiol. 2011;58(23):2432–46.
9. O'Connor CM, Whellan DJ, Lee KL, Keteyian SJ, Cooper LS, Ellis SJ, et al. Efficacy and safety of exercise training in patients with chronic heart failure: HF-ACTION randomized controlled trial. JAMA. 2009;301(14):1439–50.
10. Evans RA, Singh SJ, Collier R, Loke I, Steiner MC, Morgan MD. Generic, symptom based, exercise rehabilitation; integrating patients with COPD and heart failure. Respir Med. 2010;104(10):1473–81.
11. Vanfleteren LE, Spruit MA, Groenen MT, Bruijnzeel PL, Taib Z, Rutten EP, et al. Arterial stiffness in patients with COPD: the role of systemic inflammation and the effects of pulmonary rehabilitation. Eur Respir J. 2014;43(5):1306–15.
12. Saleh AD, Kwok B, Brown JS, Hurst JR. Correlates and assessment of excess cardiovascular risk in bronchiectasis. Eur Respir J. 2017;50(5):1701127.
13. Mesquita R, Vanfleteren LE, Franssen FM, Sarv J, Taib Z, Groenen MT, et al. Objectively identified comorbidities in COPD: impact on pulmonary rehabilitation outcomes. Eur Respir J. 2015;46(2):545–8.
14. Bolton CE, Bevan-Smith EF, Blakey JD, Crowe P, Elkin SL, Garrod R, et al. British Thoracic Society guideline on pulmonary rehabilitation in adults. Thorax. 2013;68(Suppl 2):ii1–30.
15. Sagar VA, Davies EJ, Briscoe S, Coats AJ, Dalal HM, Lough F, et al. Exercise-based rehabilitation for heart failure: systematic review and meta-analysis. Open Heart. 2015;2(1):e000163.

16. Lavie CJ, Milani RV. Cardiac rehabilitation and exercise training in secondary coronary heart disease prevention. Prog Cardiovasc Dis. 2011;53(6):397–403.
17. Evans RA, Singh SJ, Collier R, Williams JE, Morgan MD. Pulmonary rehabilitation is successful for COPD irrespective of MRC dyspnoea grade. Respir Med. 2009;103(7):1070–5.
18. Meek PM, Banzett R, Parsall MB, Gracely RH, Schwartzstein RM, Lansing R. Reliability and validity of the multidimensional dyspnea profile. Chest. 2012;141(6):1546–53.
19. York J, Jones P. Quantification of dyspnoea using descriptors: development and initial testing of the Dyspnoea-12. Thorax. 2010;65(1):21–6.
20. Maddocks M, Kon SS, Canavan JL, Jones SE, Nolan CM, Labey A, et al. Physical frailty and pulmonary rehabilitation in COPD: a prospective cohort study. Thorax. 2016;71(11):988–95.
21. Beauchamp MK, Nonoyama M, Goldstein RS, Hill K, Dolmage TE, Mathur S, et al. Interval versus continuous training in individuals with chronic obstructive pulmonary disease–a systematic review. Thorax. 2010;65(2):157–64.
22. Wisloff U, Stoylen A, Loennechen JP, Bruvold M, Rognmo O, Haram PM, et al. Superior cardiovascular effect of aerobic interval training versus moderate continuous training in heart failure patients: a randomized study. Circulation. 2007;115(24):3086–94.
23. Holland AE, Mahal A, Hill CJ, Lee AL, Burge AT, Cox NS, et al. Home-based rehabilitation for COPD using minimal resources: a randomised, controlled equivalence trial. Thorax. 2017;72(1):57–65.

Chapter 12
Acute Exacerbations of Chronic Lung Disease: Cardiac Considerations

Kate Milne and Don D. Sin

Pearls
- Cardiovascular disease and COPD commonly occur in the same patient and share both risk factors and common pathophysiologic mechanisms.
- Diagnosis of cardiovascular comorbidities in patients with COPD can be challenging and requires a low threshold for investigation in accordance with disease-specific guidelines.
- Patients with COPD and cardiovascular disease are at risk of being undertreated due to concerns regarding the safety of disease-specific therapies in comorbid patients; however, most therapies are safe.
- Increased systemic inflammation during an exacerbation of COPD is associated with cardiac dysfunction, morbidity, and mortality.
- Influenza vaccination reduces cardiovascular risk in COPD patients
- Long-acting bronchodilators are safe in patients with COPD and comorbid cardiovascular conditions. They may even reduce the risk of cardiovascular events in select patients.

Introduction

The importance of appropriately recognizing and managing patients with cardiovascular and pulmonary comorbidities is underscored by the poor outcomes described in complex comorbid patients. Patients with chronic obstructive pulmonary disease (COPD) have an increased risk, up to one-third greater than the general population,

K. Milne · D. D. Sin (✉)
University of British Columbia (UBC) Division of Respiratory Medicine (Department of Medicine) and Centre for Heart Lung Innovation, St. Paul's Hospital, Vancouver, BC, Canada
e-mail: katemilne@alumni.ubc.ca; Don.Sin@hli.ubc.ca

© Springer Nature Switzerland AG 2020
S. P. Bhatt (ed.), *Cardiac Considerations in Chronic Lung Disease*,
Respiratory Medicine, https://doi.org/10.1007/978-3-030-43435-9_12

of cardiovascular comorbidities including hypertension and diabetes [1]. Patients with COPD have higher rates of ischemic heart disease, heart failure, and arrhythmias with risks that are 2–5 times higher than those in age-matched control subjects [1, 2]. This presence of cardiovascular disease in patients with COPD leads to lower quality of life, increased rates of hospitalization, and death [3]. Patients with COPD are at a particularly high risk of cardiovascular events during acute exacerbations of COPD (AECOPD) [4]. Indeed, AECOPDs increase the risk of acute coronary events and stroke by 3–5-fold, a risk that can be mitigated by preventing exacerbations related to respiratory tract infections. Thus, understanding the common mechanisms and risk factors for COPD and cardiovascular disease, diagnostic and management challenges, and the interplay between comorbidities during episodes of an acute exacerbation of COPD is central for the clinical care of these complex patients.

COPD Exacerbations

AECOPDs are defined by an increase in patient symptoms beyond the day-to-day variation, which leads to increase in pharmacologic therapy [5]. Currently, AECOPDs are diagnosed largely based on clinical acumen, irrespective of the etiology. As there are no reliable ways of phenotyping exacerbations (e.g., infectious versus noninfectious), all AECOPDs are empirically treated with systemic corticosteroids and/or broad-spectrum antibiotics, which likely leads to their overuse in the community [5]. The treatment and outcomes for AECOPD are far from optimal. Once patients are sick enough to come to emergency departments for AECOPD, 9 out of 10 patients will be admitted for treatment for an average length of hospital stay of 10 days [6]. One in 12 of these patients will die either in hospital or within 6 months of hospital discharge; 1 in 8 patients will require noninvasive or invasive mechanical ventilation, and 1 in 3 patients will suffer another exacerbation over 3–6 months of follow-up [6]. The treatment side effects are also substantial. During therapy, more than 50% patients will experience new or worsening hyperglycemia, 12–18% will develop new or worsening of hypertension, and 12% will experience other steroid-related adverse effects including adrenal insufficiency [6]. Incredibly, treatment for AECOPD has not changed over the past 30 years. Health care providers treat everyone with AECOPD with antibiotics despite good data suggesting that fewer than 50% of the episodes are associated with bacterial infections and with prednisone even though approximately 30% of the episodes are not associated with lung or systemic inflammation!

It is widely postulated, though not completely proven, that respiratory tract infections by microbial agents are the leading cause of AECOPD [5]. By using polymerase chain reaction on spontaneous sputum samples, Bafadhel et al. found that the prevalence of "virus"-associated exacerbation was 29% (with rhinovirus being the most common) and that of "bacteria"-associated exacerbation was more than 40% [7]. However, it should be noted that many patients with COPD demonstrate evidence of bacterial colonization even during clinical stability, whereas presence of viruses is distinctly rare except during exacerbations [7]. Thus, the clinical relevance of identifying bacterial species in spontaneous sputum of patients with COPD during exacerbations is uncertain.

Exacerbations and Cardiovascular Events

The multiple potentially reciprocal mechanisms through which either an exacerbation of COPD may potentiate cardiovascular decompensation or through which cardiac dysfunction can trigger an acute exacerbation of COPD are complex (Fig. 12.1) [8]. Multiple mechanisms are triggered during an AECOPD that lead to cardiovascular dysfunction and morbidity. Platelet activation, fibrinogen production, and interleukin-6, interleukin-8, and tumor necrosis factor α levels are elevated during an acute exacerbation of COPD, and these are pro-atherothrombotic. This cascade can lead to atherosclerotic plaque rupture and acute coronary syndrome as demonstrated in Fig. 12.2. The most important pathway appears to be related to inflammation. COPD patients have chronic lung inflammation which worsens during acute exacerbations [7]. Acute coronary syndromes can be associated with an AECOPD [4]. This increased risk seems most closely associated with respiratory infection and inflammation as an exacerbation trigger [9].

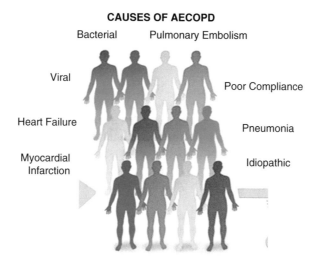

CAUSES OF AECOPD

Bacterial   Pulmonary Embolism

Viral

Poor Compliance

Heart Failure

Pneumonia

Myocardial Infarction

Idiopathic

Fig. 12.1 Causes of acute exacerbations of COPD. There are multiple causes of acute exacerbations of COPD (AECOPD). Although almost all clinically significant AECOPDs are treated with oral antibiotics and/or systemic corticosteroids, at least 30% of the AECOPDs are caused by noninflammatory, noninfectious causes. A significant number of cases are caused by cardiovascular events. In one study, approximately 20% of hospitalized AECOPDs were characterized by pulmonary edema on chest radiograph [82]

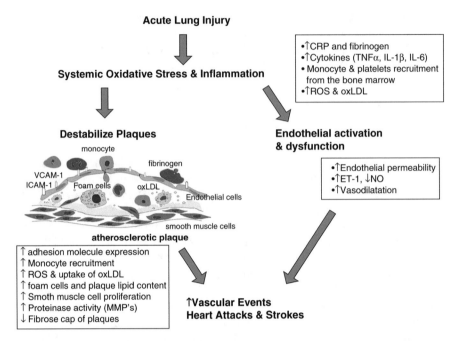

Fig. 12.2 A proposed schema of how acute exacerbations of COPD may lead to acute cardiovascular events. We propose that respiratory tract infection leads to acute lung injury, resulting in lung inflammation and oxidant stress. This causes endothelial dysfunction and acute disruption of stable atherosclerotic plaques, resulting in the conversion of stable plaques into unstable (or vulnerable) ones. Vulnerable plaques are much more likely to rupture, causing acute myocardial infarction or stroke than stable plaques [83]. Neutrophilic inflammation appears to play a central role in this process [26]

Regardless of the etiology of the AECOPD, during AECOPD events, many patients experience myocardial injury and stress. Patel et al., for instance, found that approximately 16% of patients during AECOPD experienced a marked elevation in serum troponin, a biomarker of myocardial injury, and a similar number experienced a rise in N-terminal pro b-type natriuretic peptide (NT-proBNP), a biomarker of myocardial stretch and failure. In their study, the levels of these blood cardiac biomarkers peaked at day 7 of the AECOPD event and then gradually returned to normal levels after 30–90 days post-event [10]. Increased troponins and electrocardiographic (ECG) changes have been reported in patients with COPD, in the absence of an acute coronary syndrome, which complicates making the correct diagnosis [11]. As a result, diagnosis of ST-elevation myocardial infarction (STEMI) is frequently delayed in patients with COPD [12]. Increased troponin in patients with acute exacerbation of COPD is an independent risk factor for mortality, even in the absence of acute coronary syndrome, and can be due to multiple factors [13]. The pathophysiology of increased troponin observed during an acute exacerbation of COPD may be related to the development of supply-demand mismatch to the myocardium due to tachycardia or coexisting left ventricular hypertrophy [8]. The hypoxemia and hypercapnia resulting from an acute exacerbation of COPD can also be pro-arrhythmogenic, leading to arrhythmias during an acute exacerbation of COPD which can in turn trigger heart failure decompensation [14]. Troponin may also be increased as a result of increased pulmonary pressures and right heart dysfunction during an exacerbation [8]. Natriuretic peptides are a useful tool in diagnosing acute heart failure in the setting of comorbid COPD as heart failure is unlikely with normal values (BNP < 100 pg/ml or NT-proBNP < 300 pg/ml) [15]. However, the appropriate cutoff value in patients with pulmonary disease is debated as associations between elevated plasma N-terminal proBNP (NT-proBNP) and decreased FEV_1 have been described in patients without heart failure. Elevations of BNP or NT-proBNP in patients with an acute exacerbation of COPD predict worse cardiovascular outcomes and death [8]. BNP is released from ventricular myocytes due to either volume or pressure overload and resulting myocyte stretch. Changes in intrathoracic pressure during an acute exacerbation of COPD impact venous return, cardiac function, and pulmonary pressures leading to elevation of BNP [8].

During AECOPD, patients also demonstrate endothelial dysfunction systemically as evidenced by a significant increase in pulse wave velocity of the affected blood vessels. Most importantly, the risk of myocardial infarction (MI) and stroke increases substantially during the first few days of AECOPD. One study showed that the risk of MI increased by 2.27 times the baseline rate within 1–5 days of AECOPD, whereas the risk of stroke increased by 26% [4].

The relationship between acute respiratory tract infection and cardiovascular events is particularly notable and interesting. In the largest study of its kind, Kwong et al. evaluated 364 hospitalizations for MI between May 1, 2009, and May 31, 2014, in Ontario, Canada. They obtained nasal swab data using reverse-transcriptase polymerase chain reaction (rtPCR; monoplex or multiplex assays), viral culture, direct fluorescent antibody staining, and enzyme immunoassays on influenza A and B as well as other respiratory viruses including respiratory syncytial virus, adenovirus, coronavirus, enterovirus (such as rhinovirus), parainfluenza virus, and human metapneumovirus [16]. They found that during the first 7 days of the respiratory tract infection, the risk of MI was 6-fold higher than during "control" periods (i.e., weeks when they were infection-free). The highest risk period was within 1–3 days of the respiratory tract infection (relative risk, RR, of 6.30) with the risk sharply decaying by day 8 of the infection. In this study, most (82%) of the respiratory tract infections were caused by influenza A and only 31% of the cohort had received influenza vaccination prior to the study year.

These data are consistent with other studies including that by Warren-Gash et al. who showed by using the General Practice Research Database (GPRD) in the United Kingdom (UK) that the risk of MI was 4 times higher during the first 3 days of the infection compared with controlled periods with the risk gradually decaying over time and returning to baseline levels by 30–90 days postinfection [17]. Most importantly, in a secondary prevention trial of 439 patients who had been hospitalized with an acute coronary syndrome, Phrommintikul et al. showed that influenza vaccination therapy (versus no vaccination in the control group) resulted in 30%

lower rate of combined major cardiovascular end points including death, rehospitalization for acute coronary syndrome or from heart failure, or stroke and a strong trend towards lower rate of cardiovascular mortality (hazard ratio, HR, 0.39; $p = 0.088$) [18]. It should also be noted that influenza vaccination or pneumococcal vaccination per se is not associated with any increase or decrease in cardiovascular events [9]. Thus, vaccination is safe.

The relationship between infection and cardiovascular events is not restricted to respiratory tract infections. Infection elsewhere in the body is also associated with increased risk of cardiovascular events. Minassian et al. showed using a Medicare beneficiary database that individuals who developed herpes zoster infection (i.e., shingles) experienced a 2.4-fold increase in the risk of ischemic stroke and 1.7-fold increase in the risk of MI within the first week of infection [19]. It should be noted, however, that while infection in other organ systems is associated with increased risk of cardiovascular events, the relationship between respiratory tract infections and cardiovascular events is particularly strong. For instance, Smeeth and colleagues showed using the UK GPRD database that the risk of MI in the first 3 days of a respiratory tract infection was 5.0-fold higher than that during controlled periods, whereas the relative risk for MI for urinary tract infections was only 1.7 [9]. Together these data suggest that respiratory tract infections are one of the most important triggers of MI and stroke and mitigation strategies to reduce these infections will not only decrease the risk of AECOPD but also prevent cardiovascular events.

Common Mechanisms and Risk Factors for Cardiovascular Disease and COPD

The mechanism by which AECOPD leads to cardiovascular events remains largely a mystery. COPD and cardiovascular disease such as heart failure, atrial fibrillation, and ischemic heart disease share common risk factors such as cigarette smoking and age [15]. However, independent of the risk imposed by smoking, reduced lung function, assessed by using decrease in FEV_1, has been associated with mortality due to ischemic heart disease [20]. However, whether there exists a common mechanism or link beyond shared risk factors is an ongoing subject of debate.

Systemic inflammation has been observed in patients with COPD, ischemic heart disease, and atrial fibrillation and has been proposed as a potential mechanism leading to poor clinical outcomes [21, 22]. Smoking and alterations in the lung microbiome and elastin fiber have been implicated as potential sources of ongoing inflammation [23, 24]. Other environmental exposures including air pollution, viral and bacterial respiratory infection, and oral disease are thought to increase inflammation and contribute to inflammation associated with poor cardiovascular outcomes [25]. Although the precise pathways are unknown, animal studies suggest that inhalation of small particulate matter leads to chronic lung inflammation and systemic inflammation. This chronic inflammatory state is thought to contribute to the development of atherosclerotic disease, independent of dyslipidemia [25]. A proposed model for how this may occur is presented in Fig. 12.2.

Another important consideration is the effect of lung inflammation related to respiratory tract infection on the cardiovascular system. Jaw et al. modeled the effects of respiratory tract infection on the cardiovascular system using lipopolysaccharide (LPS) stimulation directly to the airways of mice, which were prone to atherosclerosis [26]. LPS is a bioactive component of gram-negative bacterial wall and induces local inflammation by stimulating toll-like receptor 4. In this model, instillation of LPS into the airways resulted in conversion of 68% of the atherosclerotic plaques from "stable" to "vulnerable" ones. In contrast, instillation of just saline into the airways led to 12% of the plaques becoming vulnerable ($p = 0.0004$). Repeating this experiment following temporary depletion of neutrophils using Ly6G antibodies prevented conversion of stable to vulnerable plaques related to LPS exposure. Interestingly, injection of LPS intraperitoneally to mimic infection outside of the thoracic cavity did not lead to any significant destabilization of atherosclerotic plaques. Together, these data suggest that acute respiratory tract infections induce neutrophilic inflammation locally and systemically that lead to disruption of stable plaques and cause acute myocardial and cerebrovascular events. These adverse effects may be prevented by reducing neutrophilic inflammation.

Does Prevention of AECOPD Reduce the Risk of Cardiovascular Events?

As noted above, influenza vaccination is effective in reducing the risk of significant cardiovascular events in patients with and without COPD. The effects of other drugs commonly used in the treatment of COPD patients on the risk of cardiovascular events are much more uncertain and controversial. The first line of therapy for COPD patients with persistent symptoms is long-acting muscarinic antagonist (LAMA) [5]. In the Understanding Potential Long-Term Impacts on Function with Tiotropium (UPLIFT) trial, the rate of serious cardiac adverse events was 16% lower in the group that was assigned to tiotropium ($n = 2986$) over 4 years compared with the group that was assigned to placebo ($n = 3006$; $p < 0.05$). This relative reduction was largely driven by lower rates of congestive heart failure (RR, 0.59) and myocardial infarction (RR, 0.71) [27]. However, these data should be interpreted cautiously as the primary end point, the rate of decline in lung function, was no different between tiotropium and placebo and the cardiac events were not fully adjudicated; thus, misclassification of events could have occurred. In a population-based study in Ontario, Canada, Gershon et al. demonstrated that elderly patients (66 years of age and older) who were newly prescribed a LAMA or a long-acting beta-2 agonist (LABA), another class of long-acting bronchodilator, had a 31% increase in the risk of cardiovascular events [28]. Another population-based study in the UK showed similar results with use of LAMA being associated with a small increase in the risk of stroke and MI and a significant reduction in total mortality [29]. LAMA in inhalation spray format, which leads to increased drug deposition in the small airways, has been associated with increased risk of cardiovascular events compared with LAMA in a dry powder formulation, which leads to increased drug deposition in the upper and larger airways [30]. However, in the largest clinical trial of its kind involving 17,135 patients with COPD, the use of tiotropium in inhalation spray format was not associated with any significant increase in the risk of major cardiovascular adverse effects compared with tiotropium in a dry powder formulation, though in the higher tiotropium spray dose (5 μg daily), there was a trend towards increased MI (RR, 1.41; $p = 0.06$) [31]. Collectively, these data suggest that long-acting bronchodilators are safe in patients with COPD and may in select patients reduce the risk of cardiovascular events, possibly by reducing the rate of exacerbations.

Inhaled corticosteroids (ICS) in combination with a LABA are also frequently used to prevent exacerbations in COPD. In one population-based study in Saskatchewan, Canada, the use of ICS was associated with a 32% reduction in the relative risk of MI [32]. However, a systematic review of randomized controlled trials did not demonstrate any significant association between ICS use and the risk of MI or other cardiovascular end points [33]. In the largest clinical trial of its kind ($n = 16,485$), the use of ICS or ICS/LABA was not associated with cardiovascular mortality or any other serious cardiovascular adverse events compared with placebo [34]. In aggregate, these data suggest that neither ICS alone nor ICS in combination with LABA has any salutary effects on cardiovascular events in patients with COPD.

Challenges in Cardiovascular Disease and COPD

Ischemic Heart Disease

COPD patients have an increased risk of ischemic heart disease (odds ratio [OR] 2.28, 95% confidence interval [CI] 1.76–2.96, $p < 0.0001$) compared to the general population [1]. Patients with ischemic heart disease similarly have high rates of COPD; however, it is often undiagnosed [35, 36]. Patients with coexisting airflow limitation and ischemic heart disease, as opposed to ischemic heart disease alone, have both a higher burden of COPD symptoms and cardiovascular risk [37]. Recognizing COPD in ischemic heart disease is important as it has been associated with worse short- and long-term outcomes compared to patients with ischemic heart disease alone [38, 39]. Cardiovascular death accounts for a large proportion of deaths in patients with COPD, with estimates of up to 20–30% [3, 40].

Patients with COPD or ischemic heart disease may present with a variety of symptoms including dyspnea, cough, sputum production, exertional chest pain, or decreased exercise tolerance. Symptoms such as shortness of breath and decreased exercise tolerance could be present in either COPD or ischemic heart disease and require appropriate investigation in order to confirm a diagnosis [1]. In the presence of ischemic heart disease, the diagnostic criteria of COPD are not altered and spirometry is required [5]. In patients with COPD, ischemic heart disease symptoms should be investigated in accordance with established guidelines [41].

Although some therapies for ischemic heart disease and COPD have previously been scrutinized for potential harm in patients with both diseases, standard medications are thought to be safe in comorbid patients [15]. Antiplatelet therapy for ischemic heart disease should be prescribed in accordance with established guidelines in patients with COPD [41]. Beta-blockers should not be withdrawn from patients with COPD, are generally safe, and decrease mortality [42]. Although the proposed common mechanism of systemic inflammation present in both ischemic heart disease and COPD raised the question of whether statin therapy may offer a benefit in COPD alone, statin therapy does not impact acute exacerbation risk, but is indicated in ischemic heart disease [39, 43]. Following invasive therapeutic interventions for ischemic heart disease, COPD patients experience more morbidity [44]. COPD patients undergoing percutaneous coronary intervention have increased rates of revascularization and death [44]. Strategies to reduce perioperative as well as longer-term morbidity following invasive therapies for ischemic heart disease in patients with coexisting COPD will require ongoing research.

Inhaled therapies for COPD including LABA, LAMA, and ICS are safe and effective in patients with coexisting ischemic heart disease [15]. In comparing LABA-LAMA or ICS-LABA combination therapies for COPD, rates of MI, unstable angina, and revascularization did not differ between treatment groups [45]. In another study that included patients with COPD and known ischemic heart disease or risk factors for ischemic heart disease, rates of MI and unstable angina were similar between groups treated with LABA-ICS, LABA, ICS, and placebo [34]. This evidence supports the safety of inhaled COPD therapies in patients with ischemic heart disease.

Heart Failure

Similar to ischemic heart disease, heart failure is more common in patients with COPD than the general population (OR 2.57, 95% CI 1.90–3.47, $p < 0.0001$) [1]. Patients with heart failure and concomitant COPD have higher mortality rates than patients with heart failure alone (HR 1.24–1.7) [46]. Given this increased mortality risk, making the appropriate diagnosis is especially important. Heart failure and COPD share risk factors, frequently occur in the same patient, and share similar presenting symptoms such as dyspnea and functional limitation. This makes distinguishing the presence of these diseases a clinical challenge. The diagnosis of COPD requires spirometry and should be performed with a low threshold in patients with established heart failure [5]. Heart failure with reduced ejection fraction (HFrEF) can result in an up to 20% reduction in both FEV_1 and FVC; however, it does not affect the FEV1/FVC ratio, and spirometry therefore retains its diagnostic utility

[47]. Establishing a diagnosis of heart failure also requires a low threshold for investigation with echocardiogram in COPD patients [48].

Despite accepted guidelines and mortality benefit of beta-blockers in HFrEF, clinicians underprescribe these medications in patients with COPD [49]. A large retrospective study demonstrated no difference in outcomes between heart failure patients with and without COPD taking cardioselective and nonselective beta blockers [50]. Retrospective analysis of patients from the STATCOPE and MACRO studies demonstrated no decrease in lung function overtime or increase in exacerbation rate attributable to beta-blocker use in patients with COPD [51]. The benefits of beta-blockers in heart failure outweigh potential risks, even in the context of severe COPD, and should be prescribed as indicated [15, 52]. Other heart failure medications including angiotensin-converting enzyme inhibitors, mineralocorticoid receptor antagonists, and ivabradine are recommended, as appropriate, in patients with COPD [53, 54].

Although the use of ICS and roflumilast to treat COPD has not been associated with an increased risk of cardiovascular events, the safety of inhaled bronchodilators in patients with COPD and heart failure has been controversial [55, 56]. Observational studies previously identified an increased risk of hospitalization or death with short-acting beta agonists in patients with HFrEF [57, 58]. However, other studies have not identified an independent risk of mortality with long-acting beta agonists in patients with heart failure [59]. Short-acting muscarinic agents have also been associated with an increased risk of heart failure [60]. Longer-acting agents such as tiotropium, glycopyrronium, aclidinium, and umeclidinium have not been associated with an increased risk of heart failure [61–63]. The cardiovascular safety of a combination long-acting bronchodilators, including LABA-LAMA combinations, are similar to the component medications and are generally safe [45, 64]. LABA and tiotropium use in patients with heart failure and COPD has been associated with an increased risk of emergency department visit and hospitalization for heart failure [28]. It may be reasonable, taking the evidence currently available into consideration, to preferentially choose LAMA agents over LABA bronchodilators; however, there is no specific evidence that COPD must be treated differently in the setting of heart failure [65]. It is recommended that patients with heart failure being started on bronchodilators be closely followed up in the two to three weeks following bronchodilator initiation for signs and symptoms of worsening heart failure [15].

Atrial Fibrillation

Atrial fibrillation is the most common arrhythmia in the general population and in patients with COPD [2]. The risk of cardiac dysrhythmia in patients with COPD is almost double that of the general population (OR 1.94, 95% CI 1.55–2.43, $p < 0.0001$) [15]. Prevalence of atrial fibrillation in COPD varies from 4.7% to 15% and up to 30% in severe COPD [66]. The severity of airflow obstruction is related to an increased prevalence of atrial fibrillation [67]. Outcomes of patients with COPD and coexisting atrial fibrillation are worse with increased risk of hospitalization, lower quality of life, and all-cause mortality [66].

Patients with COPD and atrial fibrillation may present with dyspnea due to either disease; however, co-occurring symptoms such as palpitations or cough may help to increase suspicion for atrial fibrillation or COPD, respectively [15]. The diagnosis of COPD in patients with atrial fibrillation can be made using spirometry, similar to the setting of coexisting ischemic heart disease or heart failure [5]. Atrial fibrillation can be diagnosed with an ECG, but may require 24-hour or longer recording devices to diagnose paroxysmal atrial fibrillation. The detection of atrial fibrillation in patients with COPD is important given the risk for worse outcomes in comorbid patients as well as stroke risk reduction and highlights a potential role for screening. However, screening for asymptomatic atrial fibrillation and mechanisms by which this would most effectively be achieved in patients with COPD has not been defined.

The presence of COPD in atrial fibrillation creates a challenge for atrial fibrillation management. COPD is associated with progression from paroxysmal to permanent atrial fibrillation, unsuccessful cardioversion, and recurrence following interventional catheter ablation [68]. General recommendations regarding atrial fibrillation treatment, including rate and rhythm control strategies and anticoagulation to reduce risk of thromboembolic disease, include patients with COPD [69]. Rate control strategies using non-dihydropyridine calcium channel blockers for patients with atrial fibrillation and COPD is recommended in major guidelines [69]. Cardioselective beta-blockers are also recommended for rate control and have been associated with lower mortality [70]. Use of nonselective beta-blockers for atrial fibrillation should be avoided in patients with severe airflow obstruction and COPD, although evidence for this recommendation is limited [71]. Recommendations for anticoagulation and stroke prevention can be applied to patients with COPD and atrial fibrillation in accordance with guidelines [69].

Concerns exist regarding the pro-arrhythmogenic properties of short-acting beta-agonist bronchodilators [72]. LAMA agents have demonstrated mixed results in increasing rates of atrial fibrillation. Tiotropium does not increase cardiac arrhythmias, but glycopyrronium has been associated with increased rates of atrial fibrillation compared to placebo [63, 73]. Despite evidence of these possible increased risks, LABA, LAMA, and ICS preparations can be safely used to treat COPD in patients with atrial fibrillation [31, 74].

Non-Pharmacologic Therapies

Given the shared risk factors and suspected common pathophysiological mechanisms, a holistic approach to non-pharmacologic management and interventions is important. Smoking cessation is key in the non-pharmacologic management of both COPD and ischemic heart disease [75]. Dietary modification can play a role in improving both cardiovascular and lung health [76]. Rehabilitation programs involving supervised exercise training, education, and support are important and help to improve outcomes in COPD [77]. These programs are also important in patients with ischemic heart disease and heart failure [78, 79]. Despite the benefits of rehabilitation programs in both COPD and cardiovascular disease, the existence of comorbidities is associated with a lower referral rate to rehabilitation programs [80, 81]. There is no evidence that the presence of comorbidities negatively affects patient outcomes and complex comorbid patients should still be referred for cardio-pulmonary rehabilitation [81].

Conclusions

Systemic inflammation is common to both COPD and cardiovascular disease. Mechanisms contributing to chronic inflammation and cardiopulmonary disease development as well as the cascade of changes during acute exacerbations of COPD that can lead to decompensation of cardiovascular disease and increased morbidity and mortality are increasingly understood. Elucidating the complex mechanisms through which COPD and cardiovascular disease influence and modify each other will be important in developing therapies and strategies to reduce the burden of morbidity and mortality in these patients.

Cardiologists, respirologists/pulmonologists, internists, and primary care physicians must be attuned to the presence of coexisting cardiac and respiratory disease. Patients with cardiovascular disease and COPD should be investigated for COPD and cardiovascular disease, respectively. A low threshold for investigation is important in order to thoroughly assess presenting symptoms which these comorbidities share in common and reach the correct diagnosis. Therapeutic challenges in treating patients with COPD and cardiovascular disease including ischemic heart disease, heart failure, and atrial fibrillation have been hindered by concerns regarding the safety of disease-specific therapies in patients with complex comorbidities. However, patients with COPD and cardiovascular disease can safely be treated in accordance with major disease-specific guidelines. Given the complexity of diagnosis and management of patients with cardiovascular disease and COPD, models of care that can address the complex multimorbid patient must be developed.

References

1. Chen W, Thomas J, Sadatsafavi M, FitzGerald JM. Risk of cardiovascular comorbidity in patients with chronic obstructive pulmonary disease: a systematic review and meta-analysis. Lancet Respir Med. 2015;3:631–9.
2. Mullerova H, Agusti A, Erqou S, Mapel DW. Cardiovascular comorbidity in COPD: systematic literature review. Chest. 2013;144:1163–78.
3. Sin DD, Anthonisen NR, Soriano JB, Agusti AG. Mortality in COPD: role of comorbidities. Eur Respir J. 2006;28:1245–57.

4. Donaldson GC, Hurst JR, Smith CJ, Hubbard RB, Wedzicha JA. Increased risk of myocardial infarction and stroke following exacerbation of COPD. Chest. 2010;137:1091–7.
5. Vogelmeier CF, Criner GJ, Martinez FJ, Anzueto A, Barnes PJ, Bourbeau J, Celli BR, Chen R, Decramer M, Fabbri LM, Frith P, Halpin DM, Lopez Varela MV, Nishimura M, Roche N, Rodriguez-Roisin R, Sin DD, Singh D, Stockley R, Vestbo J, Wedzicha JA, Agusti A. Global strategy for the diagnosis, management, and prevention of chronic obstructive lung disease 2017 report. GOLD executive summary. Am J Respir Crit Care Med. 2017;195:557–82.
6. Leuppi JD, Schuetz P, Bingisser R, Bodmer M, Briel M, Drescher T, Duerring U, Henzen C, Leibbrandt Y, Maier S, Miedinger D, Muller B, Scherr A, Schindler C, Stoeckli R, Viatte S, von Garnier C, Tamm M, Rutishauser J. Short-term vs conventional glucocorticoid therapy in acute exacerbations of chronic obstructive pulmonary disease: the REDUCE randomized clinical trial. JAMA. 2013;309:2223–31.
7. Bafadhel M, McKenna S, Terry S, Mistry V, Reid C, Haldar P, McCormick M, Haldar K, Kebadze T, Duvoix A, Lindblad K, Patel H, Rugman P, Dodson P, Jenkins M, Saunders M, Newbold P, Green RH, Venge P, Lomas DA, Barer MR, Johnston SL, Pavord ID, Brightling CE. Acute exacerbations of chronic obstructive pulmonary disease: identification of biologic clusters and their biomarkers. Am J Respir Crit Care Med. 2011;184:662–71.
8. MacDonald MI, Shafuddin E, King PT, Chang CL, Bardin PG, Hancox RJ. Cardiac dysfunction during exacerbations of chronic obstructive pulmonary disease. Lancet Respir Med. 2016;4:138–48.
9. Smeeth L, Thomas SL, Hall AJ, Hubbard R, Farrington P, Vallance P. Risk of myocardial infarction and stroke after acute infection or vaccination. N Engl J Med. 2004;351:2611–8.
10. Patel AR, Kowlessar BS, Donaldson GC, Mackay AJ, Singh R, George SN, Garcha DS, Wedzicha JA, Hurst JR. Cardiovascular risk, myocardial injury, and exacerbations of chronic obstructive pulmonary disease. Am J Respir Crit Care Med. 2013;188:1091–9.
11. Chang CL, Robinson SC, Mills GD, Sullivan GD, Karalus NC, McLachlan JD, Hancox RJ. Biochemical markers of cardiac dysfunction predict mortality in acute exacerbations of COPD. Thorax. 2011;66:764–8.
12. Rothnie KJ, Smeeth L, Herrett E, Pearce N, Hemingway H, Wedzicha J, Timmis A, Quint JK. Closing the mortality gap after a myocardial infarction in people with and without chronic obstructive pulmonary disease. Heart. 2015;101:1103–10.
13. Pavasini R, d'Ascenzo F, Campo G, Biscaglia S, Ferri A, Contoli M, Papi A, Ceconi C, Ferrari R. Cardiac troponin elevation predicts all-cause mortality in patients with acute exacerbation of chronic obstructive pulmonary disease: systematic review and meta-analysis. Int J Cardiol. 2015;191:187–93.
14. Terzano C, Romani S, Conti V, Paone G, Oriolo F, Vitarelli A. Atrial fibrillation in the acute, hypercapnic exacerbations of COPD. Eur Rev Med Pharmacol Sci. 2014;18:2908–17.
15. Roversi S, Fabbri LM, Sin DD, Hawkins NM, Agusti A. Chronic obstructive pulmonary disease and cardiac diseases. An urgent need for integrated care. Am J Respir Crit Care Med. 2016;194:1319–36.
16. Kwong JC, Schwartz KL, Campitelli MA, Chung H, Crowcroft NS, Karnauchow T, Katz K, Ko DT, McGeer AJ, McNally D, Richardson DC, Rosella LC, Simor A, Smieja M, Zahariadis G, Gubbay JB. Acute myocardial infarction after laboratory-confirmed influenza infection. N Engl J Med. 2018;378:345–53.
17. Warren-Gash C, Hayward AC, Hemingway H, Denaxas S, Thomas SL, Timmis AD, Whitaker H, Smeeth L. Influenza infection and risk of acute myocardial infarction in England and Wales: a CALIBER self-controlled case series study. J Infect Dis. 2012;206:1652–9.
18. Phrommintikul A, Kuanprasert S, Wongcharoen W, Kanjanavanit R, Chaiwarith R, Sukonthasarn A. Influenza vaccination reduces cardiovascular events in patients with acute coronary syndrome. Eur Heart J. 2011;32:1730–5.
19. Minassian C, Thomas SL, Smeeth L, Douglas I, Brauer R, Langan SM. Acute cardiovascular events after herpes zoster: a self-controlled case series analysis in vaccinated and unvaccinated older residents of the United States. PLoS Med. 2015;12:e1001919.

20. Hole DJ, Watt GC, Davey-Smith G, Hart CL, Gillis CR, Hawthorne VM. Impaired lung function and mortality risk in men and women: findings from the Renfrew and Paisley prospective population study. BMJ. 1996;313:711–5; discussion 715–6.
21. Pai JK, Pischon T, Ma J, Manson JE, Hankinson SE, Joshipura K, Curhan GC, Rifai N, Cannuscio CC, Stampfer MJ, Rimm EB. Inflammatory markers and the risk of coronary heart disease in men and women. N Engl J Med. 2004;351:2599–610.
22. Gan WQ, Man SF, Senthilselvan A, Sin DD. Association between chronic obstructive pulmonary disease and systemic inflammation: a systematic review and a meta-analysis. Thorax. 2004;59:574–80.
23. Lee SH, Goswami S, Grudo A, Song LZ, Bandi V, Goodnight-White S, Green L, Hacken-Bitar J, Huh J, Bakaeen F, Coxson HO, Cogswell S, Storness-Bliss C, Corry DB, Kheradmand F. Antielastin autoimmunity in tobacco smoking-induced emphysema. Nat Med. 2007;13:567–9.
24. Sze MA, Dimitriu PA, Hayashi S, Elliott WM, McDonough JE, Gosselink JV, Cooper J, Sin DD, Mohn WW, Hogg JC. The lung tissue microbiome in chronic obstructive pulmonary disease. Am J Respir Crit Care Med. 2012;185:1073–80.
25. Van Eeden S, Leipsic J, Paul Man SF, Sin DD. The relationship between lung inflammation and cardiovascular disease. Am J Respir Crit Care Med. 2012;186:11–6.
26. Jaw JE, Tsuruta M, Oh Y, Schipilow J, Hirano Y, Ngan DA, Suda K, Li Y, Oh JY, Moritani K, Tam S, Ford N, van Eeden S, Wright JL, Man SF, Sin DD. Lung exposure to lipopolysaccharide causes atherosclerotic plaque destabilisation. Eur Respir J. 2016;48:205–15.
27. Tashkin DP, Celli B, Senn S, Burkhart D, Kesten S, Menjoge S, Decramer M, UPLIFT Study Investigators. A 4-year trial of tiotropium in chronic obstructive pulmonary disease. N Engl J Med. 2008;359:1543–54.
28. Gershon A, Croxford R, Calzavara A, To T, Stanbrook MB, Upshur R, Stukel TA. Cardiovascular safety of inhaled long-acting bronchodilators in individuals with chronic obstructive pulmonary disease. JAMA Intern Med. 2013;173:1175–85.
29. Jara M, Wentworth C 3rd, Lanes S. A new user cohort study comparing the safety of long-acting inhaled bronchodilators in COPD. BMJ Open. 2012;2:e000841.
30. Verhamme KM, Afonso A, Romio S, Stricker BC, Brusselle GG, Sturkenboom MC. Use of tiotropium Respimat Soft Mist Inhaler versus HandiHaler and mortality in patients with COPD. Eur Respir J. 2013;42:606–15.
31. Wise RA, Anzueto A, Cotton D, Dahl R, Devins T, Disse B, Dusser D, Joseph E, Kattenbeck S, Koenen-Bergmann M, Pledger G, Calverley P, TIOSPIR Investigators. Tiotropium Respimat inhaler and the risk of death in COPD. N Engl J Med. 2013;369:1491–501.
32. Huiart L, Ernst P, Ranouil X, Suissa S. Low-dose inhaled corticosteroids and the risk of acute myocardial infarction in COPD. Eur Respir J. 2005;25:634–9.
33. Loke YK, Kwok CS, Singh S. Risk of myocardial infarction and cardiovascular death associated with inhaled corticosteroids in COPD. Eur Respir J. 2010;35:1003–21.
34. Vestbo J, Anderson JA, Brook RD, Calverley PM, Celli BR, Crim C, Martinez F, Yates J, Newby DE, SUMMIT Investigators. Fluticasone furoate and vilanterol and survival in chronic obstructive pulmonary disease with heightened cardiovascular risk (SUMMIT): a double-blind randomised controlled trial. Lancet. 2016;387:1817–26.
35. Arnett DK, Goodman RA, Halperin JL, Anderson JL, Parekh AK, Zoghbi WA. AHA/ACC/HHS strategies to enhance application of clinical practice guidelines in patients with cardiovascular disease and comorbid conditions: from the American Heart Association, American College of Cardiology, and U.S. Department of Health and Human Services. J Am Coll Cardiol. 2014;64:1851–6.
36. Soriano JB, Rigo F, Guerrero D, Yanez A, Forteza JF, Frontera G, Togores B, Agusti A. High prevalence of undiagnosed airflow limitation in patients with cardiovascular disease. Chest. 2010;137:333–40.
37. Franssen FM, Soriano JB, Roche N, Bloomfield PH, Brusselle G, Fabbri LM, Garcia-Rio F, Kearney MT, Kwon N, Lundback B, Rabe KF, Raillard A, Muellerova H, Cockcroft JR. Lung function abnormalities in smokers with ischemic heart disease. Am J Respir Crit Care Med. 2016;194:568–76.

38. Behar S, Panosh A, Reicher-Reiss H, Zion M, Schlesinger Z, Goldbourt U. Prevalence and prognosis of chronic obstructive pulmonary disease among 5,839 consecutive patients with acute myocardial infarction. SPRINT Study Group. Am J Med. 1992;93:637–41.
39. van Gestel YR, Hoeks SE, Sin DD, Simsek C, Welten GM, Schouten O, Stam H, Mertens FW, van Domburg RT, Poldermans D. Effect of statin therapy on mortality in patients with peripheral arterial disease and comparison of those with versus without associated chronic obstructive pulmonary disease. Am J Cardiol. 2008;102:192–6.
40. McGarvey LP, John M, Anderson JA, Zvarich M, Wise RA, TORCH Clinical Endpoint Committee. Ascertainment of cause-specific mortality in COPD: operations of the TORCH Clinical Endpoint Committee. Thorax. 2007;62:411–5.
41. Fihn SD, Gardin JM, Abrams J, Berra K, Blankenship JC, Dallas AP, Douglas PS, Foody JM, Gerber TC, Hinderliter AL, King SB 3rd, Kligfield PD, Krumholz HM, Kwong RY, Lim MJ, Linderbaum JA, Mack MJ, Munger MA, Prager RL, Sabik JF, Shaw LJ, Sikkema JD, Smith CR Jr, Smith SC Jr, Spertus JA, Williams SV, Anderson JL, American College of Cardiology Foundation/American Heart Association Task F. 2012 ACCF/AHA/ACP/AATS/PCNA/SCAI/STS guideline for the diagnosis and management of patients with stable ischemic heart disease: a report of the American College of Cardiology Foundation/American Heart Association task force on practice guidelines, and the American College of Physicians, American Association for Thoracic Surgery, Preventive Cardiovascular Nurses Association, Society for Cardiovascular Angiography and Interventions, and Society of Thoracic Surgeons. Circulation. 2012;126:e354–471.
42. Salpeter SR, Ormiston TM, Salpeter EE, Poole PJ, Cates CJ. Cardioselective beta-blockers for chronic obstructive pulmonary disease: a meta-analysis. Respir Med. 2003;97:1094–101.
43. Criner GJ, Connett JE, Aaron SD, Albert RK, Bailey WC, Casaburi R, Cooper JA Jr, Curtis JL, Dransfield MT, Han MK, Make B, Marchetti N, Martinez FJ, Niewoehner DE, Scanlon PD, Sciurba FC, Scharf SM, Sin DD, Voelker H, Washko GR, Woodruff PG, Lazarus SC, COPD Clinical Research Network, Canadian Institutes of Health Research. Simvastatin for the prevention of exacerbations in moderate-to-severe COPD. N Engl J Med. 2014;370:2201–10.
44. Enriquez JR, Parikh SV, Selzer F, Jacobs AK, Marroquin O, Mulukutla S, Srinivas V, Holper EM. Increased adverse events after percutaneous coronary intervention in patients with COPD: insights from the National Heart, Lung, and Blood Institute dynamic registry. Chest. 2011;140:604–10.
45. Wedzicha JA, Banerji D, Chapman KR, Vestbo J, Roche N, Ayers RT, Thach C, Fogel R, Patalano F, Vogelmeier CF, FLAME Investigators. Indacaterol-glycopyrronium versus salmeterol-fluticasone for COPD. N Engl J Med. 2016;374:2222–34.
46. Rushton CA, Satchithananda DK, Jones PW, Kadam UT. Non-cardiovascular comorbidity, severity and prognosis in non-selected heart failure populations: a systematic review and meta-analysis. Int J Cardiol. 2015;196:98–106.
47. Guder G, Brenner S, Stork S, Hoes A, Rutten FH. Chronic obstructive pulmonary disease in heart failure: accurate diagnosis and treatment. Eur J Heart Fail. 2014;16:1273–82.
48. Yancy CW, Jessup M, Bozkurt B, Butler J, Casey DE Jr, Colvin MM, Drazner MH, Filippatos GS, Fonarow GC, Givertz MM, Hollenberg SM, Lindenfeld J, Masoudi FA, McBride PE, Peterson PN, Stevenson LW, Westlake C. 2017 ACC/AHA/HFSA focused update of the 2013 ACCF/AHA guideline for the management of heart failure: a report of the American College of Cardiology/American Heart Association Task Force on Clinical Practice Guidelines and the Heart Failure Society of America. J Am Coll Cardiol. 2017;70:776–803.
49. Fisher KA, Stefan MS, Darling C, Lessard D, Goldberg RJ. Impact of COPD on the mortality and treatment of patients hospitalized with acute decompensated heart failure: the Worcester Heart Failure Study. Chest. 2015;147:637–45.
50. Mentz RJ, Wojdyla D, Fiuzat M, Chiswell K, Fonarow GC, O'Connor CM. Association of beta-blocker use and selectivity with outcomes in patients with heart failure and chronic obstructive pulmonary disease (from OPTIMIZE-HF). Am J Cardiol. 2013;111:582–7.
51. Duffy S, Marron R, Voelker H, Albert R, Connett J, Bailey W, Casaburi R, Cooper JA Jr, Curtis JL, Dransfield M, Han MK, Make B, Marchetti N, Martinez F, Lazarus S, Niewoehner D, Scanlon PD, Sciurba F, Scharf S, Reed RM, Washko G, Woodruff P, McEvoy C, Aaron S, Sin

D, Criner GJ, NIH COPD Clinical Research Network and the Canadian Institutes of Health Research. Effect of beta-blockers on exacerbation rate and lung function in chronic obstructive pulmonary disease (COPD). Respir Res. 2017;18:124.
52. Creagh-Brown B. Benefits of beta blockers in chronic obstructive pulmonary disease and heart failure. BMJ. 2014;348:g3316.
53. Ekstrom MP, Hermansson AB, Strom KE. Effects of cardiovascular drugs on mortality in severe chronic obstructive pulmonary disease. Am J Respir Crit Care Med. 2013;187:715–20.
54. Bohm M, Robertson M, Ford I, Borer JS, Komajda M, Kindermann I, Maack C, Lainscak M, Swedberg K, Tavazzi L. Influence of cardiovascular and noncardiovascular co-morbidities on outcomes and treatment effect of heart rate reduction with ivabradine in stable heart failure (from the SHIFT trial). Am J Cardiol. 2015;116:1890–7.
55. White WB, Cooke GE, Kowey PR, Calverley PMA, Bredenbroker D, Goehring UM, Zhu H, Lakkis H, Mosberg H, Rowe P, Rabe KF. Cardiovascular safety in patients receiving roflumilast for the treatment of COPD. Chest. 2013;144:758–65.
56. Macie C, Wooldrage K, Manfreda J, Anthonisen N. Cardiovascular morbidity and the use of inhaled bronchodilators. Int J Chron Obstruct Pulmon Dis. 2008;3:163–9.
57. Au DH, Udris EM, Fan VS, Curtis JR, McDonell MB, Fihn SD. Risk of mortality and heart failure exacerbations associated with inhaled beta-adrenoceptor agonists among patients with known left ventricular systolic dysfunction. Chest. 2003;123:1964–9.
58. Au DH, Bryson CL, Fan VS, Udris EM, Curtis JR, McDonell MB, Fihn SD. Beta-blockers as single-agent therapy for hypertension and the risk of mortality among patients with chronic obstructive pulmonary disease. Am J Med. 2004;117:925–31.
59. Bermingham M, O'Callaghan E, Dawkins I, Miwa S, Samsudin S, McDonald K, Ledwidge M. Are beta2-agonists responsible for increased mortality in heart failure? Eur J Heart Fail. 2011;13:885–91.
60. Ogale SS, Lee TA, Au DH, Boudreau DM, Sullivan SD. Cardiovascular events associated with ipratropium bromide in COPD. Chest. 2010;137:13–9.
61. Tashkin DP, Leimer I, Metzdorf N, Decramer M. Cardiac safety of tiotropium in patients with cardiac events: a retrospective analysis of the UPLIFT(R) trial. Respir Res. 2015;16:65.
62. Verhamme KM, Afonso AS, van Noord C, Haag MD, Koudstaal PJ, Brusselle GG, Sturkenboom MC. Tiotropium Handihaler and the risk of cardio- or cerebrovascular events and mortality in patients with COPD. Pulm Pharmacol Ther. 2012;25:19–26.
63. D'Urzo AD, Kerwin EM, Chapman KR, Decramer M, DiGiovanni R, D'Andrea P, Hu H, Goyal P, Altman P. Safety of inhaled glycopyrronium in patients with COPD: a comprehensive analysis of clinical studies and post-marketing data. Int J Chron Obstruct Pulmon Dis. 2015;10:1599–612.
64. Calzetta L, Rogliani P, Matera MG, Cazzola M. A systematic review with meta-analysis of dual bronchodilation with LAMA/LABA for the treatment of stable COPD. Chest. 2016;149:1181–96.
65. Jara M, Lanes SF, Wentworth C 3rd, May C, Kesten S. Comparative safety of long-acting inhaled bronchodilators: a cohort study using the UK THIN primary care database. Drug Saf. 2007;30:1151–60.
66. Divo M, Cote C, de Torres JP, Casanova C, Marin JM, Pinto-Plata V, Zulueta J, Cabrera C, Zagaceta J, Hunninghake G, Celli B, BODE Collaborative Group. Comorbidities and risk of mortality in patients with chronic obstructive pulmonary disease. Am J Respir Crit Care Med. 2012;186:155–61.
67. Buch P, Friberg J, Scharling H, Lange P, Prescott E. Reduced lung function and risk of atrial fibrillation in the Copenhagen City Heart Study. Eur Respir J. 2003;21:1012–6.
68. de Vos CB, Pisters R, Nieuwlaat R, Prins MH, Tieleman RG, Coelen RJ, van den Heijkant AC, Allessie MA, Crijns HJ. Progression from paroxysmal to persistent atrial fibrillation clinical correlates and prognosis. J Am Coll Cardiol. 2010;55:725–31.
69. January CT, Wann LS, Alpert JS, Calkins H, Cigarroa JE, Cleveland JC Jr, Conti JB, Ellinor PT, Ezekowitz MD, Field ME, Murray KT, Sacco RL, Stevenson WG, Tchou PJ, Tracy CM,

Yancy CW, American College of Cardiology/American Heart Association Task Force on Practice G. 2014 AHA/ACC/HRS guideline for the management of patients with atrial fibrillation: a report of the American College of Cardiology/American Heart Association Task Force on Practice Guidelines and the Heart Rhythm Society. J Am Coll Cardiol. 2014;64:e1–76.

70. Bhatt SP, Wells JM, Kinney GL, Washko GR Jr, Budoff M, Kim YI, Bailey WC, Nath H, Hokanson JE, Silverman EK, Crapo J. Dransfield MT and investigators CO. beta-Blockers are associated with a reduction in COPD exacerbations. Thorax. 2016;71:8–14.

71. Mainguy V, Girard D, Maltais F, Saey D, Milot J, Senechal M, Poirier P, Provencher S. Effect of bisoprolol on respiratory function and exercise capacity in chronic obstructive pulmonary disease. Am J Cardiol. 2012;110:258–63.

72. Wilchesky M, Ernst P, Brophy JM, Platt RW, Suissa S. Bronchodilator use and the risk of arrhythmia in COPD: part 2: reassessment in the larger Quebec cohort. Chest. 2012;142:305–11.

73. Hohlfeld JM, Furtwaengler A, Konen-Bergmann M, Wallenstein G, Walter B, Bateman ED. Cardiac safety of tiotropium in patients with COPD: a combined analysis of Holter-ECG data from four randomised clinical trials. Int J Clin Pract. 2015;69:72–80.

74. Calverley PM, Anderson JA, Celli B, Ferguson GT, Jenkins C, Jones PW, Crim C, Willits LR, Yates JC, Vestbo J, TORCH Investigators. Cardiovascular events in patients with COPD: TORCH study results. Thorax. 2010;65:719–25.

75. Piepoli MF, Hoes AW, Agewall S, Albus C, Brotons C, Catapano AL, Cooney MT, Corra U, Cosyns B, Deaton C, Graham I, Hall MS, Hobbs FD, Lochen ML, Lollgen H, Marques-Vidal P, Perk J, Prescott E, Redon J, Richter DJ, Sattar N, Smulders Y, Tiberi M, van der Worp HB, van Dis I, Verschuren WM, Binno S, ESC Scientific Document Group. 2016 European Guidelines on cardiovascular disease prevention in clinical practice: The Sixth Joint Task Force of the European Society of Cardiology and Other Societies on Cardiovascular Disease Prevention in Clinical Practice (constituted by representatives of 10 societies and by invited experts) Developed with the special contribution of the European Association for Cardiovascular Prevention & Rehabilitation (EACPR). Eur Heart J. 2016;37:2315–81.

76. Jacobs DR Jr, Kalhan R. Healthy diets and lung health. Connecting the dots. Ann Am Thorac Soc. 2016;13:588–90.

77. Casaburi R, ZuWallack R. Pulmonary rehabilitation for management of chronic obstructive pulmonary disease. N Engl J Med. 2009;360:1329–35.

78. Kwan G, Balady GJ. Cardiac rehabilitation 2012: advancing the field through emerging science. Circulation. 2012;125:e369–73.

79. Ades PA, Keteyian SJ, Balady GJ, Houston-Miller N, Kitzman DW, Mancini DM, Rich MW. Cardiac rehabilitation exercise and self-care for chronic heart failure. JACC Heart Fail. 2013;1:540–7.

80. Evans RA, Singh SJ, Collier R, Loke I, Steiner MC, Morgan MD. Generic, symptom based, exercise rehabilitation; integrating patients with COPD and heart failure. Respir Med. 2010;104:1473–81.

81. Salzwedel A, Nosper M, Rohrig B, Linck-Eleftheriadis S, Strandt G, Voller H. Outcome quality of in-patient cardiac rehabilitation in elderly patients–identification of relevant parameters. Eur J Prev Cardiol. 2014;21:172–80.

82. Alotaibi NM, Chen V, Hollander Z, Hague CJ, Murphy DT, Leipsic JA, DeMarco ML, FitzGerald JM, McManus BM, Ng RT, Sin DD. Phenotyping COPD exacerbations using imaging and blood-based biomarkers. Int J Chron Obstruct Pulmon Dis. 2018;13:217–29.

83. Kullo IJ, Edwards WD, Schwartz RS. Vulnerable plaque: pathobiology and clinical implications. Ann Intern Med. 1998;129:1050–60.

Chapter 13
Lung Transplantation for Chronic Lung Disease: Cardiac Considerations

Keith M. Wille, Tyler R. Reynolds, and Victoria Rusanov

Clinical Pearls
1. Major adverse cardiovascular and cerebrovascular events (MACCE) are more common in transplant recipients than in non-transplant, noncardiac surgery patients, and lung transplant recipients have a higher MACCE risk.
2. Disorders such as significant coronary artery disease, arrhythmias, pulmonary arterial hypertension, and valvular heart disease should be identified and managed to improve the likelihood of a successful perioperative course.
3. Careful candidate selection, including a thorough assessment of cardiac function, is essential for optimizing the likelihood of survival while awaiting transplantation and minimizing the risk of cardiovascular and cerebrovascular events posttransplant.

Introduction

Lung transplantation (LT) has emerged as a viable treatment option for patients with end-stage lung disease. The development and refinement of the surgical technique, patient selection, and immunosuppression practices have resulted in both improved quality of life and overall 1-year survival rates $\geq 85\%$ for patients who otherwise would have limited treatment alternatives [1]. However, longer-term survival following LT is limited largely by chronic lung allograft dysfunction (CLAD), with

K. M. Wille (✉) · V. Rusanov
Department of Medicine, University of Alabama at Birmingham, Birmingham, AL, USA
e-mail: kwille@uabmc.edu; vrusanov@uabmc.edu

T. R. Reynolds
Louisiana State University, Baton Rouge, LA, USA

© Springer Nature Switzerland AG 2020
S. P. Bhatt (ed.), *Cardiac Considerations in Chronic Lung Disease*,
Respiratory Medicine, https://doi.org/10.1007/978-3-030-43435-9_13

5-year survival rates remaining at approximately 50% [2]. Improvements in organ availability and donor and patient management have led to a greater demand for LT. As success with LT has improved with time, criteria for the selection of appropriate LT candidates have also changed (Tables 13.1 and 13.2) [3–5]. Absolute contraindications such as severe cardiovascular disease (CVD) were established at the start of LT with the development and dissemination of consensus guidelines; however, with greater experience and advances in the treatment of CVD, centers have been more willing to consider higher-risk candidates, provided that any underlying diseases could be effectively managed and both peri- and postoperative risk remain acceptable. Since implementation of the Lung Allocation Score (LAS) in 2005, time

Table 13.1 Adult lung transplants performed by diagnostic indication (Jan 2005–Jun 2018)

Diagnosis	N (%)
IIP	13,914 (29.24)
COPD	13,201 (27.74)
CF	6996 (14.70)
ILD not IIP	3144 (6.61)
Other	3015 (6.34)
Retransplant	2045 (4.30)
A1AT	1615 (3.39)
IPAH	1268 (2.66)
Non-CF bronchiectasis	1220 (2.56)
Sarcoidosis	1173 (2.46)
Total	47,591 (100)

Adapted from 2019 International Society for Heart and Lung Transplantation Registry Data (available at http://www.ishlt.org)
A1AT alpha-1-antitrypsin, *CF* cystic fibrosis, *COPD* chronic obstructive pulmonary disease, *IIP* idiopathic interstitial pneumonia, *ILD* interstitial lung disease, *IPAH* idiopathic pulmonary arterial hypertension. Transplants performed with unknown diagnoses are excluded from this tabulation

Table 13.2 Adult heart-lung transplants performed by diagnostic indication (Jan 2005–Jun 2018)

Diagnosis	N (%)
PH not IPAH	267 (36.83)
IPAH	238 (32.83)
Other	90 (12.41)
CF	53 (7.31)
IIP	45 (6.21)
COPD	17 (2.34)
Non-CF bronchiectasis	10 (1.38)
A1AT	4 (0.55)
Retransplant	1 (0.14)
Total	725 (100)

Adapted from 2019 International Society for Heart and Lung Transplantation Registry Data (available at http://www.ishlt.org)
A1AT Alpha-1-antitrypsin, *CF* cystic fibrosis, *COPD* chronic obstructive pulmonary disease, *IIP* idiopathic interstitial pneumonia, *ILD* interstitial lung disease, *IPAH* idiopathic pulmonary arterial hypertension, *PH* pulmonary hypertension

to transplantation has decreased, wait-list mortality has decreased, and transplant volume has increased without significantly changing outcomes. The LAS was more recently modified to address disparities in wait-list urgency for patients with pulmonary arterial hypertension (PAH) [6–8]. However, access to the LT waiting list (i.e., the time from a transplant-eligible diagnosis to wait-list registration) has remained variable and can differ by underlying diagnosis [9]. Costs associated with transplantation vary considerably by diagnosis, and complications such as those requiring prolonged ventilatory support or additional interventions may drive costs associated with LT significantly higher [10].

The most recent consensus from the International Society of Heart and Lung Transplantation (ISHLT) for the selection of LT candidates, published in 2015, recognizes untreatable significant dysfunction of another major organ system (e.g., heart, liver, kidney, or brain) as an absolute contraindication to LT, unless combined organ transplantation can be performed (e.g., heart-lung, lung-liver, or lung-kidney) (Table 13.3) [5]. LT should be considered for patients with chronic, end-stage lung disease with the following characteristics: (a) high (>50%) risk of

Table 13.3 Contraindications to lung transplantation

Absolute
Recent history of malignancy
Untreatable significant dysfunction of another major organ system (unless combined organ transplantation is considered)
Uncorrected atherosclerotic and/or coronary artery disease not amenable to revascularization
Acute medical instability
Uncorrectable bleeding diathesis
Chronic infection with highly virulent and/or resistant microbes that are poorly controlled before transplant (including active *Mycobacterium tuberculosis* infection)
Significant chest wall or spinal deformity
Significant (class II or III) obesity (BMI ≥ 35 kg/m²)
Limited functional status with poor rehabilitation potential
Nonadherence to medical therapy
Absence of adequate social support
Substance abuse or dependence
Relative
Age > 65 years associated with low physiologic reserve and/or other relative contraindications
Class I obesity (BMI 30–34.9 kg/m²)
Severe malnutrition
Severe osteoporosis
Extensive prior chest surgery with lung resection
Mechanical ventilation and/or extracorporeal life support
Atherosclerotic disease burden that may result in end-organ damage post-transplant
Colonization or infection with highly resistant or highly virulent organisms
HIV, Hepatitis B or C (transplant may be considered at select centers where infection is well-controlled and end-organ disease is absent)
Uncontrolled medical conditions (such as diabetes, systemic hypertension, and gastroesophageal reflux disease)

Adapted from Weill D et al. [5]
BMI body mass index

death from lung disease within 2 years if LT is not performed, (b) high (>80%) likelihood of surviving at least 90 days after LT, (c) high (>80%) likelihood of 5-year posttransplant survival, and (d) no other available treatment options [5, 11]. Lung retransplantation has also been performed in select instances, typically for recipients who develop CLAD, with variable outcomes [2, 12–18].

A recent study examined the rates of perioperative major adverse cardiovascular and cerebrovascular events (MACCE) after noncardiac transplant surgery [19]. Using the Healthcare Cost and Utilization Project's National Inpatient Sample, Smilowitz et al. identified 49,978 hospitalizations for transplant surgery. The most common surgeries performed were renal (67.3%), liver (21.6%), and lung (6.7%), and in total, perioperative MACCE occurred in 1539 (3.1%) transplant surgeries. Transplant recipients were more likely to have perioperative MACCE as compared to patients undergoing non-transplant, noncardiac surgery (3.1% vs. 2.0%, adjusted odds ratio [OR] 1.29, 95% confidence interval [CI] 1.22–1.36; $p < 0.001$). Moreover, among hospitalizations for renal, liver, and lung transplantation, MACCE occurred in 1.7%, 5.6%, and 7.5% of recipients, respectively. As cardiovascular complications are common in LT recipients, this review will focus on cardiac considerations in the LT candidate and implications for the pre- and postoperative period.

Coronary Artery Disease

The severity of underlying coronary artery disease (CAD) may affect candidate selection for LT. Obstructive CAD (typically defined as a luminal diameter stenosis ≥70%) [20] that is not correctable by percutaneous or surgical intervention has been considered a relative contraindication to LT at most centers. At present, there are no consensus guidelines regarding the optimal preoperative CAD evaluation for LT candidates; society-endorsed practice guidelines were previously published for liver and kidney transplant candidates [21]. While methods used for CAD detection in LT candidates may vary among centers, coronary angiography remains a commonly utilized study. The prevalence of CAD in patients with end-stage lung disease referred for transplantation has ranged from 6% to 23%; however, when only the studies that defined obstructive CAD were included, the prevalence was 11% [22–27]. The rate of CAD in this population is thought to vary significantly in the literature for several reasons, including differences in the frequency of CAD risk factors among candidate diagnostic groups (CF, COPD, ILD, etc.), differences in how studies define the presence of CAD, and potentially differences in referral practices as well as racial and gender biases. Angiographic CAD has typically been defined as a luminal stenosis ≥50%; however, lesions ≥70% are more often flow-limiting and thus potentially amenable to intervention [20]. However, for LT candidates, it is unclear whether detection of CAD on preoperative angiography is predictive of postoperative complications. Further, in a large prospective trial, preoperative coronary revascularization was not associated with improved postoperative or long-term outcomes when compared with medical therapy in high-risk patients undergoing major vascular surgery [28]. As there are no prospective trials for LT candidates, whether this patient population derives any benefit from preoperative coronary angiography and subsequent revascularization remains unknown.

Patients with advanced lung disease may develop CAD as a result of recognized cardiac risk factors (including advancing age, diabetes, hyperlipidemia, hypertension, and tobacco use) and/or chronic inflammatory changes affecting the heart and lungs. For example, studies have demonstrated that COPD patients have a greater risk of cardiovascular morbidity and mortality as compared to the general population. In a study of more than 5000 patients from the Saskatchewan Health database, Huiart et al. found that cardiovascular morbidity and mortality rates were higher in the COPD cohort than in the general population (standardized rate ratios of 1.9 and 2.0, respectively) [29]. Also, CVD and specifically ischemic heart disease were more commonly reported as a cause of death, rather than COPD (19.6 vs. 15.5 per 1000 person-years). However, longer-term mortality due to cardiac disease may not significantly differ between CAD and non-CAD-designated recipients, once selected candidates undergo transplantation [30].

Using the Kaiser Permanente Medical Care Program, Sidney et al. studied the relationship between COPD and hospitalization and mortality events due to CVD end points. In their study, CVD study end points included cardiac arrhythmias, angina pectoris, acute myocardial infarction, congestive heart failure (CHF), stroke, pulmonary embolism, and a composite of the previously mentioned end points [31]. Mean follow-up time was 2.75 years for case patients and 2.99 years for control patients. The relative risk (RR) for hospitalization for the composite of all study end points was 2.09 (95% CI, 1.99–2.20), after adjustment for confounding variables that included gender, preexisting CVD end points, hypertension, hyperlipidemia, and diabetes. Moreover, the adjusted RR for mortality for the composite measure of all study end points was 1.68 (95% CI, 1.50–1.88).

Patients with fibrotic lung disease, which since 2007 has been the most common indication for lung transplantation, may also be at increased risk for CAD. Kizer et al. found that the fibrotic lung diseases were associated with an increased prevalence of CAD as compared to the nonfibrotic diseases, after adjustment for traditional CV risk factors (OR 2.18; 95% CI, 1.17–4.06) [32]. However, this association appeared to be driven largely by non-granulomatous fibrotic disease (particularly IPF). Notably, the association between the fibrotic disorders and CAD strengthened when multivessel disease was examined (OR 4.16; 95% CI, 1.46–11.9). In a series of 243 LT candidates, Snell et al. analyzed 85 patients who underwent coronary angiography and found that 32 had CAD [33]. The degree of obstruction was significant (>50% stenosis) in 16 patients and 8 patients required intervention. The incidence of CAD in patients >50 years old who were being considered for LT was 17%. Ben-Dor et al. reported a 17.8% incidence of significant CAD (defined as >70% stenosis) and a 17.8% incidence of nonsignificant CAD in their cohort of 118 patients [22]. There were no differences in demographic or CV risk factors among patients with or without significant CAD, and severity of CAD was not related to posttransplant survival over short-term follow-up. As demonstrated by this study, cardiac risk factors do not identify all LT candidates with significant CAD.

CAD is a relative contraindication to LT. However, heart-lung transplantation can be considered in select patients with both end-stage lung disease and advanced coronary disease with left ventricular dysfunction [5]. In the setting of preserved ventricular function, obstructive CAD may be addressed by percutaneous or surgical revascularization [34]. Studies have reported acceptable outcomes following percutaneous coronary intervention before transplant or simultaneous bypass grafting during the transplant procedure; however, the latter approach may not be offered to all patients, or available at all centers [22, 27, 34]. In a recent single-center retrospective study of 333 patients from 2004 to 2013, Halloran et al. found that the presence of CAD and coronary artery bypass grafting (CABG) at the time of lung transplantation did not impact overall retransplant-free survival [35].

Historically, prior CABG has been considered a contraindication to LT due to CAD severity and the technical surgical challenges of chest reentry; however, post-CABG patients are now increasingly being considered for and in select instances undergoing LT. McKellar et al. identified 292 (1.97%) out of 14,791 LT patients with a pretransplant CABG using data from the United Network for Organ Sharing Registry between 2004 and 2013. Patients most commonly underwent single right LT ($n = 181$), followed by single left LT ($n = 68$) and bilateral LT ($n = 43$). Pretransplant CABG predicted mortality at 30 days and at 1, 3, and 5 years, with hazard ratios ranging from 1.97 (95% CI, 1.23–3.16; $p < 0.01$) at 30 days to 1.38 (95% CI, 1.12–1.69; $p < 0.01$) at 5 years. However, this finding was driven principally by the increased mortality in patients that received bilateral LT [36].

Noncontrast cardiac computed tomography (CT) has received increasing attention as a less invasive method for detecting coronary artery calcification, and this technique may be helpful in select patient groups [37]. However at this time, cardiac CT has not been adequately studied in LT candidates, and therefore, its utility remains uncertain. Using a patient registry, Gaisl et al. matched 81 COPD patients with 81 non-COPD patients with a smoking history. There was no difference in coronary artery calcium scores between COPD patients (Global Initiative for Chronic Obstructive Lung Disease classification I, 5%; II, 23%; III, 16%; and IV, 56%) and controls (median difference: 68 Agatston units [95% CI, 176.5–192.5], $p = 0.90$). However, there was a higher incidence of major adverse cardiac events in the COPD cohort (RR = 2.80, $p = 0.016$) compared with controls over a median follow-up duration of 42.6 months. Cardiac ischemia and coronary artery calcification score were identified by proportional hazards modeling as independent predictors for adverse cardiac events. Another study by Nathan et al. found that CT performs moderately well for predicting CAD in IPF patients. In 57 patients with CAD (significant disease in 28.1%, mild disease in 40.3%, and none in 31.6%), the sensitivity of moderate to severe calcification for significant CAD was 81% and specificity was 85%, with an associated odds ratio of 25.2 (95% CI, 4.64–166; $p < 0.005$). There was also excellent interobserver agreement among reviewers grading the coronary calcification. CT has been studied as part of the cardiac evaluation in candidates for liver and renal transplantation with similar results [21, 38, 39]. Nevertheless, additional prospective data are needed before considering CT in place of angiography in LT candidates.

Use of extracorporeal life support, including extracorporeal membrane oxygenation (ECMO), as a bridge to lung or heart-lung transplantation has increased in recent years [40–45]. However, ECMO may limit the ability to perform a more thorough cardiac evaluation due to the underlying disease severity, inability to access the pulmonary circulation or accurately perform right heart catheterization (particularly when the internal jugular vein is accessed using a dual-lumen cannula), or inability to transport the patient for other logistic reasons. There is growing experience with ambulation while on ECMO support, which allows for more aggressive physical rehabilitation while awaiting transplantation [46–52]. Cardiac catheterizations and percutaneous intervention procedures have been performed in pediatric and adult ECMO patients, with acceptable outcomes [53–60].

In terms of management, patients with CAD may be candidates for percutaneous coronary intervention or CABG preoperatively or, in some instances, combined lung transplant and CABG. Successful revascularization of CAD has been well documented [25, 27, 34, 61, 62]; however, the type of coronary stent used in transplant candidates (bare metal or drug-eluting) and severity of CAD considered acceptable vary among transplant centers. Additionally, the timing of registration of candidates onto the transplant waiting list (and consequently the timing of transplantation) may be impacted by use of several medications common in CAD management, including the novel oral anticoagulants (NOACs), direct oral anticoagulants (DOACs), and various antiplatelet agents [63–67]. A case illustrating the ability to perform LT in a patient receiving Rivaroxaban has been reported [68]. Direct oral anticoagulant therapy was also well tolerated in heart and lung transplant recipients, but drug interactions and dosing adjustment for renal function were common [69].

In the future, expanded use of genome-wide association studies (GWAS) may one day help identify novel single-nucleotide polymorphisms (SNP) associated with CAD in patients with advanced lung disease. In a recent study that included more than 88,000 CAD cases and 162,000 controls, 25 new SNP-CAD associations were identified ($p < 5 \times 10^{-8}$, in fixed-effects meta-analysis) from 15 genomic regions, including SNPs in or near genes involved in cellular adhesion, leukocyte migration and atherosclerosis (PECAM1, rs1867624), coagulation and inflammation (PROCR, rs867186 [p.Ser219Gly]), and vascular smooth muscle cell differentiation (LMOD1, rs2820315) [70].

Diastolic Dysfunction

Poor cardiac function is generally considered a contraindication to LT. However, given the propensity for right ventricular (RV) function to improve following LT, it is typically the left ventricle (LV) that determines LT eligibility. Nevertheless, there has been increasing interest in how the presence and severity of diastolic dysfunction may affect perioperative outcomes, early graft function, and long-term survival in LT candidates.

Kato et al. studied the echocardiograms of 67 recipients before and after LT [71]. They found that RV parameters improved in all patients after LT (RV fractional area change, $36.7 \pm 5.6\%$ to $41.5 \pm 2.7\%$; RV strain, $-15.5 \pm 2.9\%$ to $-18.0 \pm 2.1\%$; RV E/e', 8.4 ± 1.8 to 7.7 ± 1.8; all $p < 0.05$). Left ventricular ejection fraction (LVEF) did not change ($58.7 \pm 6.0\%$ to $57.5 \pm 9.7\%$, $p = 0.39$); however, 20 patients (30%) had >10% LVEF decline after LT ($61.5 \pm 6.1\%$ to $47.3 \pm 4.2\%$, $p < 0.001$) and an increase in LV E/e' (11.8 ± 1.8 to 12.9 ± 2.2, $p = 0.05$). Pre-LT LV E/e' (OR 1.38, [95% CI, 1.01–1.95], $p = 0.043$) and lower pre-LT LV strain (OR 1.29, [95% CI, 1.09–1.61], $p = 0.002$) were associated with LVEF decrease after LT. The authors concluded that some recipients may experience worsening of both LV systolic and diastolic function following LT and that pretransplant LV diastolic dysfunction may increase the risk of LVEF deterioration post-LT. In a study of 65 lung transplant candidates, Nowak et al. found that mortality was higher in patients with smaller left ventricular end-systolic (LVESD) and end-diastolic (LVEDD) diameters (HR 3.03, [95% CI, 1.16–7.69], $p = 0.023$; and HR 2.9, [95% CI 1.16–7.14], $p = 0.022$, respectively) [72]. This finding was most relevant for patients with IPF, where a worse prognosis was previously related to increased pulmonary arterial pressures [73].

Pretransplant diastolic dysfunction may also be associated with an increased risk for primary graft dysfunction (PGD) following LT. In a retrospective cohort study of patients with ILD, COPD, and PAH enrolled in the Lung Transplant Outcomes Group (LTOG), Porteous et al. examined whether a higher ratio of early mitral inflow velocity (E) to early diastolic mitral annular velocity (é), which suggests worse LV diastolic function, was associated with a higher PGD risk [74]. They found that a higher E/é and E/é >8 were associated with increased PGD risk (E/é OR, 1.93 [95% CI, 1.02–3.64]; $p = 0.04$; E/é >8 OR, 5.29 [95% CI, 1.40–20.01]; $p = 0.01$). In a separate study, Perez-Teran et al. used both conventional and speckle-tracking echocardiography to examine RV function and PGD risk [75]. Patients who developed severe PGD had higher systolic pulmonary arterial pressure (48 ± 20 vs. 41 ± 18 mm Hg; $p = 0.048$), longer ischemia time (349 ± 73 vs. 306 ± 92 minutes; $p < 0.01$), and better RV function as estimated by basal free wall longitudinal strain (BLS; $-24\% \pm 9\%$ vs. $-20\% \pm 6\%$; $p = 0.039$). In a multivariate analysis adjusted for potentially confounding variables, basal free wall longitudinal strain (BLS) $\geq -21.5\%$ was independently associated with severe PGD (OR 4.56 [95% CI, 1.20–17.38]; $p = 0.026$). More recently, Li et al. studied 330 bilateral lung transplant recipients and found that mean left ventricular end-diastolic pressure (LVEDP) was higher in patients with Grade 3 PGD (16 ± 7 vs. 12 ± 5 mmHg, $p < 0.0001$). Elevation of either LVEDP >15 mmHg or mean pulmonary capillary wedge pressure >15 mmHg was associated with severe PGD (adjusted OR 3.83 [95% CI, 1.90–7.73]; $p < 0.0001$ for LVEDP and adjusted OR 4.25 [95% CI, 1.83–9.86]; $p = 0.0008$ for mean pulmonary capillary wedge pressure) [76].

Avriel et al. examined LT outcomes for patients with PAH with preoperative LV diastolic dysfunction with that of patients without diastolic dysfunction [77]. Fourteen of 44 patients (31.8%) with pretransplant diastolic dysfunction had a higher mean pulmonary arterial pressure (54.6 ± 10 mmHg vs. 47 ± 11.3 mmHg) and right atrial pressure (16.5 ± 5.2 mmHg vs. 10.6 ± 5.2 mmHg). Patients with diastolic dysfunction required extracorporeal life support more often (33% vs. 7%; $p = 0.02$), had higher APACHE II scores (21.7 ± 7.4 vs. 15.3 ± 5.3; $p = 0.02$), and trended toward fewer ventilator-free days (2.5 [IQR 6.5–32.5] vs. 17 [IQR 3–23]; $p = 0.08$). One-year survival was worse (hazard ratio [HR] 4.45; 95% CI, 1.3–22; $p = 0.02$), and diastolic dysfunction correlated with overall survival (HR 5.4; 95% CI, 1.3–22; $p = 0.02$). The authors concluded that diastolic dysfunction leads to worse survival in PAH patients following LT. However, Yadlapati et al. reported opposite findings. They studied the effect of pretransplant diastolic dysfunction on LT outcome in 111 patients at a single institution [78]. They found that echocardiographic findings of abnormal diastolic function, including A' > E' and A > E, did not predict adverse events ($p = 0.49$). Mildly elevated pretransplant pulmonary capillary wedge pressure (16–20 mmHg) and moderately or severely elevated pulmonary capillary wedge pressure (>20 mmHg) were not associated with adverse events following LT.

Atrial Arrhythmias

Atrial arrhythmias are common both in the general population and after LT. Atrial fibrillation (AF) is the most common atrial arrhythmia observed in Europe and the United States. In these regions, the estimated prevalence of AF is 1–2% in the general population; however, AF may be observed in >10% of individuals above the age of 80 years [79]. Notably, AF has been associated with poorer outcomes in preoperative patients undergoing cardiac and valvular heart surgery, and liver transplantation candidates with AF may be at an increased risk for posttransplant mortality [80–83].

Atrial arrhythmias may portend a poorer outcome in affected LT patients [84]. In a meta-analysis that included 2094 patients from 11 studies, Fan et al. found that the pooled incidence of any postoperative atrial arrhythmia following LT was 31% (95% CI, 25–37%) [85]. This prevalence is consistent with that reported in several other studies describing atrial arrhythmias post-lung transplant [86–90]. Risk factors associated with the development of a postoperative atrial arrhythmia included: age (>50 vs. ≤50 years, OR 2.73 [95% CI, 1.86–4.00], $p < 0.001$), history of atrial arrhythmia (OR 1.76 [95% CI, 1.34–2.32], $p = 0.002$), vasopressor use (OR 1.76 [95% CI, 1.34–2.32], $p < 0.001$), ILD (OR of 1.85 [95% CI, 1.27–2.71], $p = 0.001$), hypertension (OR 1.49 [95% CI, 1.12–1.97], $p = 0.006$), CAD (OR 1.58 [95% CI, 1.20–2.08], $p = 0.001$), hyperlipidemia (OR 1.52 [95% CI, 1.06–2.20], $p = 0.025$), and left atrial enlargement (OR 2.99 [95% CI, 1.91–4.67], $p < 0.001$). Female recipients (female vs. male, OR 0.44 [95% CI, 0.35–0.56], $p < 0.001$) and those with cystic fibrosis (OR 0.32 [95% CI, 0.18–0.59], $p < 0.001$) were less likely to develop a postoperative atrial arrhythmia. A separate meta-analysis of 2653 patients from 9 studies (7 of which were included in the above study) found that a postoperative atrial arrhythmia occurred in 29.8% of patients [91]. The authors concluded that atrial arrhythmias were associated with significantly higher perioperative mortality (OR 2.70 [95% CI, 1.73–4.19], $p < 0.0001$), a more frequent need for tracheostomy (OR 4.67 [95% CI, 2.59–8.44], $p < 0.0001$), and higher midterm mortality (OR 1.71 [95% CI, 1.28–2.30], $p < 0.001$). A similar review of 12 studies, published a year later, drew the same conclusion [92]. Chaikriangkrai et al. found that a new atrial arrhythmia was most likely to occur within 30 days of LT [87]. Of patients who underwent electrophysiologic studies, 80% had multiple mechanisms accounting for the atrial arrhythmia, including peri-tricuspid flutter (48%), peri-mitral flutter (36%), right atrial incisional reentry (24%), focal tachycardia from recipient pulmonary vein antrum (32%), focal pulmonary vein fibrillation (24%), and left atrial roof flutter (20%). Left atrial mechanisms were observed in 80% of electrophysiologic study patients and typically originated from the anastomotic pulmonary vein antrum [87].

LT recipients with preoperative atrial fibrillation may be at increased risk of poorer cardiovascular outcomes. In a single-center study of 235 lung transplant recipients from 2013 to 2015, Yerasi et al. found that AF patients were older (64.1 ± 9 vs. 58.3 ± 8.3 years, $p < 0.001$), had a longer ischemic time (520 ± 188 vs. 305 ± 83, $p < 0.001$), had more postoperative arrhythmias (73.7% vs. 20.8%, $p = 0.01$), and had a longer median postoperative length of stay (16 vs. 13 days, $p = 0.02$) [93]. Median total hospital length of stay during the first posttransplant year was longer for the AF patients (27 vs. 21 days, $p = 0.25$). Moreover, AF, along with pneumonia and any infection, was associated with 30-day readmission after LT [94]. Elevated pulmonary arterial pressure was associated with a lower occurrence of AF in a study of 174 patients, of whom 16% developed AF at a median 6 days posttransplant [95]. In this study, every 10-mmHg increase in pulmonary artery systolic pressure was associated with a 31% reduction in the odds of postoperative AF (OR 0.69 [95% CI, 0.49–0.98], $p = 0.035$). Bilateral LT, as opposed to single LT, may protect against long-term paroxysmal AF [96]. Garcia et al. [97] found that AF was associated with lower posttransplant survival; however, other studies of LT recipients with AF have not identified a similar association [86, 98, 99]. Pharmacologic treatment and ablation procedures have been performed following LT, with successful arrhythmia control [100–104]. However, there is one case report describing pulmonary toxicity following treatment with amiodarone for atrial arrhythmias after LT [105]. The study by Fan et al. also demonstrated an association between atrial arrhythmia and length of stay (weighted mean difference 9.72, 95% CI 5.07–14.38, $p < 0.001$) and overall survival after LT (HR 1.72, [95% CI, 1.39–2.12], $p < 0.001$).

PAH in Advanced Lung Diseases

Pulmonary arterial hypertension (PAH) secondary to advanced lung disease is associated with both disease severity and survival in LT candidates. PAH occurs in COPD, but the prevalence varies according to disease severity and the definition of PAH utilized – up to 90% of GOLD stage IV COPD patients had a mean pulmonary arterial pressure (mPAP) >20 mm Hg, and about 3–5% had a mPAP >35–40 mm Hg [106, 107]. Patients with IPF may have an even higher prevalence of PH, with 8.1% and 14.9% of IPF patients having mPAP >25 mm Hg in published series [108, 109]. The 5-year survival for COPD patients with PAH was 36% in one study [110], and IPF survival worsens in the presence of PAH [111–114].

The 6-minute walk test (6MWT) has long been recognized as a useful diagnostic tool for the assessment of PAH and the LT candidate [115, 116]. Walk distance and oxygen desaturation have been associated with lung function in ILD patients [117, 118]. More notably, the 6MWT has prognostic value for patients with group 1 PAH [119, 120], non-group 1 PAH [121], ILD [122–124], cystic fibrosis [125–127], and COPD [128–132]. In a cross-sectional analysis, Porteous et al. studied the determinants of 6-minute walk distance in 130 IPF patients undergoing lung transplant evaluation [133]. After adjustment for age, sex, race, height, and weight, the presence of right ventricular dilation was associated with a decrease of 50.9 m (95%CI, 8.4–93.3; $p = 0.02$) in walk distance. Additionally, for every 1 Wood unit increase in pulmonary vascular resistance, walk distance decreased by 17.3 m (95% CI, 5.1–29.5; $p = 0:006$). A pretransplant 6MWT >750 ft. (229 m) was associated with a shorter length of hospitalization (37 vs. 20 days, $p = 0.03$) in pediatric LT recipients [134]. The 6-minute walk distance has also been associated with recipient survival following lung transplant [135].

Doppler echocardiography (DE) has been evaluated as a surrogate for RHC for the detection of PAH. Balci et al. [136] studied 103 lung transplantation candidates who underwent both DE and RHC within a 72-hour period. Almost 90% of patients were able to undergo pulmonary artery systolic pressure (PASP) evaluation by DE. Median PASP was 45 (12–145) mm Hg by RHC and 45 (20–144) mm Hg by DE. PASP estimated by DE correlated with that measured by RHC ($r = 0.585$, $p < 0.0001$). Sensitivity, specificity, and positive and negative predictive values of PASP for the diagnosis of PAH were 85%, 67%, 87%, and 61%, respectively. PAH was present in 57% of their lung transplantation candidates.

In another study comparing echocardiography and cardiac catheterization to diagnose PAH, Nowak et al. [137] found that right ventricular systolic pressure (RVSP) ≥43 mm Hg predicted the presence of PAH (sensitivity 92.3%, specificity 81.8%, area under curve [AUC] 0.84 [95% CI, 0.67–1.0]; $p = 0.019$). Right ventricular outflow tract (RVOT) diameter ≥34 mm and tricuspid annular plane systolic excursion (TAPSE) ≤18 mm had adequate sensitivity, specificity and AUC for PAH (62.2%, 89.3%, 0.77 [95% CI, 0.66–0.89], $p = 0.01$, and 77.1%, 66.7%, 0.74 [95% CI, 0.61–0.87], $p = 0.027$, respectively). The combined use of RVSP, RVOT, and TAPSE increased both sensitivity and negative predictive value of PAH detection to 100%. PAH, defined by PASP >25 mm Hg on cardiac catheterization, was observed in 67.6% of IPF patients, 30% of COPD patients, and 75% of patients with other ILDs. Exercise pulmonary hemodynamic response has also predicted adverse clinical outcomes in patients with fibrotic lung disease [138].

Patients with PAH undergoing LT may be at risk for transient LV dysfunction in the immediate postoperative period. In a single-center study, Gupta et al. described their experience in 16 patients with World Health Organization (WHO) Group 1 PAH who underwent LT between 2008 and 2012 [139]. Five of 16 patients (31%) developed LV dysfunction after transplantation. Mean time to LV dysfunction onset was 4.2 days. Patients with dysfunction had lower right and left ventricular ejection fraction with higher LV end-diastolic volume before LT. However, all patients recovered LV function within 4 months of LT.

PAH is common in end-stage lung disease and associated with poorer short-term and intermediate-term LT outcomes. In a study of 518 patients, Andersen et al.

found that 58 (11%) had postcapillary PAH, while 211 (41%) had precapillary PAH and 249 (48%) had no PAH [140]. Precapillary and postcapillary PAH were associated with worse 90-day outcomes compared to non-PAH patients ($p = 0.003$ and 0.043, respectively). However, survival beyond 1 year was not altered by PAH. Using Organ Procurement and Transplant Network data, Singh et al. studied 2025 COPD, 2304 IPF, and 866 CF patients. The authors found that 1-year posttransplant survival for COPD patients with vs. without PAH was 76.9% vs. 86.2% ($p = 0.001$). COPD patients with PAH had a 1.74 (95% CI, 1.3–2.3; $p = 0.001$) times higher risk of mortality at 1 year post-LT. The presence of PAH did not influence post-LT survival for IPF and CF patients.

Valvular Heart Disease

The presence of significant valvular heart disease may preclude the possibility of LT, although the degree of valvular dysfunction considered significant likely differs among transplant centers and by surgical assessment. There is little published data evaluating the assessment of valvular heart disease prior to LT, and the ISHLT candidate selection guidelines do not specifically address valvular heart disease, outside of that contributing to "significant" heart dysfunction as a contraindication.

In a small series (5 patients), progression of mitral regurgitation following LT was not associated with 1-year or 5-year mortality [141]. However, the authors acknowledge that in some instances, MR progression may become clinically significant. LT may also unmask severe mitral regurgitation, as described in a patient transplanted for severe PAH, possibly due to ventricular remodeling and subsequent change in the mitral valve apparatus [142]. Aortic valve replacement has been performed for critical aortic stenosis after bilateral LT [143]. Transcatheter aortic valve implantation has been reported in a LT recipient, though this procedure may also be associated with a risk of exacerbation in IPF pretransplant [144, 145]. Valves have also been replaced for posttransplant infective endocarditis [146].

Conclusion

Lung transplantation remains an important treatment option for patients with advanced or end-stage lung disease; however, careful candidate selection is important for optimizing perioperative and long-term outcomes. The cardiac evaluation is a critical element of the pretransplant assessment. Disorders such as significant CAD, arrhythmias, PAH, and valvular heart disease should be readily identified and managed so that the chance for a successful transplant outcome is not adversely affected. Several current and emerging diagnostic techniques can assess for the presence of cardiac disease, and future research will focus on novel methods of detection and intervention to optimize the heart for LT.

References

1. Chambers DC, Yusen RD, Cherikh WS, et al. The Registry of the International Society for Heart and Lung Transplantation: thirty-fourth adult lung and heart-lung transplantation report-2017; focus theme: allograft ischemic time. J Heart Lung Transplant. 2017;36:1047–59.
2. Verleden SE, Todd JL, Sato M, et al. Impact of CLAD phenotype on survival after lung retransplantation: a multicenter study. Am J Transplant. 2015;15:2223–30.
3. Maurer JR, Frost AE, Estenne M, Higenbottam T, Glanville AR. International guidelines for the selection of lung transplant candidates. The International Society for Heart and Lung Transplantation, the American Thoracic Society, the American Society of Transplant Physicians, the European Respiratory Society. J Heart Lung Transplant. 1998;17:703–9.
4. Orens JB, Estenne M, Arcasoy S, et al. International guidelines for the selection of lung transplant candidates: 2006 update–a consensus report from the Pulmonary Scientific Council of the International Society for Heart and Lung Transplantation. J Heart Lung Transplant. 2006;25:745–55.
5. Weill D, Benden C, Corris PA, et al. A consensus document for the selection of lung transplant candidates: 2014–an update from the Pulmonary Transplantation Council of the International Society for Heart and Lung Transplantation. J Heart Lung Transplant. 2015;34:1–15.
6. Benza RL, Miller DP, Frost A, Barst RJ, Krichman AM, McGoon MD. Analysis of the lung allocation score estimation of risk of death in patients with pulmonary arterial hypertension using data from the REVEAL Registry. Transplantation. 2010;90:298–305.
7. Benza RL, Miller DP, Gomberg-Maitland M, et al. Predicting survival in pulmonary arterial hypertension: insights from the Registry to Evaluate Early and Long-Term Pulmonary Arterial Hypertension Disease Management (REVEAL). Circulation. 2010;122:164–72.
8. Miller DP, Farber HW. "Who'll be the next in line?" The lung allocation score in patients with pulmonary arterial hypertension. J Heart Lung Transplant. 2013;32:1165–7.
9. Liu Y, Vela M, Rudakevych T, Wigfield C, Garrity E, Saunders MR. Patient factors associated with lung transplant referral and waitlist for patients with cystic fibrosis and pulmonary fibrosis. J Heart Lung Transplant. 2017;36:264–71.
10. Vogl M, Warnecke G, Haverich A, et al. Lung transplantation in the spotlight: reasons for high-cost procedures. J Heart Lung Transplant. 2016;35:1227–36.
11. Verleden GM, Dupont L, Yserbyt J, et al. Recipient selection process and listing for lung transplantation. J Thorac Dis. 2017;9:3372–84.
12. Collaud S, Benden C, Ganter C, et al. Extracorporeal life support as bridge to lung retransplantation: a multicenter pooled data analysis. Ann Thorac Surg. 2016;102:1680–6.
13. Hayes D Jr, Higgins RS, Kilic A, et al. Extracorporeal membrane oxygenation and retransplantation in lung transplantation: an analysis of the UNOS registry. Lung. 2014;192:571–6.
14. Kawut SM. Lung retransplantation. Clin Chest Med. 2011;32:367–77.
15. Ren D, Kaleekal TS, Graviss EA, et al. Retransplantation outcomes at a large lung transplantation program. Transplant Direct. 2018;4:e404.
16. Revilla-Lopez E, Berastegui C, Saez-Gimenez B, et al. Lung retransplantation due to chronic lung allograph dysfunction: results from a Spanish transplant unit. Arch Bronconeumol. 2019;55:134–8.
17. Thomas M, Belli EV, Rawal B, Agnew RC, Landolfo KP. Survival after lung retransplantation in the United States in the current era (2004 to 2013): better or worse? Ann Thorac Surg. 2015;100:452–7.
18. Waseda R, Benazzo A, Hoetzenecker K, et al. The influence of retransplantation on survival for pediatric lung transplant recipients. J Thorac Cardiovasc Surg. 2018;156:2025–34. e2.
19. Smilowitz NR, Guo Y, Rao S, Gelb B, Berger JS, Bangalore S. Perioperative cardiovascular outcomes of non-cardiac solid organ transplant surgery. Eur Heart J Qual Care Clin Outcomes. 2019;5:72–8.
20. Smith SC Jr, Dove JT, Jacobs AK, et al. ACC/AHA guidelines for percutaneous coronary intervention (revision of the 1993 PTCA guidelines)-executive summary: a report of the American College of Cardiology/American Heart Association task force on practice guide-

lines (Committee to revise the 1993 guidelines for percutaneous transluminal coronary angioplasty) endorsed by the Society for Cardiac Angiography and Interventions. Circulation. 2001;103:3019–41.

21. Lentine KL, Costa SP, Weir MR, et al. Cardiac disease evaluation and management among kidney and liver transplantation candidates: a scientific statement from the American Heart Association and the American College of Cardiology Foundation: endorsed by the American Society of Transplant Surgeons, American Society of Transplantation, and National Kidney Foundation. Circulation. 2012;126:617–63.

22. Ben-Dor I, Shitrit D, Kramer MR, Iakobishvili Z, Sahar G, Hasdai D. Is routine coronary angiography and revascularization indicated among patients undergoing evaluation for lung transplantation? Chest. 2005;128:2557–62.

23. Jones RM, Enfield KB, Mehrad B, Keeley EC. Prevalence of obstructive coronary artery disease in patients undergoing lung transplantation: case series and review of the literature. Catheter Cardiovasc Interv. 2014;84:1–6.

24. Kaza AK, Dietz JF, Kern JA, et al. Coronary risk stratification in patients with end-stage lung disease. J Heart Lung Transplant. 2002;21:334–9.

25. Patel VS, Palmer SM, Messier RH, Davis RD. Clinical outcome after coronary artery revascularization and lung transplantation. Ann Thorac Surg. 2003;75:372–7; discussion 7.

26. Reed RM, Eberlein M, Girgis RE, et al. Coronary artery disease is under-diagnosed and under-treated in advanced lung disease. Am J Med. 2012;125:1228. e13–e22.

27. Seoane L, Arcement LM, Valentine VG, McFadden PM. Long-term survival in lung transplant recipients after successful preoperative coronary revascularization. J Thorac Cardiovasc Surg. 2005;130:538–41.

28. Schouten O, van Kuijk JP, Flu WJ, et al. Long-term outcome of prophylactic coronary revascularization in cardiac high-risk patients undergoing major vascular surgery (from the randomized DECREASE-V Pilot Study). Am J Cardiol. 2009;103:897–901.

29. Huiart L, Ernst P, Suissa S. Cardiovascular morbidity and mortality in COPD. Chest. 2005;128:2640–6.

30. Makey IA, Sui JW, Huynh C, Das NA, Thomas M, Johnson S. Lung transplant patients with coronary artery disease rarely die of cardiac causes. Clin Transpl. 2018;32:e13354.

31. Sidney S, Sorel M, Quesenberry CP Jr, DeLuise C, Lanes S, Eisner MD. COPD and incident cardiovascular disease hospitalizations and mortality: Kaiser Permanente Medical Care Program. Chest. 2005;128:2068–75.

32. Kizer JR, Zisman DA, Blumenthal NP, et al. Association between pulmonary fibrosis and coronary artery disease. Arch Intern Med. 2004;164:551–6.

33. Snell GI, Richardson M, Griffiths AP, Williams TJ, Esmore DS. Coronary artery disease in potential lung transplant recipients > 50 years old: the role of coronary intervention. Chest. 1999;116:874–9.

34. Koprivanac M, Budev MM, Yun JJ, et al. How important is coronary artery disease when considering lung transplant candidates? J Heart Lung Transplant. 2016;35:1453–61.

35. Halloran K, Hirji A, Li D, et al. Coronary artery disease and coronary artery bypass grafting at the time of lung transplantation do not impact overall survival. Transplantation. 2019;103(10):2190–5.

36. McKellar SH, Bowen ME, Baird BC, Raman S, Cahill BC, Selzman CH. Lung transplantation following coronary artery bypass surgery-improved outcomes following single-lung transplant. J Heart Lung Transplant. 2016;35:1289–94.

37. Budoff MJ, Achenbach S, Blumenthal RS, et al. Assessment of coronary artery disease by cardiac computed tomography: a scientific statement from the American Heart Association Committee on Cardiovascular Imaging and Intervention, Council on Cardiovascular Radiology and Intervention, and Committee on Cardiac Imaging, Council on Clinical Cardiology. Circulation. 2006;114:1761–91.

38. Ali A, Bhardwaj HL, Heuman DM, Jovin IS. Coronary events in patients undergoing orthotopic liver transplantation: perioperative evaluation and management. Clin Transpl. 2013;27:E207–15.

39. Ehtisham J, Altieri M, Salame E, Saloux E, Ollivier I, Hamon M. Coronary artery disease in orthotopic liver transplantation: pretransplant assessment and management. Liver Transpl. 2010;16:550–7.
40. Bermudez CA, Rocha RV, Zaldonis D, et al. Extracorporeal membrane oxygenation as a bridge to lung transplant: midterm outcomes. Ann Thorac Surg. 2011;92:1226–31; discussion 31–2.
41. Hoetzenecker K, Donahoe L, Yeung JC, et al. Extracorporeal life support as a bridge to lung transplantation-experience of a high-volume transplant center. J Thorac Cardiovasc Surg. 2018;155:1316–28. e1.
42. Kearns SK, Hernandez OO. "Awake" extracorporeal membrane oxygenation as a bridge to lung transplant. AACN Adv Crit Care. 2016;27:293–300.
43. Sharma NS, Hartwig MG, Hayes D Jr. Extracorporeal membrane oxygenation in the pre and post lung transplant period. Ann Transl Med. 2017;5:74.
44. Spinelli E, Protti A. Get fit for lung transplant with ambulatory extracorporeal membrane oxygenation! Respir Care. 2016;61:117–8.
45. van Berkel V. Yesterday's heroic measure is now standard procedure: extracorporeal membrane oxygenation as a bridge to lung transplant. J Thorac Cardiovasc Surg. 2018;155:1314–5.
46. Garcia JP, Kon ZN, Evans C, et al. Ambulatory veno-venous extracorporeal membrane oxygenation: innovation and pitfalls. J Thorac Cardiovasc Surg. 2011;142:755–61.
47. Hayes D Jr, Kukreja J, Tobias JD, Ballard HO, Hoopes CW. Ambulatory venovenous extracorporeal respiratory support as a bridge for cystic fibrosis patients to emergent lung transplantation. J Cyst Fibros. 2012;11:40–5.
48. Jacob S, MacHannaford JC, Chamogeorgakis T, et al. Ambulatory extracorporeal membrane oxygenation with subclavian venoarterial cannulation to increase mobility and recovery in a patient awaiting cardiac transplantation. Proc (Bayl Univ Med Cent). 2017;30: 224–5.
49. Lehr CJ, Zaas DW, Cheifetz IM, Turner DA. Ambulatory extracorporeal membrane oxygenation as a bridge to lung transplantation: walking while waiting. Chest. 2015;147: 1213–8.
50. Lindholm JA. Ambulatory veno-venous extracorporeal membrane oxygenation. J Thorac Dis. 2018;10:S670–S3.
51. Wong JY, Buchholz H, Ryerson L, et al. Successful semi-ambulatory veno-arterial extracorporeal membrane oxygenation bridge to heart-lung transplantation in a very small child. Am J Transplant. 2015;15:2256–60.
52. Abrams D, Garan AR, Brodie D. Awake and fully mobile patients on cardiac extracorporeal life support. Ann Cardiothorac Surg. 2019;8:44–53.
53. desJardins SE, Crowley DC, Beekman RH, Lloyd TR. Utility of cardiac catheterization in pediatric cardiac patients on ECMO. Catheter Cardiovasc Interv. 1999;46:62–7.
54. Guzeltas A, Kasar T, Tanidir IC, Ozturk E, Yildiz O, Haydin S. Cardiac catheterization procedures in pediatric patients undergoing extracorporeal membrane oxygenation cardiac catheterization, ECMO. Anatol J Cardiol. 2017;18:425–30.
55. Booth KL, Roth SJ, Perry SB, del Nido PJ, Wessel DL, Laussen PC. Cardiac catheterization of patients supported by extracorporeal membrane oxygenation. J Am Coll Cardiol. 2002;40:1681–6.
56. Boscamp NS, Turner ME, Crystal M, Anderson B, Vincent JA, Torres AJ. Cardiac catheterization in pediatric patients supported by extracorporeal membrane oxygenation: a 15-year experience. Pediatr Cardiol. 2017;38:332–7.
57. Burke CR, Chan T, Rubio AE, McMullan DM. Early cardiac catheterization leads to shortened pediatric extracorporeal membrane oxygenation run duration. J Interv Cardiol. 2017;30:170–6.
58. Callahan R, Trucco SM, Wearden PD, Beerman LB, Arora G, Kreutzer J. Outcomes of pediatric patients undergoing cardiac catheterization while on extracorporeal membrane oxygenation. Pediatr Cardiol. 2015;36:625–32.

59. Kato A, Lo Rito M, Lee KJ, et al. Impacts of early cardiac catheterization for children with congenital heart disease supported by extracorporeal membrane oxygenation. Catheter Cardiovasc Interv. 2017;89:898–905.

60. Guerrero-Miranda CY, Hall SA. Cardiac catheterization and percutaneous intervention procedures on extracorporeal membrane oxygenation support. Ann Cardiothorac Surg. 2019;8:123–8.

61. Castleberry AW, Martin JT, Osho AA, et al. Coronary revascularization in lung transplant recipients with concomitant coronary artery disease. Am J Transplant. 2013;13:2978–88.

62. Wild J, Arrigo M, Isenring BD, et al. Coronary artery disease in lung transplant candidates: role of routine invasive assessment. Respiration. 2015;89:107–11.

63. Capodanno D. Triple antithrombotic therapy after ACS and PCI in patients on chronic oral anticoagulation: update. Heart. 2018;104:1976.

64. Fluschnik N, Becher PM, Schnabel R, Blankenberg S, Westermann D. Anticoagulation strategies in patients with atrial fibrillation after PCI or with ACS: the end of triple therapy? Herz. 2018;43:20–5.

65. Giri J, Nathan A. Is it time to abandon dual antiplatelet therapy after percutaneous coronary intervention in patients with atrial fibrillation on anticoagulation? JACC Cardiovasc Interv. 2018;11:635–7.

66. Smith M, Wakam G, Wakefield T, Obi A. New trends in anticoagulation therapy. Surg Clin North Am. 2018;98:219–38.

67. Webster E, Gil M. Advances in anticoagulation therapy. JAAPA. 2018;31:30–5.

68. Renner TA, Zalunardo MP, Weder W, Spahn DR. Bilateral lung transplantation in a patient receiving rivaroxaban anticoagulation. J Cardiothorac Vasc Anesth. 2015;29:723–6.

69. Lichvar AB, Moore CA, Ensor CR, McDyer JF, Teuteberg JJ, Shullo MA. Evaluation of direct oral anticoagulation therapy in heart and lung transplant recipients. Prog Transplant. 2016;26:263–9.

70. Howson JMM, Zhao W, Barnes DR, et al. Fifteen new risk loci for coronary artery disease highlight arterial-wall-specific mechanisms. Nat Genet. 2017;49:1113–9.

71. Kato TS, Armstrong HF, Schulze PC, et al. Left and right ventricular functional dynamics determined by echocardiograms before and after lung transplantation. Am J Cardiol. 2015;116:652–9.

72. Nowak J, Hudzik B, Niedziela JT, et al. The role of echocardiographic parameters in predicting survival of patients with lung diseases referred for lung transplantation. Clin Respir J. 2019;13:212.

73. Nowak J, Hudzik B, Przybylowski P, et al. Prognostic value of mean, diastolic, and systolic pulmonary artery pressure in patients with end-stage lung disease referred for lung transplantation. Transplant Proc. 2018;50:2048–52.

74. Porteous MK, Ky B, Kirkpatrick JN, et al. Diastolic dysfunction increases the risk of primary graft dysfunction after lung transplant. Am J Respir Crit Care Med. 2016;193:1392–400.

75. Perez-Teran P, Roca O, Rodriguez-Palomares J, et al. Influence of right ventricular function on the development of primary graft dysfunction after lung transplantation. J Heart Lung Transplant. 2015;34:1423–9.

76. Li D, Weinkauf J, Hirji A, et al. Elevated pre-transplant left ventricular end-diastolic pressure increases primary graft dysfunction risk in double lung transplant recipients. J Heart Lung Transplant. 2019;38:710.

77. Avriel A, Klement AH, Johnson SR, de Perrot M, Granton J. Impact of left ventricular diastolic dysfunction on lung transplantation outcome in patients with pulmonary arterial hypertension. Am J Transplant. 2017;17:2705–11.

78. Yadlapati A, Lynch JP 3rd, Saggar R, et al. Preoperative cardiac variables of diastolic dysfunction and clinical outcomes in lung transplant recipients. J Transp Secur. 2013;2013:391620.

79. Heeringa J, van der Kuip DA, Hofman A, et al. Prevalence, incidence and lifetime risk of atrial fibrillation: the Rotterdam study. Eur Heart J. 2006;27:949–53.

80. Bargehr J, Trejo-Gutierrez JF, Rosser BG, et al. Liver transplantation in patients with atrial fibrillation. Transplant Proc. 2013;45:2302–6.

81. Vannucci A, Rathor R, Vachharajani N, Chapman W, Kangrga I. Atrial fibrillation in patients undergoing liver transplantation-a single-center experience. Transplant Proc. 2014;46:1432–7.

82. Rogers CA, Angelini GD, Culliford LA, Capoun R, Ascione R. Coronary surgery in patients with preexisting chronic atrial fibrillation: early and midterm clinical outcome. Ann Thorac Surg. 2006;81:1676–82.

83. Wang TK, Ramanathan T, Choi DH, Gamble G, Ruygrok P. Preoperative atrial fibrillation predicts mortality and morbidity after aortic valve replacement. Interact Cardiovasc Thorac Surg. 2014;19:218–22.

84. Roukoz H, Benditt DG. Atrial arrhythmias after lung transplantation. Trends Cardiovasc Med. 2018;28:53–61.

85. Fan J, Zhou K, Li S, Du H, Che G. Incidence, risk factors and prognosis of postoperative atrial arrhythmias after lung transplantation: a systematic review and meta-analysis. Interact Cardiovasc Thorac Surg. 2016;23:790–9.

86. Orrego CM, Cordero-Reyes AM, Estep JD, et al. Atrial arrhythmias after lung transplant: underlying mechanisms, risk factors, and prognosis. J Heart Lung Transplant. 2014;33:734–40.

87. Chaikriangkrai K, Jyothula S, Jhun HY, et al. Incidence, risk factors, prognosis, and electrophysiological mechanisms of atrial arrhythmias after lung transplantation. JACC Clin Electrophysiol. 2015;1:296–305.

88. D'Angelo AM, Chan EG, Hayanga JW, et al. Atrial arrhythmias after lung transplantation: incidence and risk factors in 652 lung transplant recipients. J Thorac Cardiovasc Surg. 2016;152:901–9.

89. Raghavan D, Gao A, Ahn C, et al. Contemporary analysis of incidence of post-operative atrial fibrillation, its predictors, and association with clinical outcomes in lung transplantation. J Heart Lung Transplant. 2015;34:563–70.

90. Henri C, Giraldeau G, Dorais M, et al. Atrial fibrillation after pulmonary transplantation: incidence, impact on mortality, treatment effectiveness, and risk factors. Circ Arrhythm Electrophysiol. 2012;5:61–7.

91. Waldron NH, Klinger RY, Hartwig MG, Snyder LD, Daubert JP, Mathew JP. Adverse outcomes associated with postoperative atrial arrhythmias after lung transplantation: a meta-analysis and systematic review of the literature. Clin Transpl. 2017;31(4):e12926.

92. Saad M, Elgendy IY, Mentias A, et al. Incidence, predictors, and outcomes of early atrial arrhythmias after lung transplant: a systematic review and meta-analysis. JACC Clin Electrophysiol. 2017;3:718–26.

93. Yerasi C, Roy SB, Olson M, et al. Outcomes of lung transplant recipients with preoperative atrial fibrillation. Asian Cardiovasc Thorac Ann. 2018;26:127–32.

94. Osho AA, Castleberry AW, Yerokun BA, et al. Clinical predictors and outcome implications of early readmission in lung transplant recipients. J Heart Lung Transplant. 2017;36:546–53.

95. Malik A, Hsu JC, Hoopes C, Itinarelli G, Marcus GM. Elevated pulmonary artery systolic pressures are associated with a lower risk of atrial fibrillation following lung transplantation. J Electrocardiol. 2013;46:38–42.

96. Lee G, Wu H, Kalman JM, et al. Atrial fibrillation following lung transplantation: double but not single lung transplant is associated with long-term freedom from paroxysmal atrial fibrillation. Eur Heart J. 2010;31:2774–82.

97. Garcia S, Canoniero M, Sattiraju S, et al. Atrial fibrillation after lung transplantation: incidence, predictors and long-term implications. J Atr Fibrillation. 2011;4:363.

98. Jesel L, Barraud J, Lim HS, et al. Early and late atrial arrhythmias after lung transplantation-incidence, predictive factors and impact on mortality. Circ J. 2017;81:660–7.

99. Mason DP, Marsh DH, Alster JM, et al. Atrial fibrillation after lung transplantation: timing, risk factors, and treatment. Ann Thorac Surg. 2007;84:1878–84.

100. Bazaz R, Salizzoni S, Bonde P, Espinoza A, Toyoda Y. A novel strategy for prevention of post-operative atrial arrhythmias in patients undergoing lung transplantation. J Heart Lung Transplant. 2010;29:713–5.

101. Szeplaki G, Szegedi N, Tahin T, Merkely B, Geller L. Successful catheter ablation of right atrial tachycardia after bilateral lung transplantation. Transplantation. 2015;99:e115–6.

102. Fournet D, Zimmermann M, Campanini C. Atrial tachycardia with recipient-to-donor atrio-atrial conduction and isthmus-dependent donor atrial flutter in a patient after orthotopic heart

transplantation. Successful treatment by radiofrequency catheter ablation. J Heart Lung Transplant. 2002;21:923–7.

103. Isiadinso I, Meshkov AB, Gaughan J, et al. Atrial arrhythmias after lung and heart-lung transplant: effects on short-term mortality and the influence of amiodarone. J Heart Lung Transplant. 2011;30:37–44.

104. Adegunsoye A, Strek ME, Garrity E, Guzy R, Bag R. Comprehensive care of the lung transplant patient. Chest. 2017;152:150–64.

105. Diaz-Guzman E, Mireles-Cabodevila E, Arrossi A, Kanne JP, Budev M. Amiodarone pulmonary toxicity after lung transplantation. J Heart Lung Transplant. 2008;27:1059–63.

106. Andersen KH, Iversen M, Kjaergaard J, et al. Prevalence, predictors, and survival in pulmonary hypertension related to end-stage chronic obstructive pulmonary disease. J Heart Lung Transplant. 2012;31:373–80.

107. Chaouat A, Bugnet AS, Kadaoui N, et al. Severe pulmonary hypertension and chronic obstructive pulmonary disease. Am J Respir Crit Care Med. 2005;172:189–94.

108. Hamada K, Nagai S, Tanaka S, et al. Significance of pulmonary arterial pressure and diffusion capacity of the lung as prognosticator in patients with idiopathic pulmonary fibrosis. Chest. 2007;131:650–6.

109. Kimura M, Taniguchi H, Kondoh Y, et al. Pulmonary hypertension as a prognostic indicator at the initial evaluation in idiopathic pulmonary fibrosis. Respiration. 2013;85:456–63.

110. Oswald-Mammosser M, Weitzenblum E, Quoix E, et al. Prognostic factors in COPD patients receiving long-term oxygen therapy. Importance of pulmonary artery pressure. Chest. 1995;107:1193–8.

111. Maher TM, Dejonckheere F, Nathan SD. Survival in idiopathic pulmonary fibrosis: perspectives from pulmonary arterial hypertension. J Manag Care Spec Pharm. 2017;23:S3–4.

112. Nathan SD. Pulmonary hypertension complicating pulmonary fibrosis: bad and ugly, but good to treat? Thorax. 2014;69:107–8.

113. Nathan SD, Shlobin OA, Ahmad S, et al. Serial development of pulmonary hypertension in patients with idiopathic pulmonary fibrosis. Respiration. 2008;76:288–94.

114. Shorr AF, Wainright JL, Cors CS, Lettieri CJ, Nathan SD. Pulmonary hypertension in patients with pulmonary fibrosis awaiting lung transplant. Eur Respir J. 2007;30:715–21.

115. Kadikar A, Maurer J, Kesten S. The six-minute walk test: a guide to assessment for lung transplantation. J Heart Lung Transplant. 1997;16:313–9.

116. Redelmeier DA, Bayoumi AM, Goldstein RS, Guyatt GH. Interpreting small differences in functional status: the Six Minute Walk test in chronic lung disease patients. Am J Respir Crit Care Med. 1997;155:1278–82.

117. Chetta A, Aiello M, Foresi A, et al. Relationship between outcome measures of six-minute walk test and baseline lung function in patients with interstitial lung disease. Sarcoidosis Vasc Diffuse Lung Dis. 2001;18:170–5.

118. Holland AE, Hill CJ, Conron M, Munro P, McDonald CF. Small changes in six-minute walk distance are important in diffuse parenchymal lung disease. Respir Med. 2009;103:1430–5.

119. Demir R, Kucukoglu MS. Six-minute walk test in pulmonary arterial hypertension. Anatol J Cardiol. 2015;15:249–54.

120. Souza R, Channick RN, Delcroix M, et al. Association between six-minute walk distance and long-term outcomes in patients with pulmonary arterial hypertension: data from the randomized SERAPHIN trial. PLoS One. 2018;13:e0193226.

121. Golpe R, Castro-Anon O, Perez-de-Llano LA, et al. Prognostic significance of six-minute walk test in non-group 1 pulmonary hypertension. Heart Lung. 2014;43:72–6.

122. Gadre A, Ghattas C, Han X, Wang X, Minai O, Highland KB. Six-minute walk test as a predictor of diagnosis, disease severity, and clinical outcomes in scleroderma-associated pulmonary hypertension: the DIBOSA study. Lung. 2017;195:529–36.

123. Swigris JJ, Olson AL, Shlobin OA, Ahmad S, Brown KK, Nathan SD. Heart rate recovery after six-minute walk test predicts pulmonary hypertension in patients with idiopathic pulmonary fibrosis. Respirology. 2011;16:439–45.

124. Ussavarungsi K, Lee AS, Burger CD. Can a six-minute walk distance predict right ventricular dysfunction in patients with diffuse parenchymal lung disease and pulmonary hypertension? Oman Med J. 2016;31:345–51.

125. Donadio MV, Heinzmann-Filho JP, Vendrusculo FM, Frasson PXH, Marostica PJC. Six-minute walk test results predict risk of hospitalization for youths with cystic fibrosis: a 5-year follow-up study. J Pediatr. 2017;182:204–9. e1.

126. Malamud AL, Ricard PE. Feasibility of the six-minute walk test for patients who have cystic fibrosis, are ambulatory, and require mechanical ventilation before lung transplantation. Phys Ther. 2016;96:1468–76.

127. Martin C, Chapron J, Hubert D, et al. Prognostic value of six minute walk test in cystic fibrosis adults. Respir Med. 2013;107:1881–7.

128. Andrianopoulos V, Wouters EF, Pinto-Plata VM, et al. Prognostic value of variables derived from the six-minute walk test in patients with COPD: results from the ECLIPSE study. Respir Med. 2015;109:1138–46.

129. Brasil Santos D, de Assis Viegas CA. Correlation of levels of obstruction in COPD with lactate and six-minute walk test. Rev Port Pneumol. 2009;15:11–25.

130. Enfield K, Gammon S, Floyd J, et al. Six-minute walk distance in patients with severe end-stage COPD: association with survival after inpatient pulmonary rehabilitation. J Cardiopulm Rehabil Prev. 2010;30:195–202.

131. Fujimoto H, Asai K, Watanabe T, Kanazawa H, Hirata K. Association of six-minute walk distance (6MWD) with resting pulmonary function in patients with chronic obstructive pulmonary disease (COPD). Osaka City Med J. 2011;57:21–9.

132. Moreira MA, Medeiros GA, Boeno FP, Sanches PR, Silva Junior DP, Muller AF. Oxygen desaturation during the six-minute walk test in COPD patients. J Bras Pneumol. 2014;40:222–8.

133. Porteous MK, Rivera-Lebron BN, Kreider M, Lee J, Kawut SM. Determinants of 6-minute walk distance in patients with idiopathic pulmonary fibrosis undergoing lung transplant evaluation. Pulm Circ. 2016;6:30–6.

134. Yimlamai D, Freiberger DA, Gould A, Zhou J, Boyer D. Pretransplant six-minute walk test predicts peri- and post-operative outcomes after pediatric lung transplantation. Pediatr Transplant. 2013;17:34–40.

135. Castleberry AW, Englum BR, Snyder LD, et al. The utility of preoperative six-minute-walk distance in lung transplantation. Am J Respir Crit Care Med. 2015;192:843–52.

136. Balci MK, Ari E, Vayvada M, et al. Assessment of pulmonary hypertension in lung transplantation candidates: correlation of doppler echocardiography with right heart catheterization. Transplant Proc. 2016;48:2797–802.

137. Nowak J, Hudzik B, Jastrze Bski D, et al. Pulmonary hypertension in advanced lung diseases: echocardiography as an important part of patient evaluation for lung transplantation. Clin Respir J. 2017;12(3):930–8.

138. Jose A, King CS, Shlobin OA, Brown AW, Wang C, Nathan SD. Exercise pulmonary haemodynamic response predicts outcomes in fibrotic lung disease. Eur Respir J. 2018;52:1801015.

139. Gupta S, Torres F, Bollineni S, Mohanka M, Kaza V. Left ventricular dysfunction after lung transplantation for pulmonary arterial hypertension. Transplant Proc. 2015;47:2732–6.

140. Andersen KH, Schultz HH, Nyholm B, Iversen MP, Gustafsson F, Carlsen J. Pulmonary hypertension as a risk factor of mortality after lung transplantation. Clin Transpl. 2016;30:357–64.

141. McCartney SL, Cooter M, Samad Z, et al. Mitral regurgitation after orthotopic lung transplantation: natural history and impact on outcomes. J Cardiothorac Vasc Anesth. 2017;31:924–30.

142. Udoji TN, Force SD, Pelaez A. Severe mitral regurgitation unmasked after bilateral lung transplantation. Pulm Circ. 2013;3:696–9.

143. Banack T, Ziganshin BA, Barash P, Elefteriades JA. Aortic valve replacement for critical aortic stenosis after bilateral lung transplantation. Ann Thorac Surg. 2013;96:1475–8.

144. Brill AK, Gloekler S, Aubert JD, Wenaweser PM, Geiser T. Transcatheter aortic valve implantation in a lung transplant recipient. Ann Thorac Surg. 2014;97:e159–60.

145. Sugizaki Y, Mori S, Nagamatsu Y, et al. Critical exacerbation of idiopathic pulmonary fibrosis after transcatheter aortic valve implantation: need for multidisciplinary care beyond "heart team". J Cardiol Cases. 2018;18:171–4.

146. Lazaro M, Ramos A, Ussetti P, et al. Aspergillus endocarditis in lung transplant recipients: case report and literature review. Transpl Infect Dis. 2011;13:186–91.

Index

© Springer Nature Switzerland AG 2020
S. P. Bhatt (ed.), *Cardiac Considerations in Chronic Lung Disease*,
Respiratory Medicine, https://doi.org/10.1007/978-3-030-43435-9

Printed in the United States
by Baker & Taylor Publisher Services